HANDBOOK FOR
Anesthesia and Co-Existing Disease

D0954508

HANDBOOK FOR
Anesthesia and Co-Existing Disease

SECOND EDITION

Robert K. Stoelting, M.D.
Professor and Chair
Department of Anesthesia
Indiana University School of Medicine
Indianapolis, Indiana

Stephen F. Dierdorf, M.D.
Professor
Department of Anesthesia
Indiana University School of Medicine
Indianapolis, Indiana

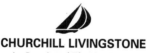

CHURCHILL LIVINGSTONE
An Imprint of Elsevier Science
New York   Edinburgh   London   Philadelphia

CHURCHILL LIVINGSTONE
An Imprint of Elsevier Science

The Curtis Center
Independence Square West
Philadelphia, Pennsylvania 19106

Library of Congress Cataloging-in-Publication Data

Handbook for Anesthesia and co-existing disease / [edited by]
Robert K. Stoelting, Stephen F. Dierdorf—2nd ed.

p. ; cm

Includes index.

ISBN 0–443–06605–1

1. Anesthesia—Complications—Handbooks, manuals, etc.
2. Therapeutics, Surgical—Handbooks, manuals, etc. I. Stoelting,
Robert K.   II. Dierdorf, Stephen F.   III. Anesthesia and
co-existing disease.
[DNLM: 1. Anesthesia—adverse effects—Outlines.
2. Anesthetics—Outlines. WO 245

A578 2002 Suppl.]
RD87 .A53 2002 Suppl.

617.9′6041—dc21   2001047236

HANDBOOK FOR ANESTHESIA AND CO-EXISTING DISEASE
ISBN 0–443–06605–1

Printed in the United States of America.

Last digit is the print number: 9 8 7 6 5 4 3 2 1

Preface

This second edition of the *Handbook for Anesthesia and Co-Existing Disease* is intended to provide a rapid and accurate source of information relevant to the impact of the pathophysiology of disease states on the perioperative management of patients. The Handbook utilizes an outline format that follows the identical chapters and headings in the fourth edition of *Anesthesia and Co-Existing Disease*, thus permitting students and practitioners to refer to corresponding areas of the more detailed information in the textbook. As such, the intent of the Handbook is to serve as a "companion" to *Anesthesia and Co-Existing Disease* and an easy cross-reference to *Anesthesia and Co-Existing Disease* and its more in-depth discussion of each disease entity. The emphasis in the Handbook is on presentation of information in table format. This design provides rapid visibility of pertinent aspects of a patient's medical condition that can be readily assessed, if needed, on site in the operating rooms or other areas of the health care facility that are remote from the individual's personal library.

We wish to thank Deanna M. Walker for her secretarial help in the preparation of the manuscript.

Robert K. Stoelting, M.D.
Stephen F. Dierdorf, M.D.

Contents

1

Ischemic Heart Disease

Ischemic heart disease, which reflects the presence of atherosclerosis in coronary arteries (coronary artery disease), is present in an estimated 30% of patients who undergo surgery annually in the United States (Stoelting RK, Dierdorf SF. Ischemic heart disease. In: Anesthesia and Co-existing Disease, 4th ed. New York, Churchill Livingstone, 2002;1–24). Angina pectoris, acute myocardial infarction, and sudden death (cardiac dysrhythmias) are often the first manifestations of ischemic heart disease. The two most important risk factors for the development of atherosclerosis involving the coronary arteries are male gender and increasing age (Table 1–1).

I. ANGINA PECTORIS

Angina pectoris occurs when there is an imbalance between coronary blood flow (supply) and myocardial oxygen consumption (demand).

A. **Diagnosis** of angina pectoris depends on the description of pain (retrosternal chest discomfort that may be perceived as pain or chest heaviness that often radiates to the neck, left arm, or mandible). Angina pectoris usually lasts several minutes, whereas a sharp pain that lasts only seconds or a dull ache that lasts for hours is rarely due to myocardial ischemia. Retrosternal chest pain exacerbated by deep breathing suggests pericarditis. Esophageal spasm can produce substernal pressure that is relieved by nitroglycerin.

  1. **Electrocardiography.** Myocardial (subendocardial) ischemia is confirmed when ST segment depression on the electrocardiogram (ECG) coincides in time with an episode of anginal chest pain.

    a. **Exercise electrocardiography** is more useful for establishing the patient's left ventricular function than for establishing the diagnosis of ischemic heart disease.

≡ Table 1–1 • Risk Factors for the Development of Ischemic Heart Disease

Male gender
Increasing age
Hypercholesterolemia
Systemic hypertension
Cigarette smoking
Diabetes mellitus
Obesity
Sedentary lifestyle
Family history (premature development of ischemic heart disease)

Exercise testing may not be possible in patients with aortic stenosis or in the presence of certain noncardiac diseases (peripheral vascular disease and claudication, lung disease, arthritis).

b. The minimum criterion for an abnormal ST segment response is at least 1 mm of depression or elevation during or within 4 minutes after exercise.

2. **Noninvasive imaging tests.** Coronary artery calcification can be measured by electron-beam computed tomography. In patients who cannot exercise, cardiac stress (increased heart rate) can be drug-induced (dobutamine) or induced by artificial cardiac pacing.

a. **Echocardiography** wall motion analysis is performed after stressing the heart by dobutamine infusion or pacing. Ventricular wall motion abnormalities induced by stress correspond to the site of myocardial ischemia.

b. **Nuclear stress imaging** using tracers (thallium, technetium) is useful for assessing coronary perfusion (coronary artery obstruction causes less tracer activity).

3. **Coronary angiography** provides the most information about the coronary arteries and is indicated in patients when angina pectoris persists despite maximal medical therapy. In many of these patients revascularization provides the best treatment for pain relief and improved prognosis.

a. The two most important prognostic determinants in patients with coronary artery disease are the anatomic extent of the atherosclerotic disease (coronary angiog-

---

≡ Table 1–2 • Treatment of Ischemic Heart Disease

Lifestyle modification
  Cessation of smoking
  Maintenance of ideal body weight
  Regular aerobic exercise
  Treatment of systemic hypertension
  Lowering of low density lipoprotein (LDL) cholesterol
Medical treatment of ischemia
  Antiplatelet drugs (low-dose aspirin)
  Antithrombin drugs
  β-Blockers
  Calcium channel blockers
  Organic nitrates
Revascularization
  Procedures requiring cardiopulmonary bypass may be
    associated with postoperative cognitive dysfunction

---

raphy) and the state of left ventricular function (ejection fraction).

  b. Plaques most likely to rupture and lead to formation of an occlusive thrombus (myocardial infarction) have a fine fibrous cap and a large lipid core containing an increased number of macrophages.

  c. Although stenosis of a coronary artery (> 70%) is typically required to produce angina pectoris, such stenoses tend to have dense fibrotic caps and are less likely to rupture than are mild to moderate coronary artery stenoses, which are generally more lipid-laden.

B. Treatment. See Table 1–2.

II. ACUTE MYOCARDIAL INFARCTION

Acute myocardial infarction (acute coronary artery syndrome) is caused most often by sudden disruption of an arteriosclerotic plaque and hemorrhage into the vessel wall, resulting in partial or total occlusion of the artery. Long-term prognosis following an acute myocardial infarction is determined principally by the severity of left ventricular dysfunction (determined 2 to 3 months after myocardial infarction), the presence and degree of residual ischemia, and the potential for malignant ventricular dysrhythmias.

▅ Table 1–3 • Diagnosis of Acute
Myocardial Infarction

Angina pectoris (new onset or change in pattern)
Anxiety
Sinus tachycardia
Hypotension
Cardiac dysrhythmias
ST segment elevation on electrocardiogram
Cardiac troponins increased
Wall motion abnormalities on echocardiography

A. **Pathophysiology.** The acute coronary artery syndrome represents a hypercoagulable state. There is increasing evidence that atherosclerosis is an inflammatory disease, and inflammation is important in the cascade of events that lead to plaque rupture.
   1. It is somewhat paradoxical that plaques that rupture and lead to occlusion of a coronary artery are rarely flow-restrictive.
   2. Flow restrictive plaques that produce angina pectoris and stimulate the development of collateral circulation tend to be "mature" and less likely to rupture.
B. **Diagnosis** of acute myocardial infarction requires the presence of at least two of three criteria: (1) clinical history of

---

▅ Table 1–4 • Treatment of Acute
Myocardial Infarction

Aspirin (administered as soon as diagnosis is made)
Morphine for analgesia
Thrombolytic therapy (streptokinase, tissue plasminogen activator)
   ideally initiated within 30–60 minutes of hospital arrival
Intracoronary stenting plus platelet glycoprotein blockade
Coronary angioplasty
Coronary artery bypass graft surgery
Adjunctive medical therapy (intravenous heparin, β-blockers,
   angiotensin-converting enzyme inhibitors)

≡ Table 1–5 • Complications of Acute Myocardial Infarction

Cardiac dysrhythmias
    Ventricular fibrillation (peak incidence during first 4 hours)
    Ventricular tachycardia
    Atrial fibrillation (most common cardiac dysrhythmia)
    Bradydysrhythmias and heart block
Pericarditis
Mitral regurgitation (ischemic injury to papillary muscles)
    Pulmonary edema
    Cardiogenic shock
Ventricular septal defect
Congestive heart failure and cardiogenic shock (may require use
    of circulatory assist devices)
Myocardial rupture
Right ventricular infarction (echocardiography facilitates diagnosis;
    treatment includes intravascular fluid replacement)
Cerebral vascular accident

angina pectoris; (2) serial ECG changes indicative of myocardial infarction; and (3) rise and fall in serum concentrations of cardiac enzyme markers (Table 1–3).
    C. Treatment. See Table 1–4.
    D. Complications of acute myocardial infarction. See Table 1–5.

III. PREOPERATIVE ASSESSMENT OF PATIENTS WITH KNOWN OR SUSPECTED HEART DISEASE

In stable patients undergoing elective major noncardiac surgery, six independent predictors of major cardiac complications have been identified (ventricular fibrillation, third-degree atrioventricular heart block, pulmonary edema, death) (Table 1–6). Perioperative risk can also be estimated on the basis of the patient's exercise tolerance (strenuous walking or climbing stairs without cardiac symptoms). The primary challenge of the preoperative assessment is to distinguish patients who require little or no preoperative testing from those for whom specialized testing is beneficial and cost-effective (exercise electrocardiography, echocardiography, radionuclide ventriculography, dipyridamole-thallium scintigraphy).

≡ **Table 1-6** • Cardiac Risk Index for Patients Undergoing Elective Major Noncardiac Surgery

High Risk Surgery
Abdominal aneurysm
Peripheral vascular
Thoracotomy
Major abdominal
Ischemic Heart Disease
History of myocardial infarction
History of positive exercise test
Current complaints of angina pectoris
Use of nitrate therapy
Q waves on ECG
Congestive Heart Failure
History of congestive heart failure
History of pulmonary edema
History of paroxysmal nocturnal dyspnea
Physical examination showing bilateral rales or S_3 gallop
Chest radiograph showing pulmonary vascular redistribution
Cerebrovascular Disease
History of stroke
History of transient ischemic attack
Insulin-dependent diabetes mellitus
Preoperative serum creatinine concentration > 2 mg/dl

Adapted from Lee TH, Marcantonio ER, Mangione CM, et al. Derivation and prospective validation of a simple index for prediction of cardiac risk of major noncardiac surgery. Circulation 1999;100:1043–9.

A. **History.** An important goal of the history is to elicit the severity, progression, and functional limitations introduced by ischemic heart disease. Limited exercise tolerance, in the absence of significant lung disease, is the most striking evidence of decreased cardiac reserve. Dyspnea following the onset of angina pectoris suggests the presence of acute left ventricular dysfunction due to myocardial ischemia. It is important to recognize the presence of incipient congestive heart failure preoperatively, as the added stress of anesthesia, surgery, fluid replacement, and postoperative pain may result in overt congestive heart failure.

1. **Silent myocardial ischemia.** It is estimated that nearly 75% of ischemic episodes in patients with symptomatic ischemic heart disease are not associated with angina pectoris, and 10% to 15% of acute myocardial infarctions are silent.

≡ Table 1–7 • Treatment of Excessive β-Blockade

Atropine 0.4–0.6 mg IV (initial treatment)
Isoproterenol 2–5 μg/min IV (titrate to desired heart rate)
Dobutamine
Calcium 500–1000 mg IV (works at sites other than β-receptors)

2. **Prior myocardial infarction.** It is common practice to delay elective operations (up to 6 months) following an acute myocardial infarction. Hemodynamic monitoring using intra-arterial and pulmonary artery catheter monitoring (alternatively echocardiography) and prompt pharmacologic treatment or fluid infusion to treat hemodynamic alterations that are not in the normal range may decrease the risk of perioperative myocardial reinfarction in high risk patients.

3. **Co-existing noncardiac diseases.** The history should elicit symptoms of relevant co-existing noncardiac diseases (peripheral vascular disease, syncope, cough, dyspnea, diabetes mellitus).

4. **Current medications.** Effective β-blockade is suggested by a resting heart rate of 50 to 60 beats/min (Table 1–7).

B. **Physical examination.** The physical examination in patients with ischemic heart disease is often normal (Table 1–8).

C. **Specialized preoperative testing.** See Table 1–9.

≡ Table 1–8 • Physical Examination Findings in Patients with Ischemic Heart Disease

Left ventricular failure (S_3 gallop)
Cerebrovascular disease (carotid bruit)
Orthostatic hypotension (effect of antihypertensive drugs)
Peripheral edema
Jugular venous distension

Table 1-9 • Specialized Preoperative Testing in Patients with Ischemic Heart Disease

Electrocardiography (exercise stress testing may not be necessary in patients with stable coronary artery disease and acceptable exercise tolerance)

Echocardiography (diagnoses left ventricular dysfunction and abnormal valve function)

Radionuclide ventriculography (determination of ejection fraction)

Thallium scintigraphy ("cold spots" denote areas of probable myocardial ischemia or infarction)

Computed tomography and magnetic resonance imaging (provide anatomic visualization of coronary artery calcification)

Positron emission tomography (demonstrates regional myocardial blood flow and metabolism)

IV. **MANAGEMENT OF ANESTHESIA IN PATIENTS WITH KNOWN OR SUSPECTED ISCHEMIC HEART DISEASE UNDERGOING NONCARDIAC SURGERY**

A. **Preoperative preparation and medication**

1. High risk patients probably benefit from optimal preoperative antiischemic and antihypertensive therapy as well as pharmacologic and psychological attempts to decrease anxiety that could evoke sympathetic nervous systemic activation with accompanying increases in systemic blood pressure and heart rate.

2. Drugs used for medical management of patients with ischemic heart disease are continued throughout the perioperative period.

B. **Intraoperative management**

1. Maintenance of the balance between myocardial oxygen requirements and myocardial oxygen delivery is probably more important than the specific anesthetic techniques or drugs selected to produce anesthesia and skeletal muscle relaxation (Table 1-10).

   a. It is important to avoid persistent, excessive increases in heart rate (> 110 beats/min) and systemic blood pressure (attempt to maintain within 20% of awake value).

   b. An increase in heart rate is more likely than systemic hypertension to produce signs of myocardial ischemia. Conceptually, a rapid heart rate increases myocardial

---

Table 1–10 • Intraoperative Events that Influence the Balance Between Myocardial Oxygen Delivery and Myocardial Oxygen Requirements

---

Decreased Oxygen Delivery
Decreased coronary blood flow
   Tachycardia
   Diastolic hypotension
   Hypocapnia (coronary artery vasoconstriction)
   Coronary artery spasm
Decreased oxygen content
   Anemia
   Arterial hypoxemia
   Shift of the oxyhemoglobin dissociation curve to the left
Increased preload (wall tension)
Increased Oxygen Requirements
Sympathetic nervous system stimulation
   Tachycardia
   Systemic hypertension
   Increased myocardial contractility
   Increased afterload

---

    oxygen requirements and decreases the time during diastole for coronary blood flow (and thus delivery of oxygen) to occur.

    c. Increased oxygen requirements produced by systemic hypertension tend to be offset by improved perfusion through pressure-dependent atherosclerotic coronary arteries.

  2. Most episodes of intraoperative myocardial ischemia on the ECG occur in the absence of hemodynamic changes, suggesting that it is unlikely this form of myocardial ischemia is preventable by the anesthesiologist.

  3. **Induction of anesthesia** in patients with ischemic heart disease is accomplished with a variety of intravenous induction drugs (ketamine is an unlikely choice) and skeletal muscle relaxants to facilitate tracheal intubation (myocardial ischemia may occur during direct laryngoscopy and tracheal intubation).

    a. Short-duration direct laryngoscopy (< 15 seconds) may be useful for minimizing the magnitude and duration of circulatory stimulation associated with tracheal intubation.

b. When the duration of direct laryngoscopy is not likely to be brief or when systemic hypertension already exists, it is reasonable to consider additional drugs to minimize pressor responses produced by direct laryngoscopy and tracheal intubation (Table 1–11).

4. **Maintenance of anesthesia** utilizes drugs selected on the basis of the patient's presumed left ventricular function.

a. In patients with normal left ventricular function, controlled myocardial depression using volatile anesthetics with or without nitrous oxide may be useful for minimizing increased sympathetic nervous system activity and subsequent increases in myocardial oxygen requirements. At the same time, drug-induced decreases in systemic blood pressure and associated decreases in coronary perfusion pressures could be detrimental. Equally acceptable for maintenance of anesthesia is the use of nitrous oxide–opioid with the addition of volatile anesthetics to treat the undesirable increases in systemic blood pressure that may accompany painful surgical stimulation.

b. In patients with severely impaired left ventricular function, the use of short-acting opioids (fentanyl, 50–100 μg/kg IV, or equivalent doses of other opioids) may be selected, as these individuals may not tolerate myocardial depression produced by volatile anesthetics.

≡ **Table 1–11** • Drugs Intended to Attenuate the Systemic Blood Pressure and/or Heart Rate Response to Tracheal Intubation

---

Laryngotracheal lidocaine

Lidocaine 1.5 mg/kg IV 90 seconds before beginning direct laryngoscopy

Nitroprusside 1–2 μg/kg IV 15 seconds before beginning direct laryngoscopy

Esmolol 100–300 μg/kg/min IV before and during direct laryngoscopy

Fentanyl 1–3 μg/kg IV 90–120 seconds before beginning direct laryngoscopy

Nitroglycerin 0.25–1.00 μg/kg/min IV to decrease the pressor response (no evidence that the incidence of intraoperative myocardial ischemia is decreased)

---

      c. Regional anesthesia is an acceptable technique for patients with ischemic heart disease recognizing that decreases in myocardial oxygen requirements produced by peripheral sympathetic nervous system blockade may be offset by decreases in systemic blood pressure (pressure-dependent flow through coronary arteries narrowed by atherosclerosis).

    5. **Choice of muscle relaxants** for administration to patients with ischemic heart disease may be influenced by the impact these drugs could have on the balance between myocardial oxygen delivery and myocardial oxygen requirements (select drugs with minimum effects on heart rate and systemic blood pressure).

    6. **Monitoring** to detect intraoperative myocardial ischemia varies greatly in sensitivity and specificity (Table 1–12).

    7. **Intraoperative treatment of myocardial ischemia** is likely to be instituted when ST segment changes reach 1 mm in patients at high risk for developing myocardial ischemia (Table 1–13).

C. Postoperative period

    1. Continuous ECG monitoring is useful for detecting postoperative myocardial ischemia, which is often asymptomatic.

    2. Postoperative pain may result in activation of the sympathetic nervous system, leading to increased myocardial oxygen requirements and myocardial ischemia. This em-

---

Table 1–12 • Monitors to Detect Intraoperative Myocardial Ischemia

Electrocardiogram
    Changes in the ST segment characterized as depression or elevation of at least 1 mm
    Depth of ST segment depression parallels the severity of myocardial ischemia
    Leads II and V_5 detect most significant ST segment changes
Pulmonary artery catheter
    Increased pulmonary capillary wedge pressure
    V waves indicative of papillary muscle dysfunction
    Guide to treatment of myocardial ischemia
Transesophageal echocardiography
    Development of new regional ventricular wall motion abnormalities occur before changes on the electrocardiogram

---

≡ Table 1–13 • Treatment of Intraoperative Myocardial Ischemia

Esmolol if heart rate is increased

Nitroprusside if systemic blood pressure is increased in the absence of evidence of myocardial ischemia

Nitroglycerin if systemic blood pressure is increased in the presence of evidence of myocardial ischemia

Ephedrine to restore perfusion through pressure-dependent atherosclerotic coronary arteries (phenylephrine is an alternative drug)

Intravenous fluid administration to restore systemic blood pressure

---

phasizes the unique importance of providing adequate postoperative pain relief to patients with ischemic heart disease.

3. Central nervous system injury manifests as subtle changes in personality, behavior, and cognitive function.

4. Peripheral nerve injury, especially brachial plexus stretch injuries, are not uncommon following cardiac surgery that requires median sternotomy (selective damage to the fibers that become the ulnar nerve may erroneously suggest compression injury of this nerve at the condylar groove).

V. HEART TRANSPLANTATION

Heart transplantation may be recommended for patients with end-stage heart failure due to dilated cardiomyopathy or ischemic heart disease. Preoperatively, the ejection fraction is often < 0.2. Irreversible pulmonary hypertension is a contraindication to heart transplantation.

A. **Management of anesthesia** for cardiac transplantation may include ketamine, benzodiazepines, or both for induction of anesthesia plus opioids to provide analgesia during surgery.

1. Volatile anesthetics, especially in high doses, may produce undesirable degrees of direct myocardial depression and peripheral vasodilation. Nitrous oxide is seldom selected because of additive depressant effects in the presence of opioids and concern about enlargement of accidental air emboli that may occur when large blood vessels are opened during the surgical procedure.

2. Following cessation of cardiopulmonary bypass, inotropic drugs such as isoproterenol may be needed to maintain myocardial contractility and the heart rate.

B. **Postoperative complications** during the early period following heart transplant surgery are most often related to sepsis (opportunistic infections) and rejection (deterioration in function). Late complications include an increased incidence of cancer.

C. **Anesthetic considerations in heart transplant recipients.** See Table 1–14.

1. **Cardiac innervation.** The transplanted heart has no sympathetic, parasympathetic, or sensory innervation.

2. **Responses to drugs.** Responses to direct-acting sympathomimetics are intact, whereas epinephrine has augmented inotropic effects. Indirect-acting sympathomimetics such as ephedrine have blunted effects in the denervated transplanted heart. Vagolytic effects of drugs such as atropine are ineffective for increasing the heart rate.

3. **Preoperative evaluation.** Heart transplant patients may present with ongoing rejection (myocardial dysfunction, accelerated coronary atherosclerosis, cardiac dysrhythmias). It is important to confirm adequate intravascular fluid volume replacement preoperatively, as heart transplant patients are preload-dependent.

4. **Management of anesthesia.** General anesthesia is usually selected, as there is a possibility of impaired responses to hypotension after spinal or epidural anesthesia. Volatile

---

≡ Table 1–14 • Anesthetic Considerations in Heart Transplant Recipients

Altered pharmacodynamic and hemodynamic responses to drugs in a denervated heart
Side effects of immunosuppressive therapy
Risks and/or presence of infection
Drug interactions
Allograft rejection
Upper gastrointestinal bleeding
Hepatobiliary and pancreatic dysfunction

anesthetics are usually well tolerated. Goals of anesthesia include avoidance of significant peripheral vasodilation and acute decreases in preload. Aseptic technique is important in view of the likely increased susceptibility of these patients to infection.

2

Valvular Heart Disease

The most frequently encountered cardiac valve lesions produce pressure overload (mitral stenosis, aortic stenosis) or volume overload (mitral regurgitation, aortic regurgitation) on the left atrium or left ventricle (Stoelting RK, Dierdorf SF. Valvular heart disease. In: Anesthesia and Co-Existing Disease, 4th ed. New York, Churchill Livingstone, 2002;25–44). Drug selections during the perioperative period for patients with valvular heart disease are based on the likely effects of drug-induced changes in cardiac rhythm, heart rate, systemic blood pressure, systemic vascular resistance, and pulmonary vascular resistance relative to the pathophysiology of the heart disease.

I. PREOPERATIVE EVALUATION

Preoperative evaluation of patients with valvular heart disease includes assessment of the (1) severity of cardiac disease, (2) degree of impaired myocardial contractility, and (3) presence of associated major organ disease (pulmonary, renal, hepatic). Recognition of compensatory mechanisms for maintaining cardiac output (increased sympathetic nervous system activity, cardiac hypertrophy) and consideration of drug therapy are important. The presence of prosthetic heart valves introduces special considerations for the preoperative evaluation of patients, especially when noncardiac surgery is planned.

A. History and physical examination. Questions designed to define the patient's exercise tolerance are useful for evaluating cardiac reserve in the presence of valvular heart disease (Table 2–1). Congestive heart failure (CHF) is a frequent companion of chronic valvular heart disease. Ideally, elective surgery is deferred until the CHF can be treated and myocardial contractility optimized. The character, location, intensity, and direction of radiation of a heart murmur provides a clue to the location and severity of the cardiac valve

Table 2–1 • New York Heart Association Classification of Patients with Heart Disease

Class	Description
I	Asymptomatic
II	Symptomatic with ordinary activity but comfortable at rest
III	Symptoms with minimal activity but comfortable at rest
IV	Symptoms at rest

lesion (Fig. 2–1). Cardiac dysrhythmias, especially atrial fibrillation, are common. Valvular heart disease and ischemic heart disease (angina pectoris) often co-exist.

B. Drug therapy. Patients with valvular heart disease are likely to be receiving digitalis preparations (heart rate control) and diuretics. An adequate digitalis effect for heart rate control is indicated by ventricular rates of < 80 beats/min. Digitalis toxicity is suggested by prolongation of the PR

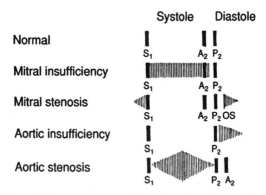

Fig. 2–1 • Timing and characteristics of cardiac murmurs in relation to systole and diastole. (From Fishman MC, Hoffman AR, Klausner RD, et al. Medicine. Philadelphia, Lippincott, 1981;42, with permission.)

interval on the electrocardiogram (ECG) and by patient complaints related to gastrointestinal dysfunction.

C. **Laboratory data.** The ECG often demonstrates characteristic changes: broad and notched P waves, left atrial enlargement, left and/or right axis deviation. On a posteroanterior chest radiograph the heart size should not exceed 50% of the internal width of the thoracic cage. Cardiac catheterization provides useful information (cardiac filling pressures, transvalvular pressure gradients) as to the severity of valvular heart disease. Arterial blood gases may reflect decreases in PaO_2 most likely due to interstitial pulmonary edema and altered ventilation-to-perfusion relations.

1. **Doppler echocardiography** is essential for noninvasive evaluation of valvular heart disease (Table 2–2).

2. Doppler echocardiography with color flow mapping allows assessment of the magnitude of valvular regurgitation.

D. **Presence of prosthetic heart valves**

1. **Assessment of prosthetic heart valve function.** Prosthetic valve dysfunction may be suggested by changes in the intensity or quality of the existing murmur or the appearance of a new murmur. Transesophageal echocardiography is utilized whenever dysfunction of the mitral valve is suspected. Cardiac catheterization permits measurement of transvalvular pressure gradients.

2. **Complications associated with prosthetic heart valves.** See Table 2–3.

3. **Management of anticoagulation in patients with prosthetic heart valves.** See Table 2–4.

■ **Table 2–2** • Doppler Echocardiography and Valvular Heart Disease

Determine significance of cardiac murmurs (most often aortic stenosis)
Identify hemodynamic abnormalities associated with physical findings (most often mitral regurgitation)
Determine transvalvular pressure gradient
Determine orifice area of cardiac valve
Determine ventricular ejection fraction
Diagnose cardiac valve regurgitation
Evaluate prosthetic cardiac valve function

≡ **Table 2–3** • Complications Associated with Prosthetic Heart Valves

Valve thrombosis
Systemic embolization
Structural failure of bioprosthetic valves
Hemolysis
Paravalvular regurgitation
Endocarditis

II. MITRAL STENOSIS

A. **Pathophysiology.** Mitral stenosis is characterized by mechanical obstruction to left ventricular filling secondary to progressive decreases in the orifice of the mitral valve, producing increases in left atrial volume and pressure. Pulmonary venous pressure is increased in association with increased left atrial pressure. The result is transudation of fluid into the pulmonary interstitial space, pulmonary edema, and dyspnea on exertion.

B. **Diagnosis.** Echocardiography is the premier noninvasive diagnostic tool for assessing the severity of mitral stenosis and calculating the valve area. Pulmonary hypertension is likely when the left atrial pressure is chronically increased above 25 mmHg. Clinically, mitral stenosis is recognized by the characteristic opening snap that occurs early during diastole and by a rumbling diastolic heart murmur best heard at the cardiac apex (Fig. 2–1).

C. **Treatment.** See Table 2–5.

D. **Management of anesthesia** (Table 2–6). The development of atrial fibrillation with rapid ventricular response rates

≡ **Table 2–4** • Management of Anticoagulation in Patients with Prosthetic Heart Valves

Continue anticoagulation for minor surgery (dental extractions)
Discontinue warfarin for 3–5 days preoperatively when major surgery is planned (substitute intravenous heparin up until 2–4 hours before surgery and continue postoperatively until effective anticoagulation is achieved with oral warfarin)
Administer low-dose heparin during pregnancy (warfarin is associated with embryopathy)

≡ Table 2–5 • Treatment of Patients with Mitral Stenosis

Prophylaxis against endocarditis
Diuretics to decrease left atrial pressure
Control heart rate (digoxin, β-blockers, calcium channel blockers), as tachycardia impairs left ventricular filling and increases left atrial pressure
Anticoagulant therapy (risk of embolization is increased)
Surgical correction (commissurotomy, valve reconstruction, mitral valve replacement) when symptoms increase or evidence of pulmonary hypertension develops

---

may greatly decrease cardiac output and produce pulmonary edema. Treatment consists of cardioversion or intravenous administration of β-antagonists such as esmolol. Digoxin is useful when more sustained but not immediate control of the heart rate is needed. Sudden decreases in systemic vascular resistance may not be tolerated, as systemic blood pressure can be maintained only by increasing the heart rate. Treatment is administration of sympathomimetic drugs, such as ephedrine (increases contractility and possibly the heart rate) or phenylephrine (does not increase heart rate but could adversely increase left ventricular afterload).

1. **Preoperative medication** is intended to decrease the likelihood of anxiety-induced tachycardia. Administration of anticholinergic drugs is controversial because of concern that adverse increases in heart rate could occur. Digoxin administered for heart rate control is continued.

≡ Table 2–6 • Anesthetic Considerations in Patients with Mitral Stenosis

Avoid sinus tachycardia or rapid ventricular response rates during atrial fibrillation
Avoid marked increases in central blood volume (as associated with overtransfusion or head-down position)
Avoid drug-induced decreases in systemic vascular resistance
Avoid events such as arterial hypoxemia and/or hypoventilation that may exacerbate pulmonary hypertension and evoke right ventricular failure

2. **Induction of anesthesia** is most often accomplished with drugs administered intravenously that are unlikely to increase the heart rate (avoid ketamine) or abruptly decrease the systemic vascular resistance.

3. **Maintenance of anesthesia** is intended to minimize the likelihood of marked, sustained changes in heart rate, systemic vascular resistance, pulmonary vascular resistance, and myocardial contractility. These goals are most likely to be achieved with the combination of nitrous oxide and opioids or low concentrations of volatile drugs. Nitrous oxide may increase pulmonary vascular resistance, especially in the presence of co-existing severe pulmonary hypertension.

4. **Monitoring.** Use of invasive monitoring depends on the complexity of the operative procedure and the magnitude of physiologic impairment produced by mitral stenosis. Asymptomatic patients without evidence of pulmonary congestion probably do not require monitoring different from that for patients without valvular heart disease.

5. **Postoperative management.** Patients with mitral stenosis are at risk for developing postoperative pulmonary edema and right ventricular failure. Mechanical support of ventilation may have to be continued, especially after major thoracic or abdominal surgery.

III. MITRAL REGURGITATION

A. **Pathophysiology.** Mitral regurgitation is characterized by left atrial volume overload and decreased forward left ventricular stroke volume, as part of the stroke volume is regurgitated through the incompetent mitral valve back into the left atrium. The frequent combination of mitral regurgitation and mitral stenosis results in increased volume and pressure work by the heart.

B. **Diagnosis.** Echocardiography confirms enlargement of the left ventricular chamber, and color-flow examination of the mitral valve establishes the pattern of disturbed flow caused by regurgitation across the mitral valve. Clinically, mitral regurgitation is recognized by the presence of a holosystolic apical murmur (Fig. 2–1). The presence of V waves on the recording of the pulmonary artery occlusion pressure reflects regurgitant flow through the mitral valve.

C. **Treatment.** Surgical replacement of the mitral valve is indicated when the ejection fraction is < 0.6. After mitral valve replacement, the dilated left ventricle is suddenly exposed to increased resistance to ventricular ejection as the low-resistance left atrial "pop off" has been removed, which may contribute to the development of CHF.

D. **Management of anesthesia** (Table 2–7). Forward left ventricular stroke volume is facilitated by modest increases in heart rate (sudden bradycardia may result in an abrupt left ventricular overload) and decreased systemic vascular resistance. Because left ventricular dysfunction usually accompanies mitral regurgitation, even minimal drug-induced myocardial depression is undesirable. Left ventricular failure may be treated with afterload reduction provided by nitroprusside and a cardiac inotrope, such as dopamine, to increase myocardial contractility.

1. **Induction of anesthesia** is most often accomplished with drugs administered intravenously, keeping in mind the importance of avoiding excessive, abrupt changes in systemic vascular resistance or decreases in heart rate (succinylcholine).

2. **Maintenance of anesthesia** is often provided with nitrous oxide plus volatile anesthetics. When myocardial function is severely compromised, as in the presence of acute mitral regurgitation due to papillary muscle dysfunction or rupture of chordae tendineae, the use of an opioid anesthetic technique, which minimizes the likelihood of drug-induced myocardial depression, may be a consideration.

3. **Monitoring** is determined by the complexity of the operative procedure and the magnitude of the physiologic impairment produced by mitral regurgitation. Transesophageal echocardiography is useful for monitoring mitral valve function, myocardial contractility, and the adequacy of intravascular fluid volume replacement. Al-

---

▤ Table 2–7 • Anesthetic Considerations in Patients with Mitral Regurgitation

Avoid sudden decreases in heart rate
Avoid sudden increases in systemic vascular resistance
Minimize drug-induced myocardial depression
Monitor the magnitude of regurgitant flow with echocardiography and/or a pulmonary artery catheter (size of V waves)

ternatively, a pulmonary artery catheter may be useful, especially if peripheral vasodilating drugs are administered in an attempt to increase the forward left ventricular stroke volume (changes in the amplitude of V waves can parallel the magnitude of mitral regurgitation). Maintenance of intravascular fluid volume with prompt replacement of blood loss is important for maintaining forward left ventricular stroke volume.

IV. MITRAL VALVE PROLAPSE

Mitral valve prolapse (billowing of the posterior mitral leaflet into the left atrium during systole) is predominantly a benign condition. Using echocardiographic criteria, the true incidence of mitral valve prolapse is low (2.4% of the population), and unexplained cerebral events cannot be demonstrated to occur more frequently than in normal patients. The risk of sudden death is not increased.

A. **Diagnosis** of mitral valve prolapse is based on echocardiography. Cardiac dysrhythmias commonly associated with mitral valve prolapse are nonspecific.

B. **Management of anesthesia** for noncardiac surgery in patients with mitral valve prolapse follows the same principles outlined for patients with mitral regurgitation (Table 2–7). An important concept is the recognition that increased left ventricular emptying or decreased left ventricular filling in these patients can accentuate mitral valve prolapse, leading to acute mitral regurgitation (Table 2–8).

1. **Preoperative evaluation** should focus on identifying patients with purely functional mitral valve prolapse

---

≡ **Table 2–8** • Perioperative Events that Increase Left Ventricular Emptying and/or Decrease Left Ventricular Filling

Increased sympathetic nervous system activity
   Tachycardia
   Increased myocardial contractility
   Cardiac dysrhythmias
Decreased systemic vascular resistance
Assumption of the upright (sitting) position
Hypovolemia

(women less than 45 years of age treated with β-blockers) versus individuals with anatomic mitral valve prolapse (older men who often manifest evidence of CHF). Premedication of patients with mitral valve prolapse should produce anxiolysis without causing tachycardia.

   a. **Antibiotic prophylaxis** is likely to be recommended, yet patients without echocardiographic evidence of mitral valve prolapse are at low risk for infective endocarditis and do not benefit from prophylactic antibiotic therapy.

   b. Antibiotic prophylaxis is not necessary for tracheal intubation or fiberoptic bronchoscopy but is probably indicated should nasotracheal intubation be planned.

2. **Selection of anesthetic technique.** Most patients with mitral valve prolapse have normal left ventricular function, and volatile anesthetics are well tolerated. Anesthetic-induced (regional or general anesthesia) decreases in systemic vascular resistance and the resulting undesirable decreases in left ventricular volume can be offset by repletion of the intravascular fluid volume prior to institution of regional anesthesia or induction of anesthesia.

3. **Induction of anesthesia** with intravenous drugs must consider the need to avoid sudden decreases in systemic vascular resistance. The myocardial depressant and peripheral vasodilating effects of barbiturates and propofol could be undesirable in patients with hemodynamically significant mitral valve prolapse. Ketamine could stimulate the sympathetic nervous system and accentuate mitral regurgitation.

4. **Maintenance of anesthesia** is designed to minimize sympathetic nervous system activation secondary to painful intraoperative stimulation (volatile anesthetics combined with nitrous oxide, opioids, or both). Unexpected cardiac dysrhythmias may occur during anesthesia, especially during operations performed in the head-up or sitting positions, presumably reflecting increased left ventricular emptying and accentuation of mitral valve prolapse. Prompt replacement of blood loss and generous intravenous fluid maintenance replacement can likely blunt any adverse effects caused by positive-pressure ventilation of the lungs.

5. **Monitoring.** The ECG is monitored for prompt detection of cardiac dysrhythmias that may occur in patients with

mitral valve prolapse. Transesophageal echocardiography is used to monitor and assess the degree of mitral regurgitation. A pulmonary artery catheter may be placed to provide information complementary to that derived from echocardiography and to permit measurement of cardiac output and calculation of systemic vascular resistance.

V. AORTIC STENOSIS

A. **Pathophysiology.** Obstruction to ejection of blood into the aorta due to a decrease in the area of the aortic valve orifice necessitates an increase in left ventricular pressure to maintain forward stroke volume. Critical aortic stenosis that is capable of causing symptoms and sudden death is characterized by transvalvular pressure gradients higher than 50 mmHg.

B. **Diagnosis.** The classic symptoms of aortic stenosis are angina pectoris, dyspnea on exertion, and syncope, which is often associated with exertion. Clinically, aortic stenosis is recognized by a characteristic systolic ejection murmur radiating into the neck that is best heard in the aortic area (second right intercostal space) (Fig. 2–1). Because many patients with aortic stenosis are asymptomatic, it is important to listen for this murmur in patients scheduled for surgery.

1. **Echocardiography** with Doppler examination of the aortic valve provides a more accurate assessment of the severity of aortic stenosis (transvalvular pressure gradients, area of aortic valve) than does clinical evaluation.

2. Cardiac catheterization and coronary angiography may be necessary when the severity of the aortic stenosis cannot be determined by echocardiography.

C. **Treatment.** Except for antibiotic prophylaxis against infective endocarditis, there is no medical therapy for aortic stenosis. The only effective treatment is surgical replacement of the diseased valve.

D. **Management of anesthesia** (Table 2–9). General anesthesia is often selected in preference to epidural or spinal anesthesia, as peripheral sympathetic nervous system blockade produced by regional anesthesia can lead to undesirable decreases in systemic vascular resistance. It is important to have available a direct-current defibrillator whenever anesthesia is administered to patients with aortic stenosis (exter-

≡ Table 2–9 • Anesthetic Considerations in Patients with Aortic Stenosis

Maintain normal sinus rhythm
Avoid bradycardia
Avoid sudden increases or decreases in systemic vascular resistance
Optimize intravascular fluid volume to maintain venous return and left ventricular filling

---

nal cardiac massage is unlikely to be effective, as it is difficult to create an adequate stroke volume across a stenotic aortic valve by mechanically compressing the patient's sternum).

1. **Preoperative medication** includes prophylactic antibiotics and titration of any sedative drugs to avoid the likelihood of decreases in systemic vascular resistance.

2. **Induction of anesthesia** in the presence of aortic stenosis can be achieved with available intravenous induction drugs, keeping in mind that bradycardia is undesirable.

3. **Maintenance of anesthesia** is most often accomplished with a combination of nitrous oxide plus volatile anesthetics or opioids. When left ventricular function is severely impaired by aortic stenosis, it is useful to avoid any additional depression of myocardial contractility with volatile anesthetics. Decreased systemic vascular resistance produced by high concentrations of volatile anesthetics is not recommended. Intravascular fluid volume is maintained by prompt replacement of blood loss and liberal administration of intravenous fluids. The onset of junctional rhythm or bradycardia during anesthesia and surgery usually requires prompt treatment with intravenous administration of atropine. Supraventricular tachycardia may require treatment with esmolol or electrical cardioversion.

4. **Monitoring** requirements are determined by the magnitude of the surgery and severity of the aortic stenosis. It may include transesophageal echocardiography, a pulmonary artery catheter, or both.

5. **Regional anesthesia** and the associated sympathetic nervous system blockade (decreased systemic vascular resistance and venous return) may be considered undesirable in patients with aortic stenosis.

VI. AORTIC REGURGITATION

A. **Pathophysiology.** The basic hemodynamic derangement of aortic regurgitation is a decrease in forward left ventricular stroke volume due to regurgitation of part of the ejected stroke volume from the aorta back into the left ventricle. The magnitude of the regurgitant volume depends on the heart rate (time available for regurgitant flow to occur) and the pressure gradient across the aortic valve (systemic vascular resistance). The magnitude of aortic regurgitation is decreased by tachycardia and peripheral vasodilation. Compared with chronic aortic regurgitation, patients with acute aortic regurgitation experience sudden increases in left ventricular volume before left ventricular hypertrophy can occur, limiting the effectiveness of compensatory mechanisms (tachycardia and increased myocardial contractility).

B. **Diagnosis.** Clinically, aortic regurgitation is recognized by the characteristic diastolic blowing murmur, best heard along the left sternal border, plus peripheral signs of a hyperdynamic circulation (widened pulse pressure, decreased diastolic blood pressure, bounding peripheral pulses) (Fig. 2–1). Echocardiography with Doppler examination of the aortic valve and aortography during cardiac catheterization are useful for confirming the diagnosis and the severity of aortic regurgitation.

C. **Treatment.** Surgical replacement of the diseased aortic valve is recommended before the onset of permanent left ventricular damage, even in asymptomatic patients. Medical therapy of aortic regurgitation is based on decreasing the left ventricular afterload with drug-induced vasodilation.

D. **Management of anesthesia** (Table 2–10). It is useful to maintain the patient's heart rate at more than 80 beats/min, as bradycardia, by increasing the duration of ventricular diastole, predisposes to acute left ventricular volume over-

---

≡ **Table 2–10 • Anesthetic Considerations in Patients with Aortic Regurgitation**

Avoid sudden decreases in heart rate
Avoid sudden increases in systemic vascular resistance
Minimize drug-induced myocardial depression

load. Abrupt increases in systemic vascular resistance can precipitate left ventricular failure, requiring treatment with peripheral vasodilators, such as nitroprusside. Modest increases in heart rate and decreases in systemic vascular resistance are reasonable goals for management of anesthesia, recognizing that these patients may be exquisitely sensitive to peripheral vasodilation.

1. **Induction of anesthesia** in the presence of aortic regurgitation can be achieved with available intravenous induction drugs (ketamine may be advantageous by virtue of its ability to increase the heart rate, but the accompanying increase in resistance to ejection of the forward left ventricular stroke volume could be undesirable).

2. **Maintenance of anesthesia** is often provided with nitrous oxide plus volatile anesthetics and/or opioids. Maintenance of the intravascular fluid volume with prompt replacement of blood loss is important for maintaining cardiac filling and ejection of an optimal forward left ventricular stroke volume. Bradycardia and junctional rhythm may require prompt treatment with intravenous administration of atropine.

3. **Monitoring.** In the presence of severe aortic regurgitation, monitoring with transesophageal echocardiography or a pulmonary artery catheter is helpful for early recognition of undesirable degrees of myocardial depression and facilitation of intravenous fluid replacement.

VII. TRICUSPID REGURGITATION

A. **Pathophysiology.** Tricuspid regurgitation is usually functional, reflecting dilation of the right ventricle due to pulmonary hypertension. Right atrial volume overload is usually well tolerated, reflecting the high compliance of the right atrium and venae cavae (minimal increases in right atrial pressure).

B. **Management of anesthesia.** Intravascular fluid volume and central venous pressure are maintained in high normal ranges to facilitate an adequate right ventricular stroke volume and left ventricular filling. Events known to increase pulmonary vascular resistance (arterial hypoxemia, hypercarbia) should be avoided. If nitrous oxide is administered, it may be helpful to monitor the central venous pressure and consider the possible role of nitrous oxide should there be unexpected increases in right atrial pressure.

3

Congenital Heart Disease

Congenital anomalies of the heart and cardiovascular system are present in 0.7% to 1.0% of all live births (Table 3–1) (Stoelting RK, Dierdorf SF. Congenital heart disease. In: Anesthesia and Co-Existing Disease, 4th ed. New York, Churchill Livingstone, 2002;45–65). Signs and symptoms of congenital heart disease are apparent during the first week of life in about 50% of afflicted neonates and before 5 years of age in virtually all remaining patients (Table 3–2). Echocardiography is the initial diagnostic step if congenital heart disease is suspected, although cardiac catheterization and selective angiocardiography are the most definitive diagnostic procedures available for use in patients with congenital heart disease. Certain complications are likely to accompany the presence of congenital heart disease (Table 3–3).

I. ACYANOTIC CONGENITAL HEART DISEASE

Acyanotic congenital heart disease is characterized by a left-to-right intracardiac shunt (Table 3–4). The ultimate result of this intracardiac shunt, regardless of its location, is increased pulmonary blood flow with pulmonary hypertension, right ventricular hypertrophy, and eventually congestive heart failure (CHF).

A. Atrial septal defect (ASD) accounts for about one third of cases of congenital heart disease detected in adults. It is two to three times more frequent in females than males. The physiologic consequences of an ASD are the same regardless of the anatomic location and reflect the shunting of blood from one atrium to the other. A systolic ejection murmur audible in the second left intercostal space may be mistaken for an innocent flow murmur. Atrial fibrillation and supraventricular tachycardia may accompany an ASD that remains uncorrected into adulthood. Transesophageal echocardiography and Doppler color-flow echocardiography are useful for detecting and determining the location of ASDs.

≡ Table 3–1 • Classification and Incidence of Congenital Heart Disease

Classification	Incidence (%)
Acyanotic Defects	
Ventricular septal defect	35
Atrial septal defect	9
Patent ductus arteriosus	8
Pulmonary stenosis	8
Aortic stenosis	6
Coarctation of the aorta	6
Atrioventricular septal defect	3
Cyanotic Defects	
Tetralogy of Fallot	5
Transposition of the great vessels	4

1. **Signs and symptoms.** ASDs initially produce no signs or symptoms and may thus remain undetected. Symptoms of a large ASD include dyspnea on exertion, supraventricular dysrhythmias, right heart failure, paradoxical embolism, and recurrent pulmonary infections. When pulmo-

≡ Table 3–2 • Signs and Symptoms of Congenital Heart Disease

Infants
Tachypnea
Failure to gain weight
Heart rate > 200 beats/min
Heart murmur
Congestive heart failure
Cyanosis
Children
Dyspnea
Slow physical development
Decreased exercise tolerance
Heart murmur
Congestive heart failure
Cyanosis
Clubbing of the digits
Squatting
Hypertension (systemic or pulmonary)

▬ Table 3–3 • Problems Commonly
Associated with Congenital
Heart Disease

Infective endocarditis
Cardiac dysrhythmias
Complete heart block
Hypertension (systemic or pulmonary)
Erythrocytosis
Thromboembolism
Coagulopathy
Brain abscess
Increased plasma uric acid concentration
Sudden death

nary blood flow is 1.5 times the systemic blood flow, the
ASD should be surgically closed to prevent right ventricular dysfunction and irreversible pulmonary hypertension.

   2. Management of anesthesia. See Table 3–5.

B. **Ventricular septal defect** (VSD) is the most common congenital cardiac abnormality in infants and children (many close
   spontaneously by 2 years of age). Echocardiography with
   Doppler flow studies confirms the presence and location of
   the VSD.

   1. Signs and symptoms. The physiologic significance of a
      VSD depends on the size of the defect and the relative
      resistance in the systemic and pulmonary circulations.
      In the presence of a large defect, pulmonary vascular
      resistance increases with time, and the direction of the
      shunt may reverse, resulting in cyanosis. Adults with
      small defects and normal pulmonary arterial pressures are
      generally asymptomatic, and pulmonary hypertension is

▬ Table 3–4 • Congenital Heart Defects
Resulting in a Left-to-Right Intracardiac
Shunt or Its Equivalent

Secundum atrial septal defect
Primum atrial septal defect (endocardial cushion defect)
Ventricular septal defect
Aorticopulmonary fenestration

≡ Table 3–5 • Management of Anesthesia in Patients with Left-to-Right Intracardiac Shunts

Prophylactic antibiotics when a cardiac valvular abnormality is present

Avoid delivery of air into the circulation as through intravenous delivery tubing

Pharmacokinetics of inhaled and injected drugs unlikely to be altered

Positive-pressure ventilation well tolerated

Avoid acute and persistent increases in systemic vascular resistance or decreases in pulmonary vascular resistance

Transient cardiac dysrhythmias or conduction disturbances may follow surgical repair

---

unlikely to develop. The murmur of a VSD is holosystolic and is loudest at the lower left sternal border.

2. **Management of anesthesia** (Table 3–5). Third-degree atrioventricular heart block may follow surgical closure if the cardiac conduction system is near the VSD.

C. **Patent ductus arteriosus** (PDA) is present when the ductus arteriosus (which arises just distal to the left subclavian artery and connects the descending aorta to the left pulmonary artery) fails to close spontaneously after birth. The PDA can usually be visualized on echocardiography, and Doppler studies confirm continuous flow into the pulmonary circulation.

1. **Signs and symptoms.** Most patients with PDA are asymptomatic, with the defect first being recognized by a continuous systolic and diastolic murmur that is detected during a routine physical examination. If pulmonary hypertension develops, surgical closure is not possible.

2. **Treatment** of PDA may be medical (cyclooxygenase inhibitors) or surgical (may be performed in neonatal intensive care units).

3. **Management of anesthesia** (Table 3–5). Anesthesia with volatile drugs is useful, as these drugs tend to lower the systemic blood pressure, lessening the danger of the PDA escaping from the vascular clamp or tearing as it is being surgically divided. Ligation of the PDA is often associated with significant systemic hypertension during the postop-

erative period, which may require treatment with intravenous nitroprusside.

D. **Aorticopulmonary fenestration** is characterized by a communication between the ascending aorta and the pulmonary artery. The resulting hemodynamic alterations resemble a PDA.

E. **Aortic stenosis.** Bicuspid aortic valves occur in 2% to 3% of the population, and an estimated 20% of these patients have other cardiovascular abnormalities such as PDA or coarctation of the aorta. Transthoracic echocardiography with Doppler flow permits accurate assessment of the severity of the aortic stenosis and of left ventricular function.

1. **Signs and symptoms.** Most patients with congenital aortic stenosis are asymptomatic until adulthood (see Chapter 2). Infants with severe aortic stenosis may present with congestive heart failure. Angina pectoris in the absence of coronary artery disease reflects the inability of coronary blood flow to meet increased myocardial oxygen requirements of the hypertrophied left ventricle. Syncope can occur when pressure gradients across the aortic valve exceed 50 mmHg.

2. Findings in patients with supravalvular aortic stenosis may include a characteristic appearance in which the facial bones are prominent, the forehead is rounded, and the upper lip is pursed. Strabismus, inguinal hernia, dental abnormalities, and moderate mental retardation are commonly present.

F. **Pulmonic stenosis** producing obstruction to right ventricular outflow is valvular in 90% of patients and supravalvular or subvalvular in the remainder. Valvular pulmonic stenosis is typically an isolated abnormality, but it may occur in association with a VSD. Echocardiography and Doppler flow studies can determine the site of the obstruction and the severity of the stenosis. Treatment of pulmonary valve stenosis is with percutaneous balloon valvuloplasty.

1. **Signs and symptoms.** In asymptomatic patients the presence of pulmonary stenosis is identified by the presence of a loud systolic ejection murmur best heard at the second left intercostal space. Dyspnea on exertion may occur, and eventually right ventricular failure with peripheral edema and ascites develops.

2. **Management of anesthesia** is designed to avoid an increase in the right ventricular oxygen requirement (as produced by tachycardia and increased myocardial con-

tractility). Decreased systemic blood pressure should be promptly treated with sympathomimetic drugs.

G. **Coarctation of the aorta** typically consists of a discrete, diaphragm-like ridge extending into the aortic lumen just distal to the left subclavian artery (postductal coarctation).

1. **Signs and symptoms.** Most adults with coarctation of the aorta are asymptomatic, and the diagnosis is made during a routine physical examination when systemic hypertension in the patient's arms is detected in association with diminished or absent femoral arterial pulses.

2. **Treatment** is surgical resection of the coarctation when transcoarctation gradients exceed 30 mmHg.

3. **Management of anesthesia.** See Table 3–6.

4. **Postoperative management.** Immediate postoperative complications include paradoxical systemic hypertension and the appearance of paraplegia. Intravenous administration of nitroprusside with or without esmolol is effective in controlling systemic blood pressure during the early postoperative period. Abdominal pain may occur postoperatively and is presumably due to sudden increases in blood flow to the gastrointestinal tract.

≡ Table 3–6 • Management of Anesthesia in Patients with Coarctation of the Aorta

Maintain perfusion to lower portion of the body during aortic cross-clamping
  Monitor systemic blood pressure above (right radial) and below (right femoral) the coarctation
  Allows evaluation of the adequacy of collateral circulation
  Mean arterial pressure in the lower extremities should probably be maintained at > 40 mmHg
Propensity for systemic hypertension during aortic cross-clamping
  Hypertension may make surgical repair more difficult
  Nitroprusside may be needed but could also decrease perfusion pressure below the coarctation
Consider risk of neurologic sequelae due to ischemia of the spinal cord
  Somatosensory evoked potentials are useful for monitoring spinal cord function and adequacy of blood flow during cross-clamping

II. CYANOTIC CONGENITAL HEART DISEASE

Cyanotic congenital heart disease is characterized by a right-to-left intracardiac shunt with an associated decrease in pulmonary blood flow and development of arterial hypoxemia (Table 3–7).

A. Tetralogy of Fallot, the most common cyanotic congenital heart defect, is characterized by a large VSD, an aorta that overrides the right and left ventricles, obstruction to right ventricular outflow, and right ventricular hypertrophy. Because the resistance to flow across the right ventricular outflow tract is relatively fixed, changes in systemic vascular resistance (drug-induced) may affect the magnitude of the shunt. A decrease in systemic vascular resistance increases the magnitude of the right-to-left shunt and and accentuates arterial hypoxemia.

    1. Diagnosis. Echocardiography is used to establish the diagnosis and to assess the presence of associated abnormalities. Cardiac catheterization further confirms the diagnosis and permits confirmation of anatomic and hemodynamic data.

    2. Signs and symptoms. See Table 3–8.

    3. Treatment of tetralogy of Fallot is complete surgical correction (closure of the VSD and relief of right ventricular outflow obstruction) when patients are very young.

    4. Management of anesthesia is based on avoiding changes that would acutely increase the magnitude of the right-to-left intracardiac shunt (Table 3–9).

        a. Preoperative preparation. Preoperatively, it is important to avoid dehydration by maintaining oral feedings or providing intravenous fluids before arrival in the operating room. Crying associated with intramuscular administration of drugs used for preoperative medication can lead to hypercyanotic attacks.

≡ Table 3–7 • Congenital Heart Defects Resulting in a Right-to-Left Intracardiac Shunt

Tetralogy of Fallot
Eisenmenger syndrome
Ebstein's anomaly (malformation of the tricuspid valve)
Tricuspid atresia
Foramen ovale

▬ **Table 3–8** • Signs and Symptoms of Tetralogy of Fallot

Ejection murmur heard along the left sternal border
Cyanosis (PaO_2 usually < 50 mmHg)
Squatting (increases systemic vascular resistance)
Hypercyanotic attacks (sudden decreases in pulmonary blood flow resulting in accentuation of arterial hypoxemia; often evoked by crying or exercise; treatment is esmolol and/or phenylephrine)
Cerebrovascular accident
Cerebral abscess
Infective endocarditis

     b. Induction of anesthesia is often with ketamine, 3 to 4 mg/kg IM or 1 to 2 mg/kg IV. The beneficial effect of ketamine is presumed to reflect a drug-induced increase in systemic vascular resistance that leads to a decrease in the magnitude of the right-to-left intracardiac shunt (PaO_2 often improves). Induction of anesthesia with volatile anesthetics such as sevoflurane is acceptable but must be accomplished with caution and careful monitoring of systemic oxygenation.

     c. Maintenance of anesthesia is often achieved with nitrous oxide in combination with ketamine. The advantage of this combination is that it preserves systemic vascular resistance. The principal disadvantage of using nitrous oxide is the associated decrease in inspired oxygen concentration. Ventilation of the patient's lungs should be controlled, but it must be appreciated

▬ **Table 3–9** • Events that Increase the Magnitude of a Right-to-Left Intracardiac Shunt

Decreased systemic vascular resistance
    Volatile anesthetics
    Histamine release
    Ganglionic blockade
    α-Adrenergic blockade
Increased pulmonary vascular resistance
Increased myocardial contractility (may accentuate infundibular obstruction to ejection of right ventricular stroke volume)

that excessive positive airway pressure may adversely increase resistance to blood flow through the lungs. Intravascular fluid volume must be maintained with intravenous fluid administration, as acute hypovolemia tends to increase the magnitude of the right-to-left intracardiac shunt. Meticulous care is taken to avoid infusion of air through the intravenous delivery tubing, as it could lead to systemic embolization of air. Phenylephrine is utilized to treat undesirable decreases in systemic blood pressure caused by decreased systemic vascular resistance.

5. **Patient characteristics following surgical repair of tetralogy of Fallot.** Ventricular cardiac dysrhythmias and atrial fibrillation or flutter are common in patients following surgical correction of tetralogy of Fallot. Right bundle branch block is frequent, but third-degree atrioventricular heart block is uncommon.

B. **Eisenmenger syndrome** describes patients with a VSD or ASD in whom the left-to-right intracardiac shunt is reversed as a result of increased pulmonary vascular resistance. Shunt reversal occurs in about 50% of patients with untreated VSD and in about 10% of patients with untreated ASD. The murmur associated with these cardiac defects disappears when Eisenmenger syndrome develops.

1. **Signs and symptoms.** See Table 3–10.
2. **Treatment.** No treatment has proven beneficial, although intravenous epoprostenol may be beneficial. Hyperviscosity may be treated with phlebotomy and isovolemic

---

Table 3–10 • Signs and Symptoms of Eisenmenger Syndrome

Arterial hypoxemia
  Cyanosis
  Erythrocytosis
  Increased blood viscosity
Decreased exercise tolerance
Atrial fibrillation
Hemoptysis (pulmonary infarction)
Thrombosis
Cerebral vascular accident
Brain abscess
Syncope
Sudden death

fluid replacement. Surgical correction of the congenital defect is contraindicated in the presence of irreversibly increased pulmonary vascular resistance. Pregnancy is discouraged in women with Eisenmenger syndrome.

3. **Management of anesthesia** for patients with Eisenmenger syndrome undergoing noncardiac surgery is based on maintenance of preoperative levels of systemic vascular resistance, recognizing that increases in right-to-left shunting are likely if sudden vasodilation (regional anesthesia) occurs. If epidural anesthesia is selected, it seems prudent not to add epinephrine to local anesthetic solutions as β-adrenergic effects from absorbed epinephrine could exaggerate decreases in systemic blood pressure and systemic vascular resistance. Minimizing blood loss with the development of hypovolemia and preventing iatrogenic paradoxical embolization are important considerations.

C. **Ebstein's anomaly** is an abnormality of the tricuspid valve in which the valve leaflets are malformed or displaced downward into the right ventricle.

1. **Signs and symptoms** (Table 3–11). Echocardiography is used to assess right atrial dilation, distortion of the tricuspid valve leaflets, and severity of tricuspid regurgitation or stenosis.

2. **Treatment** of Ebstein's anomaly is based on preventing associated complications; it includes antibiotic prophylaxis against infective endocarditis and administration of diuretics and digoxin for management of CHF. Patients

---

≡ Table 3–11 • Signs and Symptoms of Ebstein's Anomaly

Cyanosis
Congestive heart failure
Paradoxical embolization if interatrial communication
Hepatomegaly (passive congestion due to increased right atrial pressure)
Massive enlargement of right atrium
First-degree atrioventricular heart block
Paroxysmal supraventricular and ventricular tachydysrhythmias (high incidence of accessory pathways)
Brain abscess
Sudden death

with supraventricular dysrhythmias are treated pharmacologically or with catheter ablation if accessory pathways are present.

3. **Management of anesthesia.** Hazards during anesthesia in patients with Ebstein's anomaly include accentuation of arterial hypoxemia due to increases in the magnitude of the right-to-left intracardiac shunt and the development of supraventricular tachydysrhythmias.

D. **Tricuspid atresia** is characterized by arterial hypoxemia, a small right ventricle, a large left ventricle, and markedly decreased pulmonary blood flow.

1. **Treatment** of tricuspid atresia is anastomosis of the right atrial appendage to the right pulmonary artery (Fontan procedure).

2. **Management of anesthesia** for patients undergoing a Fontan procedure has been successfully achieved with opioids or volatile anesthetics. It is important to maintain an increased right atrial pressure to facilitate pulmonary blood flow (monitor the central venous pressure).

E. **Transposition of the great arteries** results in complete separation of the pulmonary and systemic circulations (survival is possible only if there is a communication between the two circulations in the form of a VSD, ASD, or PDA).

1. **Signs and symptoms.** Persistent cyanosis and tachypnea at birth may be the first clues, and CHF is often present.

2. **Treatment** includes initial interventions to create intracardiac mixing of blood (prostaglandins to maintain patency of the PDA, creation of an ASD) followed by an "arterial switch" operation (aorta is connected to the left ventricle, and the pulmonary artery is connected to the right ventricle).

3. **Management of anesthesia** is often accomplished with ketamine with or without opioids. Nitrous oxide has limited use, as it is important to administer high inspired oxygen concentrations. Dehydration must be avoided during the perioperative period, as these patients may have hematocrits > 70% (cerebral venous thrombosis).

F. **Mixing of blood between the pulmonary and systemic circulations.** Rare congenital heart defects that result in mixing of blood from the pulmonary and systemic circulations manifest as cyanosis and arterial hypoxemia of varying severity depending on the magnitude of the pulmonary blood flow (Table 3–12).

▬ Table 3–12 • Mixing of Blood Between the Pulmonary and Systemic Circulations

Truncus Arteriosus (single arterial trunk serves as the origin of the aorta and pulmonary artery)

Presents as cyanosis, arterial hypoxemia, failure to thrive, and congestive heart failure

Surgical treatment may include banding of the right and left pulmonary arteries to decrease pulmonary blood flow

Positive end-expiratory pressure may serve to decrease pulmonary blood flow and blunt symptoms of congestive heart failure

Partial Anomalous Pulmonary Venous Return (pulmonary veins empty into the right heart rather than the left heart)

Presents as fatigue, exertional dyspnea, and congestive heart failure

Angiography is the most useful technique for confirming the diagnosis

Total Anomalous Pulmonary Venous Return (all four pulmonary veins drain into the systemic venous circulation)

Presents as congestive heart failure

Positive end-expiratory pressure may serve to decrease pulmonary blood flow

Operative manipulation of the right atrium may result in obstruction to flow into the right atrium

Intravenous infusions may increase right atrial pressure and result in pulmonary edema

Hypoplastic Left Heart Syndrome (hypoplasia of the left ventricle, mitral valve, aortic valve, and ascending aorta)

Treatment is initial reconstruction of the ascending aorta using the proximal pulmonary artery followed by a Fontan procedure

Management of anesthesia includes high doses of opioids plus muscle relaxants

Ventricular fibrillation is a risk due to inadequate coronary blood flow

High PaO_2 (> 100 mmHg) implies excessive pulmonary blood flow at the expense of the systemic circulation (treatment is interventions to increase pulmonary vascular resistance as produced by respiratory acidosis)

Most frequent problem after cardiopulmonary bypass is inadequate pulmonary blood flow (PaO_2 < 20 mmHg)

☰ Table 3–13 • Mechanical Obstruction of the Trachea

Double Aortic Arch

Results in a vascular ring that can produce pressure on the trachea and esophagus

Manifests as inspiratory stridor, difficulty mobilizing secretions, and dysphagia

Treatment is surgical transection

Tracheal tube is placed beyond the area of tracheal compression

Gastric tube may cause occlusion of the trachea

Aberrant Left Pulmonary Artery

Tracheal or bronchial obstruction manifests as expiratory stridor or wheezing

Esophageal obstruction is rare

Surgical division of the aberrant left pulmonary artery is the treatment of choice

Absent Pulmonary Valve

Manifests as dilation of the pulmonary artery which can result in compression of the trachea and left mainstem bronchus

Tracheal extubation and maintenance of 4–6 mmHg continuous positive airway pressure can be used to keep the trachea distended

---

III. MECHANICAL OBSTRUCTION OF THE TRACHEA

See Table 3–13.

4

Abnormalities of Cardiac Conduction and Cardiac Rhythm

The incidence of intraoperative cardiac dysrhythmias depends on the definition (any cardiac dysrhythmia versus only potentially dangerous cardiac dysrhythmias), continuous surveillance versus casual observation, patient characteristics, and nature of the surgery (Stoelting RK, Dierdorf SF. Abnormalities of cardiac conduction and cardiac rhythm. In: Anesthesia and Co-Existing Disease, 4th ed. New York, Churchill Livingstone, 2002; 67–91). The importance of cardiac dysrhythmias relates to the effects of the specific cardiac rhythm disturbance on the cardiac output and the possible interactions of antidysrhythmia drugs with drugs administered to produce anesthesia and skeletal muscle relaxation.

I. MECHANISMS OF CARDIAC DYSRHYTHMIAS

A. **Reentry pathways** account for most premature beats and tachydysrhythmias. Pharmacologic or physiologic events may alter the crucial balance between conduction velocities and refractory periods of dual pathways, resulting in initiation or termination of reentry cardiac dysrhythmias (Table 4–1).

B. **Automaticity** refers to the slope of phase 4 depolarization of cardiac action potentials (Table 4–2). Automatic cardiac dysrhythmias [bradydysrhythmias, disturbances of atrioventricular (AV) or intraventricular conduction] are due to enhanced automaticity of a focus in the heart capable of undergoing spontaneous depolarization (repetitive firing) analogous to that of the sinoatrial (SA) node.

II. DIAGNOSIS OF CARDIAC DYSRHYTHMIAS

A. The electrocardiogram (ECG) is essential for the diagnosis of cardiac conduction and rhythm disturbances (Table 4–3).

Table 4–1 • Events Associated with Initiation of Cardiac Dysrhythmias During the Perioperative Period

Arterial hypoxemia
Electrolyte disturbances
  Potassium
  Magnesium
Acid-base disturbances
Altered activity of the autonomic nervous system
Increased myocardial fiber stretch
  Systemic hypertension
  Tracheal intubation
Myocardial ischemia
Drugs
  Catecholamines
  Volatile anesthetics
Co-existing cardiac disease
  Ventricular preexcitation (Wolff-Parkinson-White)
  Prolonged QT interval syndrome

B. Ambulatory electrocardiographic monitoring (Holter monitoring) is most useful for documenting the occurrence of life-threatening cardiac dysrhythmias, assessing the efficacy of antidysrhythmia drug therapy, and detecting the occurrence of silent (asymptomatic) ischemia.

Table 4–2 • Events that Alter the Slope of Phase 4 Depolarization

Increase Slope
Arterial hypoxemia
Hypercarbia
Acute hypokalemia
Hyperthermia
Catecholamines
Sympathomimetic drugs
Systemic hypertension
Decrease Slope
Vagal stimulation
Positive airway pressure
Acute hyperkalemia
Hypothermia

▬ Table 4–3 • Cardiac Antidysrhythmia Drugs

Indication	Side Effects
Lidocaine	
Ventricular premature beats	Accumulation with decreased hepatic blood flow
Ventricular tachydysrhythmias	Central nervous system toxicity
Recurrent ventricular fibrillation	Direct myocardial depression
	Peripheral vasodilation
Adenosine	
Supraventricular tachycardia including that associated with accessory tracts	Peripheral vasodilation (flushing)
	Dyspnea
	Angina pectoris
	Bronchospasm (theoretic)
	Denervation hypersensitivity in heart transplant patients
Verapamil	
Supraventricular tachycardia	Direct myocardial depression
Atrial fibrillation	Hypotension
Atrial flutter	Bradycardia
	Enhanced cardiac impulse transmission through accessory pathways
Digoxin	
Atrial tachydysrhythmias	Toxicity especially in the presence of renal dysfunction and/or hypokalemia
Atrial fibrillation	
Atrial flutter	
	Enhance cardiac impulse transmission through accessory pathways
Propranolol	
Atrial fibrillation	Sinus bradycardia
Atrial flutter	Direct myocardial depression
Supraventricular tachycardia	Bronchoconstriction
Ventricular tachydysrhythmias	Lethargy
Digitalis-induced ventricular dysrhythmias	
Procainamide	
Ventricular tachydysrhythmias	Direct myocardial depression
Ventricular premature beats	Hypotension

Table continued on following page

▬ Table 4–3 • Cardiac Antidysrhythmia Drugs
Continued

Indication	Side Effects
Atrial fibrillation due to accessory pathways	Peripheral vasodilation
	Paradoxical ventricular tachycardia
	Lupus erythematosus-like syndrome
	Accumulation with renal dysfunction
	Potentiation of nondepolarizing neuromuscular blocking drugs
Amiodarone	
Supraventricular tachydysrhythmias	Prolonged elimination half-time
Ventricular tachydysrhythmias	Bradycardia
	Hypotension
	Pulmonary fibrosis
	Postoperative ventilatory failure
	Skeletal muscle weakness
Prevention of recurrent atrial fibrillation	Peripheral neuropathy
Improved response to defibrillation	Hepatitis
	Cyanotic discoloration of the face
	Corneal deposits
	Thyroid dysfunction
Bretylium	
	Initial hypertension
Recurrent ventricular fibrillation	Peripheral vasodilation
Recurrent ventricular dysrhythmias	Hypotension
	Accumulation with renal dysfunction

III. TREATMENT OF CARDIAC DYSRHYTHMIAS

It is useful to consider and correct events (PaO_2, $PaCO_2$, pH, electrolytes, autonomic nervous system activity) responsible for evoking cardiac dysrhythmias before initiating antidysrhythmia drug therapy or placing an artificial cardiac pacemaker (Table 4–1).

A. **Antidysrhythmia drugs** are administered when correction of identifiable precipitating events is not sufficient to suppress cardiac dysrhythmias (Table 4–3).

1. **Lidocaine** is effective in decreasing the automaticity of ectopic cardiac pacemakers and increases the threshold for ventricular fibrillation. Supraventricular tachydysrhythmias are not suppressed by lidocaine.

2. Treatment of ventricular premature beats is with a loading dose of lidocaine, 1 to 2 mg/kg IV, followed by a continuous intravenous infusion, 1 to 4 mg/min, to maintain a therapeutic plasma concentration of 2 to 5 μg/ml. In the presence of decreased hepatic blood flow associated with general anesthesia, it may be necessary to decrease the lidocaine dose.

B. **Electrical cardioversion** is most effective for treating atrial flutter, atrial fibrillation, and ventricular tachycardia (exceptions are digitalis-induced cardiac dysrhythmias, which may be enhanced by cardioversion). The electrical discharge is delivered by means of two chest electrodes beginning at 50 to 100 joules. Intravenous sedation for this treatment is provided with drugs such as propofol, etomidate, or methohexital. Ventricular ectopy is common after cardioversion, and artificial cardiac pacing may be necessary in the event that underlying SA node dysfunction manifests after successful cardioversion.

C. **Radiofrequency catheter ablation** utilizes an electrode catheter to produce small, well demarcated areas of thermal injury that destroys the myocardial tissue critical to the initiation or maintenance of cardiac dysrhythmias (reentrant supraventricular cardiac dysrhythmia, idiopathic ventricular tachycardia).

D. **Artificial cardiac pacemakers** inserted intravenously (endocardial lead) or by the subcostal approach (epicardial or myocardial lead) are indicated for the treatment of SA node dysfunction ("sick sinus syndrome"), AV heart block (as follows cardiopulmonary bypass), neurogenic syncope, and cardiomyopathy.

1. **Programmable pacemakers** consist of a pulse generator (battery) and pacing electrode leads (Table 4–4).

2. **Pacing modes** are designated by a four letter generic code (Tables 4–5 and 4–6).

a. **DDD pacing.** Dual-chamber DDD pacemakers provide the important benefits of maintaining AV synchrony (more efficient ventricular filling and heart rate responses to exercise) and minimizing the incidence of pacemaker syndrome (weakness, orthopnea, paroxysmal nocturnal dyspnea, and pulmonary

Table 4–4 • Definition of Terms Used to Describe Artificial Cardiac Pacemakers

Term	Definition
Pulse generator	Consists of the energy source (battery) and electrical circuits necessary for pacing and sensory functions
Implanted or external	Anatomic placement of the pulse generator relative to the skin
Lead	Insulated wire connecting the pulse generator to the electrode
Electrode	Exposed metal end of electrode in contact with endocardium or epicardium (myocardium)
Endocardial pacing	Right atrium or right ventricle stimulated following transvenous insertion of the endocardial lead
Epicardial pacing	Right atrium or right ventricle stimulated following insertion of electrode into the myocardium under direct vision
Unipolar pacing	Describes placement of the negative (stimulating) electrode in the atrium or ventricle and the positive (ground) electrode distant from the heart (metallic portion of the pulse generator) in subcutaneous tissue
Bipolar pacing	Describes placement of the negative and positive electrode in the cardiac chamber being paced
Stimulation threshold	Minimal amount of current (amperes) or voltage (volts) necessary to cause contraction of the cardiac chamber being stimulated
Resistance	Measure of the combined resistance of the electrode lead–myocardial interface as calculated using Ohm's law with values for current and voltage thresholds (normal 350–1000 ohms)
R wave sensitivity	Minimal voltage of intrinsic R wave necessary to activate the sensing circuit of the pulse generator and thus inhibit or trigger the pacing circuit (an R wave sensitivity of about 3 mV on an external pulse generator maintains ventricle-inhibited pacing)
Hysteresis	Difference between intrinsic heart rate at which pacing begins (about 60 beats/min) and pacing rate (72 beats/min)

Table 4–5 ● Generic Code for Identification and Description of Pacemaker Function

First Letter (Cardiac Chamber Paced)	Second Letter (Cardiac Chamber in which Electrical Activity Is Sensed)	Third Letter (Response of Generator to Second R Wave and P Wave)	Fourth Letter (Programmable Functions of the Generator)
V—ventricle	V—ventricle	T—triggering	P—programmable (rate and/or output only)
A—atrium	A—atrium	I—inhibited	M—multiprogrammable
D—dual (atrium and ventricle)	D—dual	D—dual	C—communicating
	O—none (asynchronous)	O—none (asynchronous)	O—none (fixed function)

■ Table 4–6 • Types of Artificial Pulse Generators

_____Letter Code[a]_____				
I	II	III	IV	Description
Single-Chamber Pacing Modes				
A	O	O		Asynchronous (fixed rate) atrial pacing
V	O	O		Asynchronous (fixed rate) ventricular pacing
A	A	I		Noncompetitive (demand) atrial pacing; electrical output inhibited by intrinsic atrial depolarization (P wave)
V	V	I		Noncompetitive (demand) ventricular pacing, electrical output inhibited by intrinsic ventricular depolarization (R wave)
A	A	T		Triggered atrial pacing, electrical output triggered by intrinsic atrial depolarization (P wave)
V	V	T		Triggered ventricular pacing, electrical output triggered by intrinsic ventricular depolarization (R wave)
Dual-Chamber Pacing Modes				
D	D	D		Paces and senses in atrium and ventricle
D	D	I		Senses in both the atrium and ventricle, but only response to a sensed event is inhibition
Rate-Adaptive Pacemakers				
A	A	I	R	Single-chamber
V	V	I	R	Single-chamber
D	D	I	R	Dual-chamber
D	D	D	R	Dual-chamber

[a] See Table 4–5 for definitions of letter codes.

edema, which may reflect decreased cardiac output and hypotension due to the loss of atrial contributions to left ventricular filling).

b. **DDI pacing.** In the DDI pacing mode, there is sensing in both the atrium and the ventricle, but the only response to a sensed event is inhibition (useful in the presence of atrial tachydysrhythmias).

c. **Rate-adaptive pacemakers (AAIR, VVIR, DDIR, DDDR).** A rate-adaptive pacemaker is considered for patients who do not have appropriate chronotropic responses to increased metabolic demand (exercise).

3. **Choice of pacing mode** depends on the primary indication for the artificial pacemaker [sinus node disease requires an atrial pacemaker; AV node disease requires a dual chamber (DDD) pacemaker; need for a chronotropic response to exercise requires a rate-adaptive pacemaker].

4. **Artificial pacemaker failure.** Early pacemaker failures are usually due to electrode displacement or breakage, whereas failures that occur more than 6 months after implantation are most often due to premature battery depletion or a faulty pulse generator. Improved shielding of artificial cardiac pacemakers has largely eliminated interference from external electrical fields (automatically change or are converted to the asynchronous mode by placing a magnet externally over the pulse generator).

E. **Noninvasive transcutaneous cardiac pacing.** An alternative to emergency transvenous cardiac pacemaker placement is delivery of low-density constant-current impulses via cutaneous chest and back electrodes.

F. **Transvenous implantable cardioverter-defibrillator.** Patients with a history of ventricular tachycardia or ventricular fibrillation may benefit from implantation of devices that deliver a high energy synchronized shock when these dysrhythmias are detected.

G. **Surgery in patients with artificial cardiac pacemakers**

1. **Preoperative evaluation** includes determining the reason for placing the pacemaker and an assessment of its present function. A preoperative history of vertigo or syncope or a 10% decrease in the discharge rate of an asynchronous cardiac pacemaker (usually 70 to 72 beats/min) may reflect pacemaker dysfunction. The ECG is evaluated to confirm 1:1 capture, as evidenced by a pacemaker spike for every palpated peripheral pulse (no value in patients with intrinsic heart rates higher than the artificial cardiac pacemaker rate). Proper function of a demand pacemaker can be confirmed by demonstrating the appearance of captured beats on the ECG when the pacemaker is converted to the asynchronous mode by placing an external converter magnet over the pulse generator. A chest radiograph may be useful for confirming the absence of a break in the pacemaker electrodes.

2. **Management of anesthesia** in patients with artificial cardiac pacemakers includes monitoring to confirm contin-

ued function of the pulse generator and ready availability of equipment and drugs to maintain an acceptable intrinsic heart rate should the artificial cardiac pacemaker unexpectedly fail (Table 4–7). There is no evidence that anesthetics or events associated with the perioperative period alter the stimulation threshold for artificial cardiac pacemakers. An artificial cardiac pacemaker that is functioning normally preoperatively should continue to function intraoperatively without incident.

a. Despite improved shielding of the artificial cardiac pacemaker, it is still a reasonable recommendation to place the ground plate for the electrocautery as far as possible from the pulse generator to minimize detection of currents by the pulse generator.

b. Skeletal muscle myopotentials (fasciculations) produced by succinylcholine may inhibit a normal functioning artificial cardiac pacemaker by causing contraction of skeletal muscle groups (myopotential inhibition) interpreted as intrinsic R waves by the pulse generator. Nevertheless, clinical experience suggests that succinylcholine is generally a safe drug.

3. Anesthesia for artificial cardiac pacemaker insertion. A functioning transvenous artificial cardiac pacemaker should be in place, or a noninvasive transcutaneous cardiac pacemaker as well as drugs (atropine, isoproterenol) should be available before induction of anesthesia for permanent artificial cardiac pacemaker placement. The presence of a transvenous pacemaker predisposes patients to the risk of ventricular fibrillation from microshock levels of electrical currents.

≡ **Table 4–7 • Management of Anesthesia in Patients with Artificial Cardiac Pacemakers**

Continuous monitoring of the electrocardiogram
Continuous monitoring of a peripheral pulse
Electrical defibrillator present
External converter magnet available
Drugs prepared (atropine, isoproterenol)

IV. DISTURBANCES OF CARDIAC IMPULSE CONDUCTION

Disturbances of cardiac impulse conduction are classified according to the site of the conduction block relative to the AV node (Table 4–8). Heart block that occurs above the AV node is usually benign and transient, whereas heart block that develops below the AV node tends to be progressive and permanent.

≡ **Table 4–8 •** Classification of Heart Block

First-Degree Atrioventricular Heart Block
PR interval > 0.2 second
Usually asymptomatic
Atropine effective
Second-Degree Atrioventricular Heart Block
Mobitz type 1 (Wenckebach) (progressive prolongation of PR interval until a beat is entirely blocked)
Mobitz type 2 (sudden interruption of cardiac conduction; frequently progressive to third-degree AV heart block)
Unifascicular Heart Block
Left anterior hemiblock
Left posterior hemiblock
Right Bundle Branch Block
QRS > 0.1 second
Usually benign
Left Bundle Branch Block
QRS > 0.12 second and wide notched R waves in all electrocardiogram leads
Often associated with ischemic heart disease
Bifascicular Heart Block
Right bundle branch block plus left anterior hemiblock
Right bundle branch block plus left posterior hemiblock
No evidence that likely to progress to third-degree AV heart block during anesthesia and surgery
Third-Degree Atrioventricular (Trifascicular, Complete) Heart Block
Nodal (heart rate 45–55 beats/min)
Infranodal (heart rate 30–40 beats/min and wide QRS complexes)
Isoproterenol 1–4 μg/min IV plus atropine is a chemical pacemaker
Causes include fibrous degeneration of the cardiac conduction system, ischemic heart disease, cardiomyopathy, myocarditis, iatrogenic after cardiac surgery, drugs (digoxin), and electrolyte disturbances
Permanent artificial cardiac pacemaker

V. DISTURBANCES OF CARDIAC RHYTHM

Disturbances of cardiac rhythm are classified as supraventricular dysrhythmias (arising in the atria or AV node) or ventricular dysrhythmias (arising below the AV node) (Table 4–9).

A. Sinus tachycardia, defined as a heart rate > 120 beats/min, is due to acceleration of the normal discharge rate of the SA node.

B. Sinus bradycardia, defined as a heart rate < 60 beats/min, is due to deceleration of the normal discharge rate of the SA node.

  1. **Spinal and epidural anesthesia** may be associated with bradycardia and asystole (6.4 per 10,000 patients).

     a. **Pathophysiology.** Proposed theories for bradycardia and asystole during spinal and epidural anesthesia include reflex-induced bradycardia due to decreased venous return or unopposed parasympathetic nervous system activity resulting from spinal or epidural-induced sympathectomy.

     b. **Clinical manifestations.** Bradycardia, asystole, or both may develop suddenly or be progressive. In most patients, pulse oximetry confirms acceptable oxygen saturation prior to the onset of bradycardia, suggesting a primary cardiac mechanism. The level of sensory anesthesia is not necessarily a predictor of bradycardia, and the risk of bradycardia and asystole may persist into the postoperative period.

     c. **Treatment** is prompt pharmacologic intervention (atropine, ephedrine, epinephrine) and precordial pacing thumps.

  2. **Syncope** is most often due to vasovagal reactions (brady-dysrhythmias).

≡ Table 4–9 • Characteristic Appearance of Ventricular Premature Beats on the Electrocardiogram

---

Premature occurrence
Absence of a P wave preceding the QRS complex
Wide and often bizarre-appearing QRS complex
ST segment in a direction opposite the QRS complex
Inverted T wave
Compensatory pause after the premature beat

C. **Sinus node dysfunction** ("sick sinus syndrome") is a common cause of bradycardia (1 in 600 patients over 65 years of age) and is a frequent indication for placing an artificial cardiac pacemaker.

D. **Atrial premature and junctional premature beats** arise from an ectopic cardiac pacemaker in the atria or near the AV node. Acceleration of the heart rate, as produced by intravenous administration of atropine, usually abolishes atrial premature beats.

E. **Supraventricular tachycardia** is any tachydysrhythmia that requires atrial or AV junctional tissue for its initiation and maintenance. The term "paroxysmal atrial tachycardia" to describe supraventricular tachycardia that begins and ends abruptly is no longer recommended, as it is likely that many of these dysrhythmias arise in the AV junction and not the atrial muscle. AV nodal reentrant tachycardia (AVNRT) is the most common type of supraventricular tachycardia (average heart rate 160 to 180 beats/min) and occurs three times more often in females than males.

1. **Mechanisms** of supraventricular tachycardia are often reentry circuits. AVNRT is probably the most common cause of AV reentrant tachycardia.

2. **Treatment** of AVNRT is initially with vagal maneuvers (carotid sinus massage, Valsalva maneuver, stimulation of the posterior pharynx). If vagal maneuvers are not effective, pharmacologic treatment is directed toward blocking AV nodal conduction.

   a. **Adenosine,** an α_1-adrenergic agonist with a rapid onset and brief duration of action, is the drug of choice for the pharmacologic treatment of AVNRT. Most AVNRTs are terminated by a single intravenous adenosine dose of 6 mg. If the initial 6 mg dose is not effective, two subsequent doses of 12 mg may be administered about 2 minutes apart. Adenosine often causes flushing and in some patients is associated with angina pectoris and dyspnea. Multifocal atrial tachycardia, atrial flutter, and atrial fibrillation are not likely to respond to adenosine.

   b. **Calcium channel blocking drugs,** including verapamil (75 to 150 μg/kg IV over about 2 minutes) and diltiazem, are useful for terminating supraventricular tachycardia. An advantage of verapamil is its longer duration of action than adenosine, but its administration may cause hypotension.

F. **Atrial flutter** is a paroxysmal disturbance, usually lasting only a few minutes to hours before spontaneously converting to normal sinus rhythm or atrial fibrillation. In the presence of hemodynamically significant atrial flutter, the treatment of choice is electrical cardioversion.

G. **Atrial fibrillation,** the most common sustained cardiac dysrhythmia, is present in about 0.4% of the U.S. population (incidence increases with age). The most common underlying cardiovascular diseases associated with atrial fibrillation are systemic hypertension and ischemic heart disease. Valvular heart disease, congestive heart failure, and diabetes mellitus are independent risk factors for atrial fibrillation.

1. **Clinical manifestations** of atrial fibrillation include palpitations, pulmonary edema, fatigue, thromboembolic events (formation of thrombi due to stasis of blood in the atria), and congestive heart failure (loss of synchronized atrial contractions and rapid ventricular response rates decrease cardiac output).

   a. **Postoperative atrial tachydysrhythmias** are common during the early postoperative period (first 2 to 4 days) especially in elderly patients following cardiothoracic surgery.

   b. Thromboembolic complications (stroke) are a high risk, and prompt anticoagulant therapy with heparin is recommended to treat postoperative atrial fibrillation. In addition, the ventricular response rate is slowed pharmacologically (β-antagonists, calcium channel blocking drugs, digoxin) or with electrical cardioversion.

2. **Treatment** of chronic atrial fibrillation is intended to restore and sustain normal sinus rhythm.

   a. **Electrical cardioversion** is the most effective method for converting atrial fibrillation to normal sinus rhythm. Before undergoing elective direct-current cardioversion, patients are fasted (6 hours), electrolyte imbalances are corrected, and toxic drug levels are excluded as the cause of the cardiac dysrhythmia. Digoxin may be withheld on the morning of the scheduled cardioversion. Anesthesia for elective cardioversion is with short-acting intravenous drugs (propofol, etomidate) plus supplemental oxygen.

   b. **Drug therapy** for atrial fibrillation often includes digoxin, which exerts a vagotonic effect on the AV node. β-antagonists and calcium channel blocking drugs may be useful, but unlike digoxin, they exert negative inotropic effects.

   c. **Anticoagulation** usually includes oral warfarin, although aspirin may be sufficient in those considered to be at low risk for thromboembolic complications

H. **Junctional rhythm** is due to the activity of an ectopic cardiac pacemaker in the tissues surrounding the AV node (P wave precedes, follows, or is obscured by the QRS complex). Intravenous administration of atropine is the initial treatment for a hemodynamically significant junctional rhythm.

I. **Wandering atrial** pacemaker reflects the presence of multiple atrial ectopic pacemakers. Intravenous administration of atropine is usually effective if the cardiac dysrhythmia is hemodynamically significant.

J. **Ventricular ectopy (ventricular premature beats)** arise from single (unifocal) or multiple (multifocal) ectopic cardiac pacemaker sites located below the AV node. Characteristic findings on the electrocardiogram (ECG) serve to identify ventricular premature beats (Table 4–9). A vulnerable period exists during diastole (R on T phenomenon) when a ventricular premature beat may initiate repetitive ventricular responses, including ventricular tachycardia or ventricular fibrillation.

   1. **Prognosis** depends on the presence and severity of left ventricular dysfunction. Ventricular premature beats occur in most patients experiencing acute myocardial infarctions. The most common conditions in which ventricular premature beats predispose to life-threatening ventricular dysrhythmias include myocardial ischemia, valvular heart disease causing pressure or volume overload on the ventricles, cardiomyopathies, a prolonged QT interval on the ECG, and the presence of electrolyte abnormalities, especially hyperkalemia.

   2. **Treatment.** Ventricular premature beats should be treated when they are frequent (> 6 beats/min), are multifocal, occur in salvos of three or more, or take place during the vulnerable period on the T wave, as these characteristics are associated with an increased incidence of ventricular tachycardia and fibrillation. The first step in the treatment of ventricular premature beats is elimination of the underlying cause, such as arterial hypoxemia or other events associated with excessive sympathetic nervous system activity. If ventricular premature beats persist despite correction of the underlying cause,

or they are hemodynamically significant, the initial drug of choice is lidocaine, 1 to 2 mg/kg IV. This initial dose of lidocaine may be followed with a continuous infusion, 1 to 4 mg/min IV, to maintain therapeutic blood concentrations and continued suppression of the ectopic ventricular pacemaker. Lidocaine is not effective in suppressing ventricular premature beats caused by mechanical irritation of the heart, such as an intracardiac catheter.

K. Ventricular tachycardia is present when three or more consecutive ventricular premature beats occur at a calculated heart rate of > 120 beats/min. The QRS complexes on the ECG are widened, reflecting aberrant intraventricular conduction of the cardiac impulses, and there are no P waves. Ventricular tachycardia is common after acute myocardial infarction and in the presence of inflammatory disease of the heart. Digitalis toxicity may manifest as ventricular tachycardia.

1. **Torsade de pointes,** an unusual form of ventricular tachycardia, is initiated by a ventricular premature beat in the presence of abnormal ventricular repolarization characterized by prolongation of the QT interval on the ECG (see "Congenital Long QT Syndrome").

2. **Treatment** of hemodynamically significant ventricular tachycardia consists of prompt electrical cardioversion. If ventricular tachycardia is well tolerated hemodynamically, it is acceptable to administer intravenous lidocaine.

L. Ventricular fibrillation is the most common cause of sudden cardiac death, and most victims have underlying ischemic heart disease.

1. **Treatment** of ventricular fibrillation is electrical defibrillation. When ventricular fibrillation is refractory to electrical treatment, administration of amiodarone, lidocaine, or bretylium may improve responses to defibrillation.

2. External cardiac compression alone may be as effective as external cardiac compressions combined with mouth-to-mouth ventilation during the period before electrical defibrillation can be applied.

VI. VENTRICULAR PREEXCITATION SYNDROMES

A. The presence of alternate ("accessory") pathways that function as electrically active muscular bridges that bypass the normal AV nodal conduction of cardiac impulses creates

---

≡ Table 4–10 • Clinical Manifestations of Wolff-Parkinson-White Syndrome

Symptomatic tachydysrhythmias (typically begin during early adulthood and may first manifest during the perioperative period)

Sudden death (presumably due to ventricular fibrillation)

Electrocardiographic findings

  Delta wave (earlier than normal deflection due to ventricular preexcitation)

  AV tachycardia

    Orthodromic (narrow complex QRS tachycardia)

    Antidromic (wide complex QRS tachycardia)

  Atrial fibrillation

  Atrial flutter

---

the potential for reentrant tachycardia. It is estimated that accessory AV pathways for conduction of cardiac impulses between the atria and ventricles are present in 0.1% to 0.3% of the population.

  B. Wolff-Parkinson-White (WPW) syndrome. The most prominent manifestation of ventricular preexcitation by cardiac impulses traveling via accessory pathways is the WPW syndrome.

    1. Clinical manifestations. See Table 4–10.

    2. Treatment. See Table 4–11.

    3. Management of anesthesia. See Table 4–12.

≡ Table 4–11 • Treatment of Wolff-Parkinson-White Syndrome

Orthodromic AV reciprocating tachycardia (narrow complex)

  Vagal maneuvers (carotid sinus massage, Valsalva maneuver, stimulation of posterior pharynx)

  Adenosine 6–12 mg IV if vagal maneuvers unsuccessful

  Verapamil if adenosine unsuccessful

Antidromic AV reciprocating tachycardia (wide complex)

  Procainamide 10 mg/kg IV if systolic blood pressure > 90 mmHg

  Electrical cardioversion if systolic blood pressure < 90 mmHg

Atrial fibrillation

  Procainamide

  Electrical cardioversion if hemodynamic instability

≡ **Table 4–12 • Management of Anesthesia in Patients with Wolff-Parkinson-White Syndrome**

Continue preoperative antidysrhythmia drugs

Avoid events associated with increased sympathetic nervous system activity (anxiety, hypovolemia)

Avoid drugs that enhance anterograde conduction of cardiac impulses through accessory pathways (digoxin, verapamil)

Availability of drugs known to be effective for treatment of tachydysrhythmias and/or electrical cardioversion

Intravenous induction of anesthesia with propofol

Establish adequate depth of anesthesia before initiating direct laryngoscopy and tracheal intubation

Volatile anesthetics to suppress sympathetic nervous system activity during maintenance of anesthesia

Monitoring influenced by complexity of surgery

VII. CONGENITAL LONG QT SYNDROME

A. The congenital long QT syndrome (Romano Ward syndrome) is an autosomal dominant disorder that usually presents as syncope during childhood or the teenage years. It is characterized by recurrent bouts of rapid polymorphic ventricular tachycardia known as **torsade de pointes.** Sud-

≡ **Table 4–13 • Management of Anesthesia in Patients with Congenital Long QT Syndrome**

Preoperative electrocardiography to rule out syndrome in patients with a family history of sudden death

Consider preoperative establishment of β-blockade or performance of a left stellate ganglion block

Induction of anesthesia with propofol is acceptable

Consider effects of volatile anesthetics on QTc interval

Avoid events known to prolong QTc interval

    Increased sympathetic nervous system activity (anxiety, tracheal intubation, surgical stimulation, presence of tracheal tube on awakening during emergence)

    Acute hypokalemia (iatrogenic hyperventilation)

Esmolol for treatment of acute ventricular dysrhythmias

Electrical defibrillator immediately available

Consider administration of phenytoin during the postoperative period

den death is a risk, especially as part of the sudden infant death syndrome. The hallmark of the long QT syndrome is prolongation of the QTc interval (> 460 to 480 ms) on the ECG.

B. Treatment. Suppression of sympathetic nervous system activity with β-adrenergic antagonists or left thoracic sympathectomy via a supraclavicular approach is the recommended treatment. A temporary measure is left stellate ganglion block, which is intended to abolish the sympathetic nervous system imbalance that exists between the left and right cardiac sympathetic nerves.

C. Management of anesthesia. See Table 4–13.

5

Systemic Hypertension

Systemic hypertension (140/90 mmHg or higher) is the most common circulatory derangement affecting approximately 24% of adults in the United States (Stoelting RK, Dierdorf SF. Systemic hypertension. In: Anesthesia and Co-Existing Disease, 4th ed. New York, Churchill Livingstone, 2002;93–104). Systemic hypertension is a significant risk factor for the development of ischemic heart disease and a major cause of congestive heart failure, cerebral vascular accident (stroke), arterial aneurysm, and end-stage renal disease (Fig. 5–1).

I. PATHOPHYSIOLOGY

Systemic hypertension is characterized as essential hypertension when a cause for the increased blood pressure cannot be identified and as secondary hypertension when the etiology is known.

A. **Essential hypertension,** which accounts for more than 95% of all cases of hypertension, is characterized by a familial incidence and inherited biochemical abnormalities (Table 5–1).

B. **Secondary hypertension** is most often due to renal artery stenosis (renovascular hypertension). Primary aldosteronism produces secondary hypertension associated with hypokalemia.

II. TREATMENT OF ESSENTIAL HYPERTENSION

The standard goal of pharmacologic therapy is to decrease systemic blood pressure to less than 140/90 mmHg (Table 5–2).

A. **Patient selection.** Patients with concomitant risk factors (hypercholesterolemia, diabetes mellitus, tobacco abuse, family history, age > 60 years) and evidence of target-organ damage (angina pectoris, prior myocardial infarction, left ventricular hypertrophy, cerebrovascular disease, nephropathy, reti-

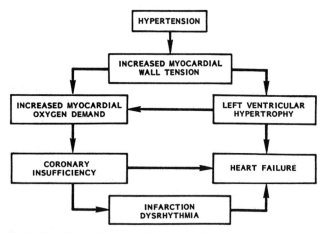

Fig. 5–1 • Chronic increases in systemic blood pressure initiates a series of pathophysiologic changes that may culminate in congestive heart failure.

≡ Table 5–1 • Conditions Associated with Systemic Hypertension

Increased sympathetic nervous system activity
Sodium and water retention
Hypercholesterolemia
Insulin resistance
Obesity
Alcohol and tobacco use
Sleep-disordered breathing (obstructive sleep apnea)
Glucose intolerance
Ischemic heart disease and angina pectoris
Left ventricular hypertrophy
Congestive heart failure
Cerebrovascular disease
Peripheral vascular disease
Renal insufficiency

━ **Table 5–2** • Beneficial Effects of Treatment
Resulting in Normalization of Systemic
Blood Pressure

Decreased incidence of cerebrovascular accidents
Decreased morbidity and mortality associated with ischemic heart
disease
Slowing or prevention of progression to more severe systemic
hypertension and development of congestive heart failure and
renal failure

nopathy, peripheral vascular disease) are most likely to benefit from pharmacologic therapy.

B. **Lifestyle modifications** of proven value for lowering systemic blood pressure include weight reduction or prevention
of weight gain, moderation of alcohol intake, increased physical activity, and cessation of tobacco use. The antihypertensive efficacy of dietary salt restriction is questionable.

C. **Pharmacologic therapy.** A large variety of antihypertensive
drugs are available, many of which present unique, potentially significant side effects (Table 5–3). The choice of antihypertensive therapy may be influenced by the presence of
cardiovascular risk factors and evidence of target organ disease (Table 5–4).

III. TREATMENT OF SECONDARY HYPERTENSION

Treatment of secondary hypertension is surgical for identifiable
causes of secondary hypertension (renal artery stenosis, pheochromocytoma). It is medical when surgery is not possible.

IV. HYPERTENSIVE CRISIS

Hypertensive crisis is defined as an acute diastolic blood pressure > 130 mmHg.

A. The need for emergency treatment of a hypertensive crisis
is determined more by the rate of increase in systemic blood
pressure than the absolute systemic blood pressure.

B. **Pharmacologic therapy.** Patients with evidence of acute or
ongoing target-organ damage (encephalopathy, congestive
heart failure, renal insufficiency) require prompt pharmacologic intervention to lower the systemic blood pressure (decrease the mean arterial pressure < 20% during the first
2 hours).

Text continued on page 70

Table 5-3 • Antihypertensive Drugs, Associated Side Effects, Special Considerations

Drugs	Side Effects	Special Considerations
Diuretics		
Thiazides	Hypokalemia Hyperuricemia Glucose intolerance Hypercholesterolemia Hypertriglyceridemia Sexual dysfunction Alkalosis	May enhance digitalis toxicity May precipitate acute gout May be ineffective in renal failure
Loop diuretics	Same as for thiazides	Effective in renal failure May precipitate gout or enhance digitalis toxicity Hyponatremia especially in elderly patients
Potassium-Sparing Drugs		
Amiloride Spironolactone	Hyperkalemia Sexual dysfunction Gynecomastia	
Adrenergic Antagonists		
β-adrenergic antagonists	Bradycardia Bronchospasm Congestive heart failure Hypertriglyceridemia Mask hypoglycemia	Do not use in patients with asthma or chronic obstructive pulmonary disease Do not use in patients with congestive heart failure, sick sinus syndrome, or heart block

Drug	Side Effects	Special Considerations
Centrally Acting Drugs		
Methyldopa	Sedation Sexual dysfunction	Use cautiously in patients with diabetes mellitus and peripheral vascular disease Abrupt discontinuation may result in rebound sympathetic nervous system stimulation
Reserpine	Drowsiness Dry mouth Fatigue	Rebound hypertension may occur when abruptly discontinued May cause liver damage May cause hemolytic anemia (Coombs' test) Decreases anesthetic requirements Do not use in patients with a history of mental depression
Clonidine	Fatigue Nasal congestion Sexual dysfunction Sedation Bradycardia Xerostomia	Decreases anesthetic requirements Decreases anesthetic requirements Abrupt discontinuation may result in rebound hypertension May be an analgesic alone or in combination with neuraxial opioids
α_1-Adrenergic Antagonists		
Prazosin	First-dose syncope Orthostatic hypotension Fluid retention	Use cautiously in elderly patients Unlikely to elicit reflex tachycardia Hypotension during neuraxial blockade may be exaggerated as compensatory vasoconstriction is blocked

Table continued on following page

Table 5–3 • Antihypertensive Drugs, Associated Side Effects, Special Considerations *Continued*

Drugs	Side Effects	Special Considerations
Combined α- and β-Adrenergic Antagonists		
Labetalol	Bronchospasm Orthostatic hypotension Fatigue	Use cautiously in patients with asthma or chronic obstructive pulmonary disease Use cautiously in patients with congestive heart failure, sick sinus syndrome, or heart block
Vasodilators		
Hydralazine	Tachycardia Headache Fluid retention Sodium retention Positive antinuclear antibody	May precipitate angina pectoris in patients with ischemic heart disease Lupus syndrome may occur
Minoxidil	Hypertrichosis	May cause or aggravate pleural effusion
Angiotensin-Converting Enzyme Inhibitors		
Benazepril Captopril Enalapril Lisinopril Moexipril	Cough Rhinorrhea Angioedema Rash Hyperkalemia Proteinuria	May be associated with hemodynamic instability and hypotension during general anesthesia especially if large fluid shifts are associated with the surgical procedure May cause neutropenia in patients with autoimmune collagen diseases

Angiotensin II Receptor Antagonists

Irbesartan
Losartan
Valsartan

Dizziness

May cause reversible acute renal failure in patients with renal artery stenosis
May cause fetal toxicity
Nonsteroidal antiinflammatory drugs may antagonize antihypertensive effects

Calcium Channel Blocking Drugs

Congestive heart failure
Hypotension
Heart block
Syncope
Hepatic dysfunction

May cause reversible renal failure in patients with renal artery stenosis
May cause fetal toxicity

Verapamil

Bradycardia

Use cautiously in patients with congestive heart failure

Adapted from Oparil S, Calhoun DA. High blood pressure. Sci Am Med 2000;1–16.

Table 5–4 • Determinants of Initial Drug Choice for
Treatment of Essential Hypertension

Diuretics or β-adrenergic antagonists (patients without presence
of cardiovascular risk factors or evidence of target organ
damage)

Angiotensin-converting enzyme inhibitors [patients with diabetes
mellitus or history of congestive heart failure (systolic
dysfunction)]

β-Adrenergic antagonists lacking intrinsic sympathomimetic
activity (patients with a history of prior myocardial infarction)

Diuretics or calcium channel-blocking drugs (elderly patients with
isolated systolic hypertension)

---

1. **Nitroprusside,** 0.5 to 10.0 μg/kg/min IV, is the drug of
   choice for treating hypertensive emergencies. Placing an
   intra-arterial catheter to monitor systemic blood pressure
   continuously may be recommended during treatment
   with nitroprusside.
2. **Nitroglycerin** is an appropriate choice for treating a hypertensive crisis in the presence of myocardial ischemia
   or cocaine overdose.

V. MANAGEMENT OF ANESTHESIA IN PATIENTS WITH ESSENTIAL HYPERTENSION

A. **Preoperative evaluation** (Table 5–5). Despite the desire to
   render patients normotensive before elective surgery, there
   is no evidence that the incidence of postoperative complications is increased when hypertensive patients (diastolic
   blood pressure < 110 mmHg) undergo an elective operation.
   It is not uncommon for the systemic blood pressure measured on admission to the hospital to be high ("white coat
   syndrome"), reflecting patient anxiety at this time in the
   preoperative period.
   1. **Evidence of end-organ damage.** Patients with essential
      hypertension are always suspect for incipient congestive
      heart failure and are presumed to have ischemic heart
      disease until proven otherwise. Symptoms of cerebrovas-
      cular disease may be reflected by dizziness or syncope
      with changes in head position, as may be necessary for
      direct laryngoscopy using tracheal intubation and subse-
      quent positioning for surgery.

▬ Table 5–5 • Management of Anesthesia in Hypertensive Patients

Preoperative Evaluation
Determine adequacy of systemic blood pressure control
Review pharmacology of drugs being administered to control
  systemic blood pressure (orthostatic hypotension, bradycardia,
  sedation, anesthetic requirements)
Evaluate for evidence of end-organ damage
  Angina pectoris
  Left ventricular hypertrophy
  Congestive heart failure
  Cerebrovascular disease
  Stroke
  Peripheral vascular disease
  Renal insufficiency
Induction of Anesthesia
Anticipate exaggerated systemic blood pressure changes
Limit duration of direct laryngoscopy
Maintenance of Anesthesia
Administer volatile anesthetics to blunt hypertensive responses
Monitor for myocardial ischemia
Postoperative Management
Anticipate periods of systemic hypertension
Maintain monitoring of end-organ function

2. **Antihypertensive drug therapy.** There is no evidence that antihypertensive drug therapy adversely alters the course or conduct of anesthesia, although many of these drugs interfere with autonomic nervous system function. A compelling reason to continue antihypertensive drug therapy throughout the perioperative period is the risk of rebound hypertension should these drugs (especially β-adrenergic antagonists and clonidine) be abruptly discontinued during the immediate preoperative period. Antihypertensive drugs that act independently of the autonomic nervous system [angiotensin-converting enzyme (ACE) inhibitors] do not seem to be associated with rebound hypertension should treatment be abruptly discontinued.

   a. **ACE inhibitors.** Despite the acceptance of the concept that antihypertensive drug therapy should be continued throughout the perioperative period, there is a risk that hemodynamic instability and hypotension may occur during anesthesia in patients being treated with ACE inhibitors, especially if the surgery is associated with major body fluid shifts.

    b. Titrating and decreasing the doses of anesthetic drugs and maintenance of intravascular fluid volume during surgery are important for minimizing the incidence and/or magnitude of hypotension attributed to ACE inhibitors.

B. Induction of anesthesia is often achieved with rapidly acting intravenous drugs (exception ketamine) (Table 5–5).

    1. Direct laryngoscopy for tracheal intubation may result in exaggerated increases in systemic blood pressure in patients with essential hypertension, even if these patients have been treated with antihypertensive drugs and rendered normotensive preoperatively. Evidence of myocardial ischemia on the electrocardiogram of patients with ischemic heart disease is most likely to occur in association with increases in systemic blood pressure and heart rate that accompany direct laryngoscopy and tracheal intubation.

    2. Attenuating the circulatory responses evoked by direct laryngoscopy and tracheal intubation is a consideration (Table 5–6).

C. Maintenance of anesthesia. The goal during maintenance of anesthesia is to adjust the depth of anesthesia in appropriate

---

☰ Table 5–6 • Methods to Attenuate Circulatory Responses Evoked by Direct Laryngoscopy and Tracheal Intubation

---

Establish a surgical level of anesthesia with volatile anesthetics
Administer a short-acting opioid before initiating direct laryngoscopy
    Alfentanil 15–30 μg/kg IV or remifentanil 1 μg/kg IV at the time of administration of intravenous induction drugs
    Fentanyl 50–150 μg/kg IV or sufentanil 10–30 μg/kg IV about 3 minutes before anticipated induction of anesthesia
Brief duration (< 15 seconds) of direct laryngoscopy
Supplemental therapy
    Laryngotracheal lidocaine 2 mg/kg
    Lidocaine 1.5 mg/kg IV
    Esmolol 100–200 mg IV
    Nitroprusside 1 μg/kg IV

directions to minimize wide fluctuations in systemic blood pressure (Table 5–5). Management of intraoperative blood pressure lability with the anesthetic technique may be more important than preoperative control of hypertension. Regional anesthesia is acceptable for hypertensive patients, recognizing that the need for high sensory levels of anesthesia and associated sympathetic nervous system denervation could unmask unsuspected hypovolemia.

1. **Intraoperative hypertension** in response to painful stimulation is likely in previously hypertensive patients—even in those previously rendered normotensive with drug therapy. Volatile anesthetics are useful for attenuating sympathetic nervous system activity, which is responsible for pressor responses. Continuous intravenous infusions of nitroprusside are alternatives to volatile anesthetics for maintaining normotension during the intraoperative period. Labetalol may be useful for blunting systemic blood pressure and heart rate responses evoked by painful stimulation.

2. **Intraoperative hypotension** that occurs during the maintenance of anesthesia may be treated by decreasing the delivered concentrations of volatile anesthetics, increasing the infusion rates of crystalloid or colloid solutions, or administering sympathomimetic drugs (pharmacologic effect is maintained despite suppressant effects of antihypertensive drugs on sympathetic nervous system activity).

3. **Monitoring** is influenced by the complexity of the surgery and the presence or absence of left ventricular dysfunction (transesophageal echocardiography is useful for monitoring left ventricular function and the adequacy of intravascular volume replacement).

D. **Postoperative management.** Systemic hypertension during the early postoperative period (often in the postanesthesia care unit) is a likely response in patients with a preoperative diagnosis of essential hypertension. The development of postoperative systemic hypertension warrants prompt assessment (pain, fluid overload) and treatment (opioids, hydralazine, labetalol, nitroprusside) to minimize the risks of myocardial ischemia, congestive heart failure, stroke, and bleeding.

6

Congestive Heart Failure

Congestive heart failure (CHF) is a major health problem in the United States (affects about 1% of adults), and despite advances in therapy the mortality remains high (Stoelting RK, Dierdorf SF. Congestive heart failure. In: Anesthesia and Co-Existing Disease, 4th ed. New York, Churchill Livingstone, 2002;105–115). The principal cause of CHF is impairment of the heart's ability to fill or empty the left ventricle (Table 6–1). Treatment to prevent or delay the progression of left ventricular dysfunction (progressive dilation and remodeling of the left ventricle) may be quite different from treatment intended to relieve symptoms and improve the patient's quality of life. Indeed, the short-term relief of symptoms attributed to CHF may have little relation to the progression of cardiac dysfunction over time. Symptoms of CHF are only weakly related to the severity of left ventricular dysfunction, although the magnitude of the dysfunction is closely linked to mortality.

I. MANIFESTATIONS OF LEFT VENTRICULAR DYSFUNCTION

A decrease in ventricular systolic wall motion reflects systolic dysfunction, whereas ventricular diastolic dysfunction is characterized by increased end-diastolic pressure in a chamber of normal size.

A. Systolic heart failure. Systemic hypertension and cardiac valve disease may produce chronic pressure or volume overloads that alter the structure and function of the left ventricle.

1. **Diagnosis.** A decreased ejection fraction (< 0.45 with or without symptoms of CHF) is a hallmark of chronic left ventricular dysfunction. Chest radiographs are not sensitive for assessing the size or function of the left ventricle, whereas the electrocardiogram (ECG) of patients with

---

**≡ Table 6–1 • Causes of Congestive
Heart Failure**

Cardiac valve abnormalities
  Mitral stenosis
  Aortic stenosis
Impaired myocardial contractility
  Ischemic heart disease
  Cardiomyopathy
Systemic hypertension
Pulmonary hypertension (cor pulmonale)

---

significant left ventricular dysfunction is almost always abnormal (including ventricular dysrhythmias).

2. A decrease in diastolic compliance, manifesting as impaired filling of the left ventricle during diastole, may be part of any type of left ventricular dysfunction.

B. **Diastolic heart failure.** Symptomatic CHF in patients with normal or near-normal left ventricular systolic function is most likely due to diastolic dysfunction (ventricle has decreased compliance and cannot fill adequately at normal diastolic pressures).

1. **Diagnosis.** Clinical signs and symptoms do not reliably differentiate systolic dysfunction from diastolic dysfunction (Table 6–2).

2. **Treatment** of diastolic CHF is empirical (diuretics, normal sinus rhythm, correction of precipitating factors such as acute myocardial ischemia and systemic hypertension) as no drugs have been documented to improve diastolic distensibility selectively.

**≡ Table 6–2 • Differentiation of Diastolic Dysfunction
from Systolic Dysfunction**

Absence of cardiomegaly on chest radiography
Presence of a normal ejection fraction
Signs of systemic or pulmonary venous congestion in the
  presence of a left ventricular chamber of normal size

≡ Table 6–3 • Hemodynamic Parameters of Ventricular Function

Cardiac Output
Output < 2.5 L/min/m^2 in presence of CHF
Increased arterial to venous oxygen content difference
Adaptive mechanisms for maintaining cardiac output
    Frank-Starling relation (increase in stroke volume that
      accompanies progressive increases in the left or right
      ventricular end-diastolic volume)
    Inotropic state (velocity of contraction developed by cardiac
      muscle, V_{max})
    Afterload
    Heart rate
    Myocardial hypertrophy and dilation
    Sympathetic nervous system activity
    Humoral-mediated responses
Ejection Fraction
Decreased by impaired myocardial contractility, increased
  afterload, or asynchrony of left ventricular contraction
End-Diastolic Pressure
Increased in presence of CHF (left ventricular end-diastolic
  pressure > 12 mmHg and right ventricular end-diastolic
  pressure > 5 mmHg)
Left ventricular end-diastolic pressure parallels left atrial pressure
  in the absence of mitral valve disease
Left ventricular end-diastolic pressure parallels pulmonary artery
  end-diastolic pressure in the absence of increased pulmonary
  vascular resistance or mitral valve disease

II. HEMODYNAMIC PARAMETERS OF VENTRICULAR FUNCTION

The hemodynamic parameters of ventricular function likely to be altered by CHF include cardiac output, ejection fraction, and ventricular end-diastolic pressure (Table 6–3).

III. DIAGNOSIS OF CONGESTIVE HEART FAILURE

A. The diagnosis of CHF is based on the history, physical examination, and interpretation of laboratory and diagnostic tests (Table 6–4).

B. **Signs and symptoms.** See Table 6–5.

    1. The pathophysiologic hallmarks of CHF are decreased cardiac output, increased ventricular end-diastolic pres-

▬ Table 6–4 • Diagnosis of Congestive
Heart Failure

Decreased cardiac output and cardiac reserve
  Fatigue
  Confusion
  Prerenal azotemia (disproportionate increases in blood urea
    nitrogen concentrations relative to the serum creatinine
    concentrations)
Moist rales in lungs often in association with tachypnea
Compensatory increases in sympathetic nervous system activity
  Resting tachycardia (unexplained during preoperative period
    suggests congestive heart failure particularly if patients are
    elderly and/or have known heart disease)
  Peripheral vasoconstriction
Third heart sound (S_3 gallop or ventricular diastolic gallop)

▬ Table 6–5 • Signs and Symptoms of Congestive
Heart Failure

Left Ventricular Failure
Dyspnea (increased stiffness of lungs due to interstitial pulmonary
  edema)
Orthopnea (inability of a failing left ventricle to handle increased
  venous return associated with the recumbent position)
Paroxysmal nocturnal dyspnea (awakens patient from sleep; must
  be differentiated from anxiety-provoked hyperventilation)
Acute pulmonary edema [ultimate manifestation of left ventricular
  failure; often accompanied by signs of sympathetic nervous
  system stimulation (systemic hypertension, tachycardia,
  vasoconstriction); treatment includes morphine to decrease
  venous return to the heart and furosemide]
Chest radiography [radiographic signs of left ventricular failure
  include perivascular edema (hilar and perihilar haze), septal
  edema (Kerley's lines), alveolar edema (butterfly pattern), and
  pleural effusion; radiographic patterns of pulmonary congestion
  may persist for 1–4 days after normalization of cardiac filling
  pressures]
Right Ventricular Failure
Systemic venous congestion (distension of external jugular veins
  above the level of clavicles of a patient in the sitting position)
Organomegaly (liver typically first organ to become engorged with
  blood, right upper quadrant tenderness, ascites)
Peripheral edema (dependent and pitting in the presence of
  jugular venous distension)

sures, peripheral vasoconstriction, and metabolic acidosis.

2. Left ventricular failure results in signs and symptoms of pulmonary edema, whereas right ventricular failure results in systemic venous hypertension and associated pulmonary edema.

IV. THERAPEUTIC GOALS IN THE MANAGEMENT OF CONGESTIVE HEART FAILURE

A. Pharmacologic therapy. See Table 6–6.

1. Short-term therapeutic goals in patients with CHF are to relieve symptoms of circulatory congestion, increase tissue perfusion, and improve quality of life. Long-term therapeutic goals are to prolong life by slowing or reversing the progressive left ventricular dysfunction (ventricular remodeling) that results in the dilated ventricular chamber and low ejection fraction that is characteristic of CHF.

2. Angiotensin-converting enzyme (ACE) inhibitors alleviate symptoms related to CHF and prolong survival.

3. Digoxin has not been shown to benefit patients with asymptomatic left ventricular dysfunction. Sensitivity to digoxin can be increased during the perioperative period if there is an associated decrease in renal function.

   a. **Prophylactic administration of digitalis** to patients scheduled for an elective operation without evidence of CHF is controversial (risk of toxicity versus evidence that the incidence of atrial fibrillation following thoracic or abdominal surgery in treated elderly patients is

---

≡ Table 6–6 • Pharmacologic Therapy of Congestive Heart Failure

Angiotensin-converting enzyme inhibitors (conserve potassium by decreasing secretion of aldosterone)

Diuretics (relieve circulatory congestion and accompanying pulmonary and peripheral edema; potassium supplementation may be needed; excessive doses may result in hypovolemia)

Vasodilators (nitroprusside or nitroglycerin act to decrease resistance to left ventricular ejection and increase venous capacitance)

Digitalis (enhances inotropy and decreases activation of the sympathetic nervous system)

decreased). There are no data to support discontinuing digoxin preoperatively, especially if the drug is being administered for heart rate control.

b. **Digitalis toxicity** during the preoperative period is suspected in patients who complain of anorexia or nausea, especially if hypokalemia is also present.

c. **Cardiac manifestations of digitalis toxicity** include cardiac dysrhythmias (ventricular premature beats, atrioventricular heart block, ventricular fibrillation).

d. **Treatment of digitalis-induced cardiac dysrhythmias** includes correction of predisposing events (hypokalemia), suppression of cardiac dysrhythmias (lidocaine, phenytoin), and placement of a temporary transvenous pacemaker if complete heart block is present.

e. **Plasma digitalis concentrations** > 3 ng/ml usually reflect toxic drug concentrations.

f. **Surgery in the presence of digitalis toxicity.** See Table 6–7.

B. **Nonpharmacologic management.** Recurrent episodes of CHF due to left ventricular ischemia may be treated with angioplasty or bypass surgery. Increasingly severe symptoms in the presence of cardiac valve lesions may be alleviated by surgical replacement of the diseased valve.

1. **Ventricular assist devices** (extracorporeal membrane oxygenation, implantable pulsatile devices) are mechanical

---

≡ Table 6–7 • Surgery in the Presence of Digitalis Toxicity

Proceed only if surgical disease is life-threatening

Avoid events or drugs (ketamine) that stimulate the autonomic nervous system

Volatile anesthetics are reasonable choices

Avoid hyperventilation of the lungs (iatrogenic hypokalemia)

Ready availability of drugs to treat cardiac dysrhythmias
  Lidocaine 0.5–1.5 mg/kg IV for ventricular irritability
  Phenytoin 20 mg/min IV for supraventricular dysrhythmias
  Atropine for bradycardia due to excessive parasympathetic nervous system activity

Temporary transvenous cardiac pacemaker if bradycardia persists despite appropriate drug therapy

Electrical cardioversion to treat supraventricular dysrhythmias may lead to ventricular fibrillation

pumps that take over the function of the damaged ventricle and facilitate restoration of normal hemodynamics and end-organ blood flow.

2. Bleeding, right-sided heart failure, venous air embolism, thromboembolism, infection, and progressive multisystem organ failure are the most common causes of morbidity and mortality associated with the use of left ventricular assist devices.

C. **New management approaches.** The steady progression of CHF and high mortality despite conventional pharmacologic therapy has led to interest in the possible efficacy of alternative drug therapy [β-adrenergic antagonists (metoprolol) and calcium channel-blocking drugs (felodipine, amlodipine) with vasodilating effects].

V. SURGERY IN THE PRESENCE OF CONGESTIVE HEART FAILURE

See Table 6–8.

≡ **Table 6–8 •** Surgery in the Presence of Congestive Heart Failure

---

Do not perform elective operations (presence of congestive heart failure is the single most important factor for predicting postoperative cardiac morbidity)

Dehydration or fluid overload during the preoperative period may predispose to congestive heart failure in predisposed patients

Ketamine for induction of anesthesia (etomidate and opioids are alternative selections)

Volatile anesthetics may produce unacceptable direct myocardial depression (exaggerated in the presence of congestive heart failure and with concomitant administration of nitrous oxide)

Opioids may be used for maintenance of anesthesia

Positive-pressure ventilation may decrease pulmonary congestion and improve arterial oxygenation (avoid hyperventilation and associated iatrogenic hypokalemia in patients being treated with digitalis)

Invasive monitoring may be justified (intra-arterial, cardiac filling pressures, echocardiography)

Inotropic support of cardiac output (dopamine, dobutamine)

Consider possible drug interactions (sympathomimetics and calcium may enhance digitalis effects)

Regional anesthesia is acceptable for peripheral operations

7

Cardiomyopathies

Cardiomyopathies are a diverse group of disorders character-
ized by progressive, life-threatening congestive heart failure
(Table 7–1) (Stoelting RK, Dierdorf SF. Cardiomyopathies.
In: Anesthesia and Co-Existing Disease, 4th ed. New York, Churchill
Livingstone, 2002;117–126). The etiology of cardiomyopathies is di-
verse and may include a genetic basis (Table 7–2).

I. IDIOPATHIC DILATED CARDIOMYOPATHY

Idiopathic dilated cardiomyopathy is a primary myocardial disease of unknown cause characterized by left ventricular or biven-
tricular dilation, impaired myocardial contractility, decreased
cardiac output, and increased ventricular filling pressures (Table
7–1). Ventricular cardiac dysrhythmias and sudden death are
common in affected individuals.

A. Clinical presentation. See Table 7–3.

B. Treatment. See Table 7–4.

C. Management of anesthesia

1. Goals during the management of anesthesia in patients
   with idiopathic dilated cardiomyopathy include avoidance of drug-induced myocardial depression (volatile anesthetics), maintenance of normovolemia, and prevention
   of increases in ventricular afterload. Regional anesthesia
   is an alternative to general anesthesia in selected patients.

2. Excessive cardiovascular depression in response to induction of anesthesia in patients with a history of alcohol
   abuse may reflect unsuspected idiopathic dilated cardiomyopathy.

3. Surgical stimulation that produces undesirable increases
   in heart rate or systemic vascular resistance may be treated
   with β-antagonists such as esmolol, keeping in mind the
   potential for these drugs to cause cardiac depression.

4. Intraoperative hypotension is logically treated with vasopressors such as ephedrine, which provide some degree
   of β-stimulation.

Table 7–1 • Classification of Cardiomyopathies on Morphologic and Hemodynamic Bases

Parameter	Criteria, by Type of Cardiomyopathy			
	Dilated	Restrictive	Hypertrophic	Obliterative
Morphology	Biventricular dilation	Decreased ventricular compliance	Hypertrophy of left ventricle and usually interventricular septum	Thickened endocardium or mural thrombi
Ventricular volume	Marked increase	Normal to modest increase	Normal to modest decrease	Modest decrease
Ejection fraction	Marked decrease	Normal to modest decrease	Marked increase	Normal to modest decrease
Ventricular compliance	Normal to modest decrease	Marked decrease	Marked decrease	Marked decrease
Ventricular filling pressure	Marked increase	Marked increase	Normal to modest increase	Modest increase
Stroke volume	Marked decrease	Normal to modest decrease	Normal to modest increase	Normal to modest decrease

▬ Table 7–2 • Etiology of Cardiomyopathies

Idiopathic
Ischemic
Infectious
    Viral (human immunodeficiency virus)
    Bacterial
Toxic
    Alcohol
    Daunorubicin
    Doxorubicin
    Cocaine
Systemic
    Muscular dystrophy
    Myotonic dystrophy
    Collagen vascular disease
    Sarcoidosis
    Pheochromocytoma
    Acromegaly
    Thyrotoxicosis
    Myxedema
Infiltrative
    Amyloidosis
    Hemochromatosis
    Primary or metastatic tumors
Nutritional
Familial (genetic)

▬ Table 7–3 • Clinical Presentation of Idiopathic Dilated Cardiomyopathy

Congestive heart failure
Angina pectoris
Ejection fraction < 0.25
Pulmonary capillary wedge pressure > 20 mmHg
Cardiac index < 2.5 L/min/m^2
Systemic hypotension
Pulmonary hypertension
Functional mitral and/or tricuspid regurgitation
Cardiac dysrhythmias
Systemic embolization

▀ Table 7–4 • Treatment of Idiopathic
Dilated Cardiomyopathy

Vasodilator therapy (angiotensin-converting enzyme inhibitors)
Anticoagulation (warfarin)
Automatic cardioverter-defibrillator (decreases risk of sudden
  death in patients with congestive heart failure who have
  survived a prior cardiac arrest)
Digitalis
Heart transplantation

---

5. Intravenous infusion of crystalloid solutions or blood
   should be guided by cardiac filling pressures to decrease
   the likelihood of volume overload. A pulmonary artery
   catheter facilitates early recognition of the need for inotropic support or administration of peripheral vasodilating drugs.

II. RESTRICTIVE CARDIOMYOPATHY

Restrictive cardiomyopathy is the least common of the cardiomyopathies, with cardiac amyloidosis and the idiopathic variety
being the most common etiologies. Increased stiffness of the
myocardium causes pressure within the ventricle or ventricles
to increase precipitously with only small increases in volume.

A. **Clinical presentation** of restrictive cardiomyopathy may resemble that of constrictive pericarditis (Table 7–1). In advanced cases, all signs of congestive heart failure are present
   except cardiomegaly. Thromboembolic complications and
   cardiac conduction disturbances (atrial fibrillation) are
   common.
B. **Treatment.** See Table 7–5.

▀ Table 7–5 • Treatment of
Restrictive Cardiomyopathy

Diuretics
Amiodarone (treat atrial fibrillation)
External cardiac pacemaker
Implantable defibrillator
Anticoagulation
Cardiac transplantation (not if due to systemic disorders)

C. **Management of anesthesia** for patients with restrictive cardiomyopathy utilizes the same principles as for patients with cardiac tamponade (maintain intravascular fluid volume, avoid abrupt bradycardia, maintain normal sinus rhythm). The presence of anticoagulation may influence the decision to select regional anesthesia.

III. HYPERTROPHIC CARDIOMYOPATHY

Hypertrophic cardiomyopathy is a common (1 in 500 individuals) genetic malformation of the heart.

A. **Clinical presentation.** The clinical course varies widely, with most individuals remaining asymptomatic throughout life; some have symptoms of congestive heart failure, and others die suddenly presumably from ventricular tachydysrhythmias, often in the absence of previous symptoms (Tables 7–1, 7–6). Marked left ventricular hypertrophy makes these patients particularly vulnerable to myocardial ischemia, especially when endocardial blood flow is decreased owing to excessive pressure in the left ventricle.

B. **Sudden death** is a recognized complication of hypertrophic cardiomyopathy (the risk parallels the magnitude of the hypertrophy).

C. **Treatment** of patients with hypertrophic cardiomyopathy is undertaken recognizing that these individuals are at risk for sudden death and so must be treated aggressively.

1. **Medical therapy.** β-Adrenergic blocking drugs and verapamil have been used extensively in the treatment of

---

≡ Table 7–6 • Clinical Presentation of Hypertrophic Cardiomyopathy

Angina pectoris (relieved by assumption of the recumbent position that decreases left ventricular outflow obstruction)
Syncope (may represent aborted sudden death)
Tachydysrhythmias
Congestive heart failure
Massive cardiac hypertrophy (echocardiography may reveal a slit-like left ventricular chamber)
Ejection fraction > 0.8
Cardiac murmurs reflecting left ventricular outflow obstruction (confused with aortic or mitral valve disease)
Sudden death

hypertrophic cardiomyopathy. In patients with hypertrophic cardiomyopathy who are considered to be at high risk for sudden death from ventricular tachydysrhythmias, the available therapeutic options include amiodarone and an implantable cardioverter-defibrillator.

   a. Management of atrial fibrillation. Atrial fibrillation often develops in individuals with hypertrophic cardiomyopathy and is associated with an increased risk of thromboembolism, congestive heart failure, and sudden death.

   b. Amiodarone is considered the most effective antidysrhythmia drug to prevent recurrence of atrial fibrillation.

  2. Surgical therapy. Surgical reduction of the outflow gradient is usually achieved by removing a small amount of cardiac muscle from the ventricular septum (myotomy-myectomy). Intraoperative echocardiography is useful for determining the extent of surgical resection and defining mitral valve structure. A marked decrease in the intraventricular systolic and end-diastolic pressures is the most tangible consequence of surgery.

  3. Nonsurgical techniques to relieve left ventricular outflow obstruction. Dual-chamber pacing may be associated with decreases in the outflow gradient and symptomatic improvement in patients with hypertrophic cardiomyopathy who are unresponsive to medical therapy.

D. Management of anesthesia in patients with hypertrophic cardiomyopathy is directed toward minimizing left ventricular outflow obstruction (Table 7–7). Overall, the risk associated with general anesthesia seems acceptable in patients with hypertrophic cardiomyopathy. However, anesthesia and surgery in patients with previously unrecognized hypertrophic cardiomyopathy may manifest intraoperatively as hypotension and as sudden increases in the intensity of a systolic murmur, typically in association with acute hemorrhage or drug-induced vasodilation.

  1. Preoperative medication ideally decreases anxiety and the associated activation of the sympathetic nervous system. Administration of atropine is questionable, as tachycardia could increase left ventricular outflow obstruction. Expansion of the intravascular fluid volume during the preoperative period is useful for maintaining the intraoperative stroke volume and minimizing the adverse effects of positive-pressure ventilation of the patient's lungs.

▬ Table 7–7 • Factors that Influence
Left Ventricular Outflow
Obstruction in Patients with
Hypertrophic Cardiomyopathy

Events that Increase Outflow Obstruction
Increased myocardial contractility
    β-Adrenergic stimulation (catecholamines)
    Digitalis
    Tachycardia
Decreased preload
    Hypovolemia
    Tachycardia
    Vasodilators (nitroprusside, nitroglycerin)
    Positive-pressure ventilation
Decreased afterload
    Hypotension
    Vasodilators
    Hypovolemia
Events that Decrease Outflow Obstruction
Decreased myocardial contractility
    β-Adrenergic blockade (esmolol)
    Volatile anesthetics (halothane)
    Calcium entry blockers
Increased preload
    Hypervolemia
    Bradycardia
Increased afterload
    α-Adrenergic stimulation (phenylephrine)
Hypervolemia

---

2. **Induction of anesthesia** with intravenous drugs (except ketamine) is acceptable, remembering the importance of avoiding sudden drug-induced decreases in systemic vascular resistance. The duration of direct laryngoscopy should be brief to minimize activation of the sympathetic nervous system (consider administration of volatile anesthetics or β-adrenergic blockers before initiating direct laryngoscopy).

3. **Maintenance of anesthesia** is designed to produce mild depression of myocardial contractility (volatile anesthetics plus nitrous oxide) and at the same time preserve intravascular fluid volume. Invasive monitoring of systemic blood pressure and cardiac filling pressures is help-

ful. Transesophageal echocardiography and Doppler color flow imaging provides useful information, particularly with respect to intraoperative left ventricular and mitral valve function as well as intravascular fluid volume.

   a. Hypotension due to decreased preload or afterload is treated with phenylephrine (predominant α-adrenergic activity) and prompt replacement of blood loss.

   b. Hypertension is treated with increased concentrations of volatile anesthetics.

4. **Parturients** with hypertrophic cardiomyopathy seem to tolerate pregnancy and delivery despite pregnancy-induced decreases in systemic vascular resistance and the risk of impaired venous return caused by uterine compression of the inferior vena cava.

   a. Parturients with hypertrophic cardiomyopathy may present major challenges, as events such as catecholamine release and "bearing down" (Valsalva maneuver) may increase left ventricular outflow obstruction.

   b. Epidural anesthesia has been utilized successfully in these parturients with emphasis on central venous pressure monitoring and maintaining euvolemia or slight hypervolemia. Should hypotension unresponsive to fluid administration occur following institution of regional anesthesia, phenylephrine may be preferred to increase the afterload.

   c. Pulmonary edema has been observed in parturients with hypertrophic cardiomyopathy following delivery. Treatment may include a fluid bolus to increase venous return and esmolol to slow the heart rate, decrease myocardial contractility, and allow prolonged diastolic filling times to decrease the left ventricular outflow obstruction.

IV. OBLITERATIVE CARDIOMYOPATHY

Obliterative cardiomyopathy may be considered a variant of restrictive cardiomyopathy. It is characterized by marked decreases in ventricular compliance (Table 7–1).

V. PERIPARTUM CARDIOMYOPATHY

See Table 7–8.

A. Diagnosis of peripartum cardiomyopathy is based on the onset of unexplained left ventricular dysfunction during the

Table 7–8 • Defining Characteristics of Peripartum Cardiomyopathy

---

Onset of left ventricular dysfunction during the last month of pregnancy or within 5 months following delivery
Absence of an identifiable cause
Absence of known heart disease prior to the last month of pregnancy
Left ventricular dysfunction demonstrated by echocardiography

---

limited period surrounding parturition. It may be difficult to differentiate between subtle symptoms of congestive heart failure and the dyspnea, fatigue, and peripheral edema associated with pregnancy.

B. **Treatment** is designed to alleviate symptoms of congestive heart failure (diuretics, vasodilators, digoxin). Angiotensin-converting enzyme inhibitors are teratogenic during pregnancy but are useful for treatment following delivery.

C. **Prognosis** appears to depend on normalization of left ventricular size and function within 6 months after delivery.

D. **Management of anesthesia** in parturients with peripartum cardiomyopathy requires assessment of cardiac status and careful planning for providing analgesia and/or anesthesia for delivery. Continuous intravenous infusions of remifentanil and/or propofol may be considered.

8

Cor Pulmonale and Pulmonary Hypertension

Cor pulmonale is right ventricular enlargement that develops secondary to pulmonary hypertension (Stoelting RK, Dierdorf SF. Cor pulmonale and pulmonary hypertension. In: Anesthesia and Co-Existing Disease, 4th ed. New York, Churchill Livingstone, 2002;127–133).

I. COR PULMONALE

A. Cor pulmonale is the third most common cardiac disorder in persons older than 50 years of age, after ischemic heart disease and hypertensive heart disease. It is estimated that 10% to 30% of patients admitted to the hospital with congestive heart failure (CHF) exhibit cor pulmonale. Chronic obstructive pulmonary disease (COPD) with associated loss of pulmonary capillaries and arterial hypoxemia leading to pulmonary vascular vasoconstriction is the most likely cause of cor pulmonale.

B. **Signs and symptoms** (Table 8–1). Clinical manifestations of cor pulmonale are often nonspecific and tend to be obscured by co-existing COPD. The rate at which right ventricular dysfunction develops depends on the magnitude of the increase in the pulmonary artery pressure and the rapidity with which this increase occurs. Right ventricular failure may occur with an abrupt increase in the pulmonary artery pressure due to pulmonary embolism, whereas a gradual increase in the pulmonary artery pressure, as due to COPD, may not produce right ventricular failure. In patients with COPD, acute right ventricular failure may develop during a pulmonary infection.

C. **Treatment** of cor pulmonale is intended to decrease the workload of the right ventricle by decreasing pulmonary vascular resistance (Table 8–2). This goal is best achieved by returning the PaO_2, $PaCO_2$, and arterial pH to normal ranges, assuming

---

≡ Table 8–1 • Signs and Symptoms of Cor Pulmonale

Dyspnea

Effort-related syncope

Increased pulmonary artery pressure (pulmonary hypertension considered moderate when mean pulmonary artery pressure > 35 mmHg)

Normal pulmonary artery occlusion pressure

Functional tricuspid regurgitation (Doppler ultrasonography)

Right ventricular failure (increased jugular venous pressure, hepatosplenomegaly, peripheral dependent edema)

Right ventricular and right atrial hypertrophy (chest radiography and electrocardiography)

---

that pulmonary artery and arteriolar vasoconstriction is reversible.

  D. **Management of anesthesia.** It is recommended that elective operations in patients with cor pulmonale be postponed until the reversible components of co-existing COPD are treated (Table 8–3). Arterial blood gases and pH are often measured to provide guidelines for management intraoperatively and postoperatively.

   1. **Preoperative medication** should not include drugs that are likely to produce excessive depression of ventilation. The depressant effects of anticholinergic drugs on mucociliary activity and the possible impairment of clearance of secretions may outweigh the advantages of including these drugs in the preoperative medication.

≡ Table 8–2 • Treatment of Cor Pulmonale

Supplemental oxygen (PaO_2 > 60 mmHg)

Diuretics

Digitalis (risk of toxicity increased in the presence of arterial hypoxemia, acidosis, and electrolyte imbalances)

Vasodilators

Anticoagulants (warfarin or antiplatelet drugs)

Antibiotics (pulmonary infections further increase pulmonary vascular resistance)

Heart-lung transplantation

☰ Table 8–3 • Preoperative Preparation of Patients with Cor Pulmonale

Elimination and control of acute and/or chronic pulmonary infections
Reversal of bronchospasm
Improvement of secretion clearance
Expansion of collapsed or poorly ventilated alveoli
Hydration
Correction of electrolyte imbalance

2. **Induction of anesthesia** is usually accomplished with intravenous drugs, taking care to avoid an abrupt decrease in systemic vascular resistance. Bronchospasm and increased systemic and pulmonary vascular resistance may accompany tracheal intubation in the presence of minimal concentrations of anesthetic drugs.

3. **Maintenance of anesthesia** is usually with volatile anesthetics combined with adjuvant drugs. Nitrous oxide may produce pulmonary artery vasoconstriction and further increases in pulmonary vascular resistance (monitor the right atrial pressures and discontinue nitrous oxide if pressures increase).

   a. Positive-pressure ventilation may increase pulmonary vascular resistance (distends alveoli), but this potential adverse effect is usually more than offset by improved arterial oxygenation. Excessive hyperventilation may produce metabolic alkalosis and hypokalemia with the risk of digitalis toxicity in patients being treated with this drug.

   b. Regional anesthetic techniques are appropriate considerations for superficial surgery or operations on the extremities of patients with cor pulmonale (high sensory levels may adversely decrease systemic vascular resistance in the presence of fixed increases in pulmonary vascular resistance).

4. **Monitoring** patients with cor pulmonale is influenced by the invasiveness of the operation. A right atrial catheter provides useful information regarding right ventricular function and the safety of intravenous infusions of fluids. An abrupt increase in right atrial pressure during the intraoperative period signals right ventricular dysfunction and

increased pulmonary vascular resistance (arterial hypoxemia, hypoventilation, nitrous oxide).

II. PRIMARY PULMONARY HYPERTENSION

Primary pulmonary hypertension is characterized by a sustained increase in pulmonary artery pressure (mean pulmonary artery pressure > 25 mmHg at rest) in the absence of demonstrable causes (left-sided cardiac valve disease, congenital heart disease, COPD, connective tissue disease, thromboembolic disease).

A. Pulmonary vascular disease with features similar to those of primary pulmonary hypertension can occur in patients with portal hypertension, acquired immunodeficiency syndrome (AIDS), or a history of cocaine abuse and in those who take

---

Table 8–4 • Diagnostic Classification of Pulmonary Hypertension

Pulmonary Hypertension Associated with Diseases of the Respiratory System or Arterial Hypoxemia
Chronic obstructive pulmonary disease
Interstitial pulmonary fibrosis
Cystic fibrosis
Chronic alveolar hypoxemia (altitude)
Pulmonary Venous Hypertension
Mitral valve disease
Chronic left ventricular dysfunction
Pulmonary veno-occlusive disease
Pulmonary Hypertension Due to Chronic Thrombotic and/or Embolic Disease
Thromboembolic obstruction of proximal pulmonary arteries
Obstruction of distal pulmonary arteries
Pulmonary Arterial Hypertension
Primary pulmonary hypertension (sporadic, familial)
Pulmonary arterial hypertension related to collagen vascular diseases (scleroderma, lupus erythematosus, rheumatoid arthritis)
Pulmonary arterial hypertension related to congenital systemic-to-pulmonary shunts (Eisenmenger syndrome, AIDS, drugs, toxins)
Pulmonary Hypertension Due to Disorders Directly Affecting the Pulmonary Vasculature
Inflammatory
Pulmonary capillary hemangiomatosis

AIDS, acquired immunodeficiency syndrome.
Adapted from Gaine S. Pulmonary hypertension. JAMA 2000;284:3160–8.

≡ Table 8–5 • Diagnosis of Primary Pulmonary Hypertension

Dyspnea
Fatigability
Angina pectoris and syncope with exertion
Symptoms of Raynaud's phenomenon
Echocardiography (rules out congenital, valvular, and myocardial disease)
Arterial hypoxemia (ventilation-to-perfusion imbalance, decreased cardiac output, shunting through a patent foramen ovale)
Pulmonary artery occlusion pressure (usually normal)

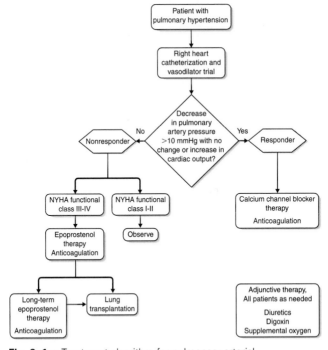

Fig. 8–1 • Treatment algorithm for pulmonary arterial hypertension. (From Gaine S. Pulmonary hypertension. JAMA 2000;284:3160–8. Copyrighted 2000, American Medical Association, with permission.)

appetite suppressant drugs (serotonin uptake inhibitor drugs).

1. The hemodynamic stresses of pregnancy (including the immediate postpartum period) are poorly tolerated by women with primary pulmonary hypertension.
2. The median period of survival after diagnosis is 2.5 years, and most patients succumb to progressive right-side heart failure (sudden death may occur).

B. **Classification.** A treatment-based classification of pulmonary hypertension divides the disease into five distinct categories (Table 8–4).

C. **Diagnosis** of primary pulmonary hypertension may be difficult, as many of the early signs and symptoms are nonspecific or subtle (Table 8–5).

D. **Treatment.** See Figure 8–1.

E. **Management of anesthesia** follows the same principles as for patients with cor pulmonale.

Pericardial Diseases

Clinicopathologic responses to pericardial injury are characterized as acute pericarditis, pericardial effusion, and constrictive pericarditis (Stoelting RK, Dierdorf SF. Pericardial diseases. In: Anesthesia and Co–Existing Diseases, 4th Ed. New York, Churchill Livingstone, 2002;135–142). Cardiac tamponade is a possibility whenever pericardial fluid accumulates under pressure.

I. ACUTE PERICARDITIS

See Table 9–1.

A. **Diagnosis** of acute pericarditis is based on the presence of chest pain (worsens with inspiration), pericardial friction rub, and changes on the electrocardiogram (ECG) (diffuse ST segment elevation).

B. **Treatment.** Symptomatic relief of pain due to acute pericarditis is often provided with oral analgesics. Corticosteroids usually relieve symptoms of acute pericarditis.

C. **Relapsing pericarditis** may follow acute pericarditis due to any cause.

D. **Pericarditis after cardiac surgery** presents as acute pericarditis and is presumed to be infective or autoimmune.

II. PERICARDIAL EFFUSION AND CARDIAC TAMPONADE

A. **Signs and symptoms.** The physiologic effects of pericardial effusions depend on whether the fluid is under increased pressure. Central venous pressure readings are accurate reflections of intrapericardial pressures.

1. **Cardiac tamponade** manifests as a spectrum of hemodynamic abnormalities of varying severity (may mimic pulmonary embolism).

a. **Clinical manifestations.** See Table 9–2.

b. Cardiac output is maintained so long as pressures in the central veins exceed right ventricular end–diastolic pressures.

≡ Table 9-1 • Causes of Acute Pericarditis with or without Pericardial Effusion

Infectious
  Viral
  Bacterial
  Fungal
  Tuberculosis (often associated with acquired immunodeficiency syndrome, or AIDS)
Postmyocardial infarction (Dressler syndrome)
Posttraumatic (cardiac surgery, pacemaker lead, pressure monitoring catheters)
Metastatic disease
Drug–induced (minoxidil, procainamide)
Mediastinal radiation
Systemic diseases
  Rheumatoid arthritis
  Systemic lupus erythematosus
  Scleroderma

---

2. **Loculated pericardial effusions** may selectively compress one or more chambers of the heart, producing localized cardiac tamponade.

B. **Diagnosis.** Echocardiography is the most accurate and practical method for the diagnosis of pericardial effusions and cardiac tamponade. Computed tomography and magnetic resonance imaging are also useful for detecting pericardial effusions and pericardial thickening.

≡ Table 9-2 • Clinical Manifestations of Cardiac Tamponade

Increased central venous pressure
Activation of the sympathetic nervous system (tachycardia and vasoconstriction)
Equalization of right and left atrial pressures and right ventricular end-diastolic pressures at about 20 mmHg (exception may be accumulation of blood and clots over the right ventricle, as may follow cardiac surgery)
Paradoxical pulse (decrease > 10 mmHg in systolic blood pressure during inspiration)
Hypotension (low cardiac output)

C. **Treatment.** Removal of fluid (pericardiocentesis) is the definitive treatment of cardiac tamponade.

D. **Temporizing measures** are designed to maintain stroke volume until definitive surgical treatment of cardiac tamponade can be instituted.

1. **Expansion of intravascular fluid volume** can be achieved by intravenous infusion of colloid or crystalloid solutions to increase right atrial pressures.

2. **Catecholamines.** Continuous intravenous infusions of isoproterenol or other catecholamines may be effective as a temporizing measure for increasing myocardial contractility and heart rate.

3. **Correction of metabolic acidosis** caused by low cardiac output in the presence of cardiac tamponade is treated with intravenous administration of sodium bicarbonate.

E. **Management of anesthesia.** Institution of general anesthesia and positive–pressure ventilation of the patient's lungs in the presence of cardiac tamponade that is hemodynamically significant can result in life–threatening hypotension (anesthetic–induced vasodilation, direct myocardial depression, decreased venous return).

1. Pericardiocentesis performed with local anesthesia is often preferred for the initial management of patients who are hypotensive owing to low cardiac output produced by cardiac tamponade.

2. When it is not possible to relieve intrapericardial pressure causing cardiac tamponade before the induction of anesthesia, the goal is to maintain cardiac output. Ketamine is useful for induction and maintenance of anesthesia, as it increases myocardial contractility, systemic vascular resistance, and heart rate. Continuous monitoring of systemic blood pressure and central venous pressure is often initiated before induction of anesthesia. Maintenance of increased central venous pressure with generous administration of intravenous fluids is indicated to maintain venous return. Continuous intravenous infusions of catecholamines, such as isoproterenol, dopamine, or dobutamine, may be useful for maintaining cardiac output until the cardiac tamponade can be relieved by surgical drainage.

III. CONSTRICTIVE PERICARDITIS

A. **Signs and symptoms.** Increased venous pressure in patients who do not have other symptoms of heart disease suggests

Table 9–3 • Clinical Features that Differentiate Constrictive Pericarditis from Cardiac Amyloidosis and Idiopathic Restrictive Cardiomyopathy

Clinical Feature	Constrictive Pericarditis	Cardiac Amyloidosis	Idiopathic Restrictive Cardiomyopathy
Early diastolic sound (S_3 or "pericardial knock")	Frequent	Occasional	Occasional
Late diastolic sound (S_4)	Rare	Frequent	Frequent
Atrial enlargement	Mild or absent	Marked	Marked
Atrioventricular or interventricular conduction defect	Rare	Frequent	Frequent
QRS voltage	Normal or low	Low	Normal or high
Mitral or tricuspid regurgitation	Rare	Frequent	Frequent
Paradoxical pulse	Frequent but usually mild	Rare	Rare
Exaggerated variation in mitral and tricuspid flow velocity with respiration	Usual	Rare	Rare

the presence of constrictive pericarditis. Constrictive pericarditis is similar to cardiac tamponade in that both conditions impede diastolic filling of the heart and result in increased central venous pressure and ultimately decreased cardiac output.

B. **Diagnosis.** Many features considered characteristic of constrictive pericarditis may also be present in patients with cardiac amyloidosis and idiopathic restrictive cardiomyopathy (Table 9–3).

C. **Treatment** of constrictive pericarditis is surgical stripping and removal of both layers of the adherent constricting pericardium, which may result in massive bleeding from the epicardial surfaces of the heart.

D. **Management of anesthesia.** In the absence of hypotension caused by increased intrapericardial pressure, anesthetic drugs and techniques that do not excessively depress myocardial contractility, decrease systemic blood pressure, slow the heart rate, or interfere with venous return are most likely to be helpful. Preoperative optimization of intravascular fluid volume is important in these patients. Cardiac dysrhythmias are common during surgical removal of adherent pericardium.

10

Aneurysms of the Thoracic and Abdominal Aorta

Diseases of the aorta are most often aneurysmal, whereas occlusive diseases are most likely to occur in peripheral arteries (Stoelting RK, Dierdorf SF. Aneurysms of the thoracic and abdominal aorta. In: Anesthesia and Co-Existing Disease, 4th ed. New York, Churchill Livingstone, 2002;143–155). The initiating event in aortic dissection is a tear in the intima through which blood surges into a false lumen, separating the intima from the adventia for various distances.

I. ANEURYSMS OF THE THORACIC AORTA

A. **Classification.** See Figure 10–1.

B. **Etiology.** See Table 10–1.

C. **Signs and symptoms.** See Table 10–2.

D. **Diagnosis.** Computed tomography is the most commonly used noninvasive technique to diagnose thoracic aortic disease. Magnetic resonance imaging, unlike computed tomography, does not require injection of contrast medium. Transesophageal echocardiography with color Doppler imaging is used to diagnose thoracic aortic disease. Aortography is usually required for patients undergoing elective operations on the thoracic aorta.

E. **Preoperative evaluation.** Because myocardial infarction, respiratory failure, and stroke are the principal causes of morbidity and mortality after operations on the thoracic aorta, preoperative assessment of the function of these organ systems is recommended. A history of cigarette smoking and the presence of chronic obstructive pulmonary disease are important predictors of respiratory failure after thoracic aorta surgery.

F. **Indications for surgery.** See Table 10–3.

G. **Unique risks of surgery.** Surgical resection of a thoracic aortic aneurysm and to a lesser extent an abdominal aortic

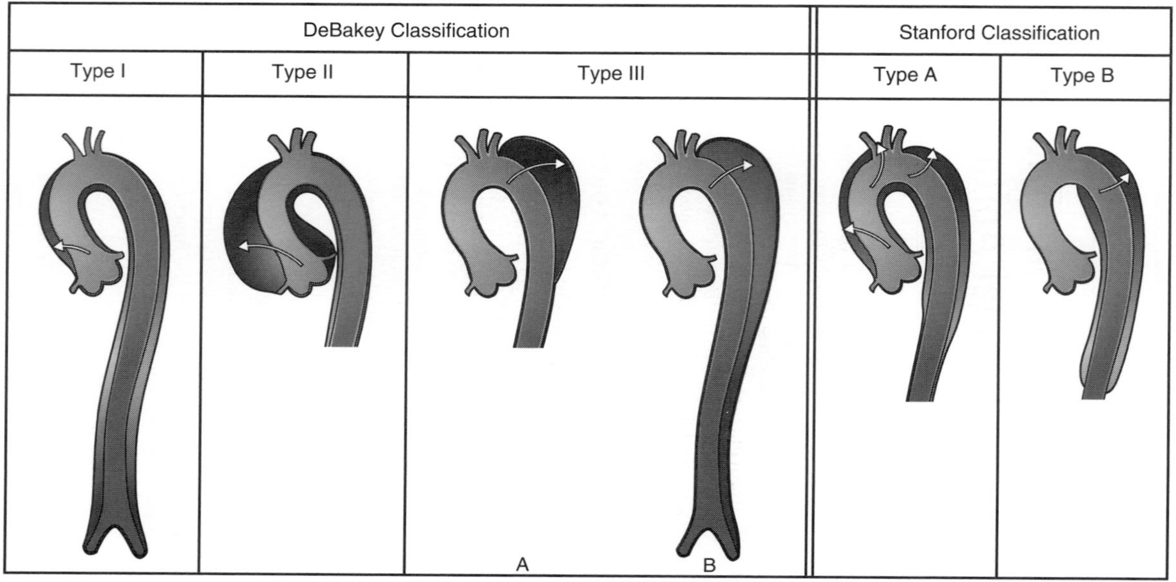

DeBakey Classification			Stanford Classification	
Type I	Type II	Type III	Type A	Type B

A   B

Fig. 10–1 • *See legend on opposite page*

☰ Table 10–1 • Etiology of Thoracic Aortic Dissection

Systemic hypertension
Congenital disorders of connective tissue
  Marfan syndrome
  Ehlers-Danlos syndrome
Deceleration injuries to the chest
Blunt trauma
Pregnancy
Iatrogenic (site of aortic cannulation or where aorta has been
  cross-clamped)

aneurysm is associated with the risk of spinal cord ischemia (paraplegia) and adverse hemodynamic responses due to cross-clamping the thoracic aorta (Figs. 10–2 , 10–3, 10–4).

1. **Anterior spinal artery syndrome** manifests as flaccid paralysis of the lower extremities. Bowel and bladder dysfunction are common, but sensation and proprioception are usually spared.

   a. **Risk factors.** Because the main mechanism of paraplegia associated with cross-clamping the descending aorta lies in spinal cord ischemia and reperfusion, the duration of cross-clamping is influential. A brief period of thoracic aortic cross-clamping (< 30 minutes), the use of partial circulatory assistance or a shunt, or both may decrease the likelihood of this complication.

   b. **Spinal cord blood flow.** The anatomy of the blood supply to the spinal cord (one anterior spinal artery and two posterior spinal arteries) is the reason cross-clamping the thoracic aorta may introduce the risk of spinal cord ischemia. The tenuous collateral anastomo-

Fig. 10–1 • The two most widely used classifications of aortic dissections are the DeBakey classification (types 1, II, IIIa, IIIb) and the Stanford classification (types A and B). (From Kouchoukos NT, Dougenis D. Surgery of the thoracic aorta. N Engl J Med 1997; 336:1876–88. Copyright 1997 Massachusetts Medical Society, with permission.)

⊒ Table 10–2 • Signs and Symptoms of Aneurysms of the Thoracic Aorta

Excruciating chest pain
Diminution or absence of peripheral pulses
    Stroke
    Paraplegia
    Ischemia of extremities
Vasoconstricted and hypertensive
Acute aortic regurgitation
Myocardial infarction
Cardiac tamponade

sis of the anterior spinal artery in the midthoracic region places segments of the spinal cord in jeopardy during aortic cross-clamping or hypotension. If the artery of Adamkiewicz arises from the part of the aorta that is cross-clamped, pressures in the anterior spinal artery may be much less than pressures in the distal aorta.

2. **Hemodynamic responses to aortic cross-clamping** are associated with severe homeostatic disturbances in virtually all organ systems in the body, reflected by expected decreases in blood flow distal to the aortic clamp (85% to

⊒ Table 10–3 • Indications for Surgery in the Presence of Thoracic Aorta Dissection

Ascending aorta (replacement of the ascending aorta and aortic valve with a composite graft)
Aortic arch (resection of thoracic aorta from the proximal origin of the innominate artery to the distal origin of the left subclavian artery; hypothermic cardiopulmonary arrest for 30–40 minutes; neurologic deficits are the major complications)
Descending thoracic aorta [treated initially with medical therapy that includes nitroprusside and β-adrenergic antagonists; surgery when there are signs of impending rupture (persistent pain, hypotension) or ischemia (renal failure, paraplegia)]

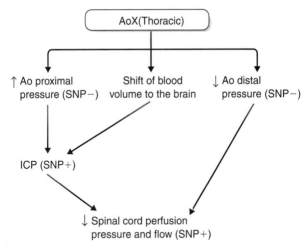

Fig. 10–2 • Spinal cord blood flow and perfusion pressure during thoracic aortic occlusion with or without sodium nitroprusside (SNP) infusion. (From Gelman S. The pathophysiology of aortic cross-clamping and unclamping. Anesthesiology 1995;82:1026–60. © 1995, Lippincott Williams & Wilkins, with permission.)

94% decrease in spinal cord blood flow and renal blood flow with thoracic aorta cross-clamping) and substantial increases in blood flow above the occlusion (Figs. 10–2, 10–3, 10–4). Systemic hypertension is the most dramatic and consistent component of the hemodynamic response to aortic cross-clamping. The level of aortic cross-clamping is important for the degree and pattern of hemodynamic changes (minimal with infrarenal aortic cross-clamping and dramatic with supraceliac aortic cross-clamping)

   a. Pharmacologic interventions intended to offset the hemodynamic effects of aortic cross-clamping includes administration of vasodilators (nitroprusside, nitroglycerin).

   b. Effects of vasodilators on distal perfusion pressures may be undesirable.

3. Hemodynamic responses to aortic unclamping include a marked, sudden decrease in systemic vascular resistance

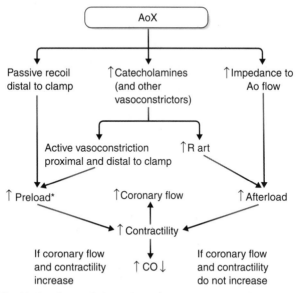

Fig. 10–3 • Systemic hemodynamic responses to aortic cross-clamping. *Different patterns are possible, see Fig. 10–2. (From Gelman S. The pathophysiology of aortic cross-clamping and unclamping. Anesthesiology 1995;82:1026–60. © 1995, Lippincott Williams & Wilkins, with permission.)

with profound hypotension (Fig. 10–5). Correction of metabolic acidosis does not significantly influence the degree of hypotension while unclamping the aorta.

H. **Management of anesthesia** in patients undergoing thoracic aneurysm resection requires special considerations for monitoring arterial blood pressure, neurologic function, and intravascular fluid volume, as well as pharmacologic interventions to control systemic hypertension during the period of aortic cross-clamping (Table 10–4). Proper monitoring is more important than the actual drugs selected for anesthesia in patients undergoing resection of a thoracic aortic aneurysm.

I. **Postoperative management.** Amelioration of pain (intrathecal or epidural opioids and local anesthetics) is essential for

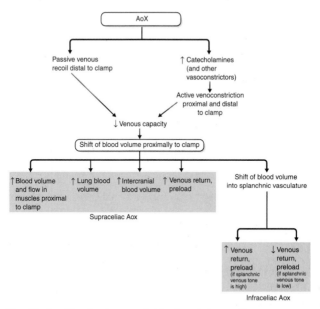

Fig. 10–4 • Blood volume redistribution during aortic cross-clamping. (From Gelman S. The pathophysiology of aortic cross-clamping and unclamping. Anesthesiology 1995;82:1026–60. © 1995, Lippincott Williams & Wilkins, with permission.)

patient comfort and to facilitate coughing and maneuvers designed to prevent atelectasis. Inclusion of local anesthetics in solutions placed in the epidural space may delay recognition of the anterior spinal artery syndrome. Cardiac, ventilatory, and renal failure may manifest during the immediate postoperative period. Systemic hypertension is common and may require treatment with nitroglycerin, nitroprusside, and labetalol.

II. MYOCARDIAL CONTUSION

Myocardial contusion is most often due to deceleration injuries caused by the sudden impact of the anterior chest wall against the automobile steering wheel. Because of its immediate subster-

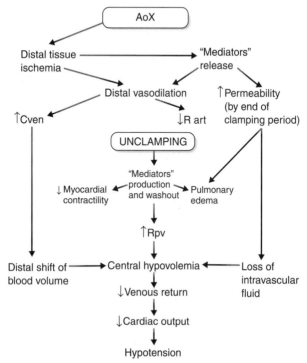

Fig. 10–5 • Systemic hemodynamic responses to aortic unclamping. (From Gelman S. The pathophysiology of aortic cross-clamping and unclamping. Anesthesiology 1995;82:1026–60. © 1995, Lippincott Williams & Wilkins, with permission.)

nal location, the right ventricle is more likely than the left ventricle to be injured.

A. Signs and symptoms. Chest pain (unrelieved by nitroglycerin) and changes on the electrocardiogram (ECG) resembling myocardial infarction should prompt questions about recent chest trauma. The most important complications of myocardial contusion are cardiac dysrhythmias. Blunt trauma may injure cardiac valves (regurgitation) and the lungs (hemorrhage into the tracheobronchial tree).

≡ Table 10–4 • Management of Anesthesia for
Resection of Thoracic Aneurysms

Monitoring Systemic Blood Pressure
Catheter in right upper extremity (occlusion of the aorta proximal
    to the left subclavian artery would prevent recording blood
    pressure from the left arm)
Loss of arterial blood pressure tracings from an artery in the right
    arm occurs if the innominate artery is occluded
Catheter in the right arm and femoral artery permits assessment
    of cerebral perfusion pressure and perfusion pressure to the
    kidneys
Common recommendation is to maintain mean arterial pressure
    near 100 mmHg in the upper part of the body and > 50 mmHg
    in the portion of the body distal to the aortic cross-clamp
Monitoring Neurologic Function
Somatosensory evoked potentials do not warn of spinal cord
    ischemia
Motor evoked potentials reflect anterior spinal cord function
Monitoring Cardiac Function
Transesophageal echocardiography
Pulmonary artery catheter
Monitoring Intravascular Fluid Volume
Important for protecting lungs and kidneys
Diuretics to maintain urine flow during aortic cross-clamping
Induction and Maintenance of Anesthesia
Selective endobronchial intubation (minimize magnitude of
    iatrogenic shunt restricting blood flow to the collapsed lung
    and/or application of 5–10 cmH$_2$O continuous positive airway
    pressure to the dependent lung)
Volatile anesthetics and opioids

B. **Diagnosis.** Cardiac contusion is best recognized clinically by
   echocardiography, which shows localized areas of impaired
   wall motion. Concentrations of circulating cardiac enzymes
   may also be increased.

C. **Treatment** of myocardial contusion is symptomatic and includes monitoring the ECG to detect cardiac dysrhythmias.

III. ANEURYSM OF THE ABDOMINAL AORTA

A. **Diagnosis** of an abdominal aneurysm is based on the presence of a pulsating abdominal mass. Abdominal ultrasonog-

raphy, computed tomography, and magnetic resonance imaging confirm the presence and size of the aneurysm.

B. Treatment of an abdominal aneurysm is elective resection and replacement with a prosthetic graft for any aneurysm > 5 cm in diameter (mortality < 5%, with death usually related to myocardial infarction).

C. Preoperative evaluation. Co-existing diseases, particularly coronary artery disease, are important to identify preoperatively in an attempt to minimize postoperative complications (postoperative myocardial infarctions are responsible for most postoperative deaths following elective resection of an abdominal aortic aneurysm). Other co-existing diseases that may influence the decision to proceed with elective resection of an abdominal aortic aneurysm include chronic obstructive pulmonary disease (vital capacity and forced expiratory vol-

---

≡ **Table 10–5** • Management of Anesthesia for Abdominal Aneurysm Resection

---

Monitor the intravascular fluid volume, cardiac, pulmonary, and renal function
    Intra-arterial catheter
    Pulmonary artery catheter
    Echocardiography
    Urine output
    Body temperature
Volatile drugs and opioids with or without nitrous oxide
Consider continuous epidural anesthesia in combination with general anesthesia (anticoagulation may influence decision)
Maintain cardiac filing pressures 3–5 mmHg above preclamp level during period of cross-clamping
Diuretics (mannitol or furosemide) if urine output < 50 ml/hr
Dopamine (3 μg/kg/min IV) (unproven efficacy)
Deepen anesthesia or administer vasodilators if systemic hypertension accompanies infrarenal aortic cross-clamping (myocardial performance and circulatory variables usually remain acceptable when aorta is cross-clamped at this level)
Transient hypotension (about 40 mmHg) not uncommon when aorta is unclamped (minimize by volume loading to higher cardiac filling pressures before cross-clamp release and/or gradual release of aortic cross-clamp; sodium bicarbonate is not reliably effective; hypotension lasting > 4 minutes suggests unrecognized bleeding or inadequate intravascular fluid volume replacement)

≡ Table 10–6 • Postoperative Management of Patients Following Abdominal Aneurysm Resection

---

Monitor for the development of cardiac, ventilatory, and renal failure

Assess graft patency

Provide adequate analgesia (essential for early tracheal extubation)

Treat systemic hypertension (may reflect overzealous intraoperative hydration and/or postoperative hypothermia with compensatory vasoconstriction) with antihypertensive drugs (nitroglycerin, nitroprusside, labetalol, hydralazine)

---

ume in 1 second $<$ 50% of normal) and marginal renal function (serum creatinine $>$ 3 mg/dl).

  D. **Rupture of an abdominal aortic aneurysm** is suggested by hypotension, back pain, and a pulsatile abdominal mass. Exsanguination is not the rule because of clotting and the tamponade effect of the retroperitoneum.

   1. So long as the patient is conscious and has adequate peripheral perfusion, euvolemic resuscitation is deferred until the rupture is surgically controlled in the operating room. Euvolemic resuscitation and increasing the systemic blood pressure without surgical control of bleeding from the ruptured aneurysm may lead to loss of retroperitoneal tamponade, with further bleeding, hypotension, and death.

   2. In any patient who is unstable with a suspected ruptured abdominal aortic aneurysm, immediate operation and control of the proximal portion of the aorta is mandatory (time is not available for confirmatory testing or optimizing the patient's preoperative condition).

  E. **Management of anesthesia** must consider the high incidence of ischemic heart disease, systemic hypertension, chronic obstructive pulmonary disease, diabetes mellitus, and renal dysfunction in these often elderly patients (Table 10–5).

  F. **Postoperative management.** See Table 10–6.

11

Peripheral Vascular Disease

Peripheral arterial disease results in compromised blood flow to the extremities, especially the legs (Stoelting RK, Dierdorf SF. Peripheral vascular disease. In: Anesthesia and Co-Existing Disease, 4th ed. New York, Churchill Livingstone, 2002;157–168). Chronic impairment of blood flow to the extremities is most often due to atherosclerosis, whereas embolism is most likely to be responsible for acute arterial occlusion (Table 11–1). Vasculitis may also be responsible for compromised blood flow to the extremities (Table 11–1).

I. PERIPHERAL ATHEROSCLEROSIS

Peripheral atherosclerosis (arteriosclerosis obliterans) that occurs in the extremities resembles atherosclerosis in the aorta, coronary arteries, and extracranial vessels.

- **A. Risk factors** associated with the development of peripheral atherosclerosis are similar to those that cause ischemic heart disease (diabetes mellitus, essential hypertension, tobacco abuse, dyslipidemia, hyperhomocysteinemia, family history).
- **B. Signs and symptoms.** Intermittent claudication and rest pain are the principal symptoms of peripheral atherosclerosis. Decreased or absent arterial pulses are the most reliable physical finding associated with peripheral arterial disease.
- **C. Diagnosis.** Doppler ultrasonography and the resulting pulse volume waveform are used to identify arterial vessels with stenotic lesions.
- **D. Treatment.** Medical therapy of peripheral arterial disease includes establishing an exercise program and identifiying and treating risk factors for atherosclerosis.
  1. **Revascularization** procedures (endovascular interventions or surgical reconstruction) are indicated in patients with disabling claudication, ischemic rest pain, or impending limb loss.

▬ Table 11–1 • Peripheral Vascular Disease

---

*Chronic Peripheral Arterial Occlusive Disease (**Atherosclerosis**)*
Distal abdominal aorta or iliac arteries
Femoral arteries
Subclavian steal syndrome
*Acute Peripheral Arterial Occlusive Disease (**Embolism**)*
Systemic Vasculitis
Takayasu's arteritis (pulseless disease)
Thromboangiitis obliterans (Buerger's disease)
Wegener's granulomatosis
Temporal arteritis
Polyarteritis nodosa
Other Vascular Syndromes
Schönlein-Henoch purpura
Raynaud's phenomenon
Moyamoya disease
Kawasaki disease
Coronary-subclavian steal syndrome
Klippel-Trenaunay syndrome
Behçet's disease

---

    2. **Surgical procedures.** The operative procedures used for
vascular reconstruction depend on the location (aortobi-
femoral bypass, axillobifemoral bypass, femorofemoral
bypass, infrainguinal bypass) and severity of the peripheral arterial stenosis. Amputation is utilized for patients
with advanced limb ischemia in whom revascularization procedures are not possible or have failed.

      a. The operative risk during reconstructive peripheral
vascular surgery, as for abdominal aortic aneurysm
resection, is primarily related to the presence of associated atherosclerotic vascular disease, particularly
ischemic heart disease and cerebrovascular disease.

      b. Mortality following revascularization surgery is usu-
ally secondary to myocardial infarction in patients
who manifested preoperative evidence of ischemic
heart disease, congestive heart failure, or a preoperative history of coronary artery bypass grafting.

  E. **Management of anesthesia** for surgical revascularization
of the lower extremities incorporates many of the same
principles described for management of patients with abdominal aneurysms (see Chapter 10).

1. The popularity of general anesthesia is in part due to the controversy surrounding the performance of regional anesthesia, especially placing an epidural catheter, in the presence of drug-induced anticoagulation. Nevertheless, placing an epidural catheter before instituting heparin anticoagulation has not been associated with untoward neurologic events. Epidural anesthesia may influence the outcome beneficially (attenuates stress-induced hypercoagulability) in high risk patients following major peripheral vascular surgery.

2. Infrarenal aortic cross-clamping and unclamping in the presence of peripheral vascular disease is associated with minimal hemodynamic derangements, presumably reflecting the presence of a collateral circulation. For this reason it is acceptable to use a central venous pressure catheter in lieu of a pulmonary artery catheter. Monitoring left ventricular function and the intravascular fluid volume may also be facilitated by use of transesophageal echocardiography.

3. Heparin is commonly administered before applying the aortic cross-clamp, presumably to decrease the risk of thromboembolic complications. Nevertheless, distal emboli, especially to the kidneys, most likely reflect dislodgement of atheroembolic debris from the diseased aorta.

4. Spinal cord damage associated with surgical revascularization of the legs is unlikely (special monitoring is not necessary).

F. **Postoperative management** includes provision of analgesia (neuraxial opioids) and treatment of fluid and electrolyte disorders. Attenuation of postoperative increases in heart rate and serum norepinephrine concentrations may be prevented by treatment with dexmedetomidine.

G. **Subclavian steal syndrome** reflects occlusion of the subclavian or innominate artery proximal to the origin of the vertebral artery by an atherosclerotic lesion resulting in reversal of flow (steal) from the brain (syncope). Pulses in the ipsilateral arm are often absent or diminished, and the systolic blood pressure is likely to be at least 20 mmHg lower.

II. ACUTE ARTERIAL OCCLUSION

Acute arterial occlusion differs from the gradual development of occlusion caused by atherosclerosis and most often reflects systemic emboli that originate from the heart (mural thrombi in the left ventricle in the presence of an acute myocardial infarction or atrial fibrillation).

A. Signs and symptoms. Acute arterial occlusion is associated with sudden onset of intense pain, paresthesia, motor weakness distal to the site of occlusion, loss of palpable peripheral pulses, cool skin, and sharply demarcated skin color changes.

B. Diagnosis is confirmed by arteriography.

C. Treatment is surgical embolectomy and administration of heparin.

III. SYSTEMIC VASCULITIS

Systemic vasculitis manifests in nonspecific ways that suggest connective tissue disease, sepsis, or malignancy (Table 11–2).

A. Takayasu's arteritis is a chronic, progressive occlusive vasculitis that causes narrowing, thrombosis, or aneurysms of systemic arteries (pulseless disease) and pulmonary arteries. The definitive diagnosis is made on the basis of contrast angiography.

  1. Signs and symptoms. See Table 11–3.

  2. Treatment of Takayasu's arteritis is with corticosteroids.

  3. Management of anesthesia must consider the drugs used to treat this disease (supplemental corticosteroids may be needed) and multiple organ system involvement by vasculitis. During the preoperative evaluation it is useful to establish the effect of changes in head position on cerebral function (hyperextension could compromise flow through the carotid arteries shortened as a result of the vascular inflammatory process).

≡ Table 11–2 • Signs and Symptoms of Systemic Vasculitis

Fever
Fatigue
Weight loss
Neuropathy
Increased erythrocyte sedimentation rate
Anemia
Hypoalbuminemia

≡ Table 11–3 • Signs and Symptoms of Takayasu's Arteritis

Central Nervous System
Vertigo
Visual disturbances
Syncope
Seizures
Cerebral ischemia or infarction
Cardiovascular System
Multiple occlusions or peripheral arteries
Ischemic heart disease
Cardiac valve dysfunction
Cardiac conduction defects
Lungs
Pulmonary hypertension
Ventilation-to-perfusion mismatch
Kidneys
Renal artery stenosis
Musculoskeletal System
Ankylosing spondylitis
Rheumatoid arthritis

---

    a. **Choice of anesthesia.** Regional anesthesia has been utilized successfully despite concerns about the presence of anticoagulation and the impact of hypotension on perfusion pressure to vital organs. Regardless of the techniques and drugs selected to produce anesthesia, the priority must be to maintain adequate arterial perfusion pressures during the intraoperative period.

    b. **Monitoring.** Systemic blood pressure may be difficult to measure noninvasively in the upper extremities. Despite a theoretical concern, placing a catheter in the radial artery may be useful. Placing a pulmonary artery catheter or transesophageal echocardiography probe is acceptable as reflected by the magnitude of the surgery.

B. **Thromboangiitis obliterans (Buerger's disease)** is an inflammatory vasculitis leading to occlusion of small and medium-size arteries and veins in the extremities. Diagnosis is confirmed by biopsy of an active vascular lesion.

    1. **Signs and symptoms.** Upper or lower extremity claudication reflects involvement of arteries by this disease.

Raynaud's phenomenon and superficial vein thrombosis are common.

2. **Treatment** includes smoking cessation. Surgical revascularization is usually not an option because of involvement of small distal vessels.

3. **Management of anesthesia** requires avoidance of events that might damage already ischemic extremities (positioning to avoid pressure points on extremities and maintenance of body temperature). Noninvasive monitoring of systemic blood pressure is preferred, as placing a catheter in a diseased artery is a concern. If a regional anesthetic is selected, it may be prudent to omit epinephrine from the local anesthetic solution to avoid any possibility of accentuating co-existing vasospasm.

C. **Wegener's granulomatosis** is characterized by the formation of necrotizing granulomas in inflamed vessels, which are present in multiple organ systems (Table 11–4). Treatment of Wegener's granulomatosis with cyclophosphamide produces dramatic remissions in nearly all patients.

▬ Table 11–4 • Signs and Symptoms of Wegener's Granulomatosis

Central Nervous System
Cerebral arterial aneurysms
Peripheral neuropathy
Respiratory Tract and Lungs
Sinusitis
Laryngeal stenosis
Epiglottic destruction
Ventilation-to-perfusion mismatch
Pneumonia
Hemoptysis
Bronchial obstruction
Cardiovascular System
Cardiac valve destruction
Disturbances of cardiac impulse conduction
Myocardial ischemia
Infarction of the tips of digits
Kidneys
Hematuria
Azotemia
Renal failure

1. **Management of anesthesia** in patients with Wegener's granulomatosis requires an appreciation of the widespread organ involvement (myocardial ischemia, renal failure, peripheral neuropathy) associated with this disease and the potentially adverse effects of cyclophosphamide (depression of the immune system, anemia, decreased plasma cholinesterase activity). Avoidance of trauma during direct laryngoscopy is important, as bleeding from granulomas and dislodgement of friable ulcerated tissues can occur. A smaller than expected endotracheal tube may be required if the glottic opening is narrowed by granulomatous changes. Arteritis that is likely to involve peripheral vessels may limit the ability to place an indwelling arterial catheter for monitoring the systemic blood pressure.

2. **Choice of anesthesia.** A careful neurologic examination is helpful before the decision is made to recommend regional anesthesia. Conceivably, volatile anesthetics could be associated with exaggerated myocardial depression when the disease process involves the myocardium and cardiac valves.

D. **Temporal arteritis** is an inflammation of the arteries of the head and neck, manifesting most often as headache, tenderness of the scalp, or jaw claudication. Prompt initiation of treatment with corticosteroids is indicated in patients with visual symptoms to prevent blindness.

E. **Polyarteritis nodosa** is a vasculitis that most often occurs in women 20 to 60 years of age and commonly in association with hepatitis B antigenemia and allergic reactions to drugs. Renal failure is the most common cause of death.

1. **Diagnosis and treatment.** Biopsy is needed for diagnosis. Treatment is with corticosteroids and cyclophosphamide.

2. **Management of anesthesia** should take into consideration the likelihood of renal or cardiac disease and the implications of co-existing systemic hypertension. Supplemental corticosteroids may be indicated.

F. **Schönlein-Henoch purpura** affects arterioles and capillaries in the skin, kidneys, gastrointestinal tract, and large joints in children.

G. **Kawasaki disease** (mucocutaneous lymph node syndrome) occurs primarily in children, manifesting as fever, conjunctivitis, inflammation of the mucous membranes, swollen erythematous hands and feet, truncal rashes, and cervical lymphadenopathy. **Management of anesthesia** should consider the possibility of intraoperative myocardial ischemia and cerebral hemorrhage.

IV. RAYNAUD'S PHENOMENON

Raynaud's phenomenon is episodic vasospastic ischemia of the digits that affects females more than males.

A. **Classification.** Raynaud's phenomenon is categorized as primary (Raynaud's disease) or secondary when it is associated with other diseases, most often scleroderma, systemic lupus erythematosus, and other related immunologic disorders.

B. **Etiology.** Mechanisms postulated to cause Raynaud's phenomenon include increased sympathetic nervous system activity (questionable because sympathectomy does not predictably produce beneficial effects), heightened digital vascular reactivity to vasoconstrictive stimuli, circulating vasoactive hormones, and decreased intravascular pressure.

C. **Diagnosis.** Noninvasive vascular tests that may be utilized to evaluate patients with Raynaud's disease include digital pulse volume recordings and measurement of the digital systolic blood pressure and digital blood flow. Raynaud's phenomenon is the initial complaint in most patients with CREST syndrome (calcinosis, Reynaud's phenomenon, esophageal dysmotility, sclerodactyly, telangiectasia).

D. **Treatment** includes protecting the hands and feet from exposure to cold. Calcium channel blocking drugs and sympathetic nervous system antagonists such as prazosin can be used to treat Raynaud's phenomenon. Stellate ganglion block may improve blood flow and increase the temperature of the ipsilateral hand.

E. **Management of anesthesia.** Maintenance of body temperature and increasing the ambient temperature of the operating rooms seems logical. Cannulation of an artery to monitor systemic blood pressure is balanced against the theoretical risk of increasing ischemia in the affected extremity. Regional anesthesia is acceptable for peripheral operations in patients with Raynaud's phenomenon, but it may be prudent not to include epinephrine in the local anesthetic solutions, as catecholamines could provoke undesirable vasoconstriction.

V. MOYAMOYA DISEASE

Moyamoya disease is a progressive cerebrovascular occlusive disease of the internal carotid arteries and anterior and middle cerebral arteries that affects children and young adults. The characteristic symptoms of the disease are transient ischemic attacks causing hemiparesis or weakness of the limbs.

A. **Treatment** may include surgical procedures designed to augment collateral cerebral blood flow.

B. **Management of anesthesia** is influenced by the need to preserve cerebral blood flow relative to cerebral metabolic oxygen requirements. Cerebral blood flow is optimized by maintaining normocarbia, avoiding systemic hypotension, and promptly replacing intravascular fluid losses to maintain normovolemia. Volatile anesthetics seem a logical choice based on the theoretical value of drug-induced cerebral vasodilation.

VI. CORONARY-SUBCLAVIAN STEAL SYNDROME

Coronary-subclavian steal syndrome occurs when incomplete stenosis of the left subclavian artery leads to reversal of blood flow (steal) through a patent internal mammary artery graft. It manifests as angina pectoris and decreased systolic blood pressure of at least 20 mmHg in the ipsilateral arm.

VII. KLIPPEL-TRENAUNAY SYNDROME

Klippel-Trenaunay syndrome is characterized by port-wine hemangiomas associated with spinal cord arteriovenous malformations. Spinal or regional anesthesia is an unlikely choice.

VIII. BEHÇET'S DISEASE

Behçet's disease is a chronic relapsing inflammatory disorder of unknown cause that manifests as oral aphthous ulcers, painful genital ulcers, and uveitis. Bowel symptoms may mimic Crohn's disease and ulcerative colitis, whereas the neurologic symptoms may resemble those of multiple sclerosis.

12

Deep-Vein Thrombosis and Pulmonary Embolism

Deep-vein thrombosis (usually involving a leg vein) and associated pulmonary embolism represent a leading cause of postoperative morbidity (Stoelting RK, Dierdorf SF. Deep-vein thrombosis and pulmonary embolism. In: Anesthesia and Co-Existing Disease, 4th ed. New York, Churchill Livingstone, 2002;169–176). An embolus is a fragment of thrombus that breaks off and travels in the blood until it lodges at a site of vascular narrowing (pulmonary vasculature if in a vein and distal small artery if in an artery). Factors that predispose to thromboembolism are multiple but often include events likely to be associated with anesthesia and surgery (Table 12–1).

I. DEEP-VEIN THROMBOSIS

A. Venous thrombi that form below the knees or in the arms rarely give rise to significant pulmonary emboli, whereas thrombi that extend into the iliofemoral venous system can produce life-threatening pulmonary embolism.

B. **Diagnosis**

1. Superficial thrombophlebitis, as may follow an intravenous infusion, is rarely associated with pulmonary embolism (intense inflammation leads to rapid and total occlusion of the vein). Treatment of superficial vein thrombosis is conservative (elevation, heat, antibiotics if infection is suspected).

2. Deep-vein thrombosis is often asymptomatic, and clinical signs are unreliable (Fig. 12–1). Compression ultrasonography is highly sensitive for detecting proximal vein thrombosis (popliteal or femoral vein). Most postoperative venous thrombi arise in the calves; but in at least 20% of patients who have undergone surgical procedures and in 40% to 50% of patients with skeletal muscle trauma, thrombi can originate in proximal veins.

■ Table 12–1 • Factors Predisposing
to Thromboembolism

Venous stasis
    Recent surgery (includes outpatient surgery)
    Trauma
    Lack of ambulation
    Pregnancy
    Low cardiac output (congestive heart failure, myocardial
       infarction)
    Stroke
Abnormality of venous wall
    Varicose veins
    Drug-induced irritation
Hypercoagulable state
    Surgery (stress response)
    Estrogen therapy (oral contraceptives)
    Cancer (malignant cells contain a cysteine proteinase that
      activates factor X)
    Deficiencies of endogenous anticoagulants (antithrombin III,
      protein C, protein S)
    Inflammatory bowel disease
History of previous thromboembolism
Morbid obesity
Advanced age

---

      a. Left untreated, deep-vein thrombosis extends into
      larger, more proximal veins in 20% to 30% of patients;
      and this extension may be responsible for subsequent
      fatal pulmonary emboli.
      b. **Thrombophilia** refers to a tendency to experience re-
      current venous thromboembolism.
    C. **Treatment.** Anticoagulation is the first-line treatment for all
    patients with the diagnosis of deep-vein thrombosis as well
    as for those with proximal vein involvement (Table 12–2).
      1. **Restoration of venous patency** by surgical thrombectomy
      may be attempted in selected patients (limb viability
      threatened by an acute iliofemoral thrombosis). Inferior
      vena cava filters may be placed in patients who experience
      recurrent pulmonary embolism despite anticoagulant
      therapy or in whom anticoagulant therapy is contraindi-
      cated.

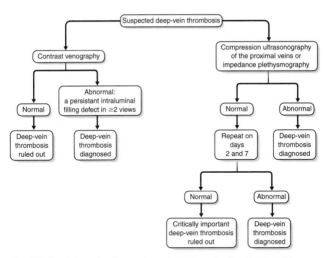

Fig. 12–1 • Steps in diagnosis and treatment of patients with suspected deep-vein thrombosis. (From Ginsberg JS. Management of venous thromboembolism. N Engl J Med 1996;335:1816–28. Copyright 1996 Massachusetts Medical Society, with permission.)

≡ Table 12–2 • Pharmacologic Treatment of Deep-Vein Thrombosis

Heparin (initial treatment administered as a continuous intravenous infusion or as subcutaneous injections to maintain the activated partial thromboplastin time 1.5 to 2.5 times the control value)

Warfarin (initiated within 24 hours of heparin therapy with the INR maintained between 2.0 and 3.0)

Discontinue heparin after about 4 days and if the INR ratio is > 2.0 for two consecutive days

Oral anticoagulants may be continued for 3 months

INR, international normalized ratio reflecting the prothrombin time.

2. **Complications of anticoagulation** include major bleeding (5% of patients treated with heparin). Approximately 3% of patients treated with heparin develop immune-mediated thrombocytopenia.

D. **Prevention of venous thromboembolism.** The presence of clinical risk factors identifies patients with the most to gain from prophylactic measures and patients who should receive antithrombotic prophylaxis during periods of increased susceptibility, such as postoperatively or postpartum (Table 12–3). The presence of malignant disease increases the risk of thrombotic complications.

1. Small subcutaneous doses of heparin (minidose heparin given in a dose of 5000 units two or three times daily) prevent deep-vein thrombosis in patients at moderate risk following abdominal or orthopedic surgery.

2. **Regional anesthesia.** The incidence of postoperative deep-vein thrombosis and pulmonary embolism is decreased in patients who have undergone total hip replacement or knee replacement with spinal or epidural anesthesia. Presumably, the early beneficial effects of regional anesthesia compared with general anesthesia (long-term outcome not altered by choice of anesthesia) are due to vasodilation that maximizes venous blood flow and to the ability to provide optimal postoperative analgesia with associated early ambulation.

E. **Postthrombotic syndrome** occurs as a long-term complication of proximal vein thrombosis that manifests as chronic leg pain associated with edema, stasis pigmentation, induration, and skin ulceration.

II. PULMONARY EMBOLISM

A. **Diagnosis** (Tables 12–4, 12–5). The most consistent manifestation of pulmonary embolism is the acute onset of dyspnea. Transthoracic echocardiography is particularly useful in critically ill patients suspected of having pulmonary embolism. It can help identify right ventricular pressure overload as well as myocardial infarction, dissection of the aorta, or pericardial tamponade. Perfusion lung scanning is the most useful test to rule out clinically important acute pulmonary embolism (Fig. 12–2).

1. Arterial blood gases may remain normal, whereas arterial hypoxemia and hypocapnia (stimulation of airway irritant receptors causes hyperventilation) are not specific for pulmonary embolism.

Table 12–3 • Risk and Predisposing Factors for the Development of Deep-Vein Thrombosis after Surgery or Trauma

Event	Low Risk	Moderate Risk	High Risk
General surgery	< 40 Years old Operation < 60 minutes	> 40 Years old Operation > 60 minutes	> 40 Years old Operation > 60 minutes Prior deep-vein thrombosis Prior pulmonary embolus Extensive trauma Major fractures Knee or hip replacement
Orthopedic surgery			
Trauma		Extensive soft tissue injury	Major fractures Multiple trauma sites
Medical conditions	Pregnancy	Postpartum period Myocardial infarction Congestive heart failure	Stroke
Incidence of deep-vein thrombosis without prophylaxis	2%	10%–40%	40%–60%
Symptomatic pulmonary embolism	0.2%	1%–8%	5%–10%
Fatal pulmonary embolism	0.002%	0.1%–0.4%	1%–5%

Table continued on following page

Table 12-3 • Risk and Predisposing Factors for the Development of Deep-Vein Thrombosis after Surgery or Trauma *Continued*

Event	Low Risk	Moderate Risk	High Risk
Recommended steps to minimize deep-vein thrombosis	Graduated compression stockings Early ambulation	External pneumatic compression Minidose heparin Intravenous dextran	External pneumatic compression Minidose heparin Intravenous dextran Warfarin Intracaval filters

Adapted from: Weinmann EE, Salzman EW. Deep-vein thrombosis. N Engl J Med 1994;331:1630–42.

≡ **Table 12–4** • Differential Diagnosis of Pulmonary Embolism

Pneumonia
Asthma
Exacerbation of chronic obstructive pulmonary disease
Pulmonary edema
Thoracic aorta dissection
Pericardial tamponade
Myocardial infarction
Pneumothorax
Anxiety

2. The electrocardiogram is mainly used to help distinguish between massive pulmonary embolism and myocardial infarction.
3. Manifestations of pulmonary embolism during anesthesia are nonspecific and often transient (Table 12–6).
B. **Treatment.** See Table 12–7.
C. **Management of anesthesia** for surgical treatment of life-threatening pulmonary embolism is designed to support vital organ function and to minimize anesthetic-induced myocardial depression. Monitoring arterial and cardiac filling pressures is recommended. Fluid administration is adjusted to optimize the right ventricular stroke volume. It may be necessary to support cardiac output with continu-

≡ **Table 12–5** • Signs and Symptoms of Pulmonary Embolism

Signs/Symptoms	Incidence (%)
Acute dyspnea	80–85
Tachypnea (> 20 breaths/min)	75–85
Pleuritic chest pain	65–70
Nonproductive cough	50–60
Accentuation of pulmonic valve S_2	50–60
Rales	50–60
Tachycardia (> 100 beats/min)	45–65
Fever (38°–39°C)	40–50
Hemoptysis	39

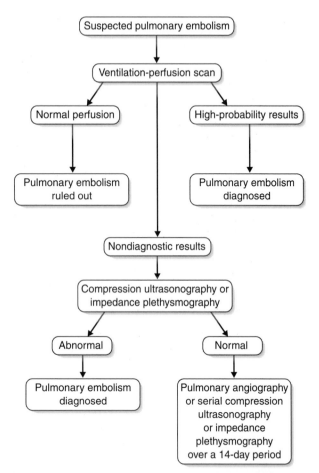

Fig. 12–2 • Steps in the diagnosis of patients with clinically suspected pulmonary embolism. (From Ginsberg JS. Management of venous thromboembolism. N Engl J Med 1996;334:1816–28. Copyright 1996 Massachusetts Medical Society, with permission.)

≡ Table 12–6 • Manifestations of Pulmonary Embolism During Anesthesia

---

Unexplained arterial hypoxemia, hypotension, tachycardia, bronchospasm

Electrocardiogram and central venous pressure may reflect an abrupt onset of right ventricular dysfunction

Increased alveolar-to-arterial difference for carbon dioxide

Echocardiography reveals acute dilation of right atrium, right ventricle, pulmonary artery

---

ous infusions of catecholamines (isoproterenol, dopamine, dobutamine) during surgery.

   1. Induction and maintenance of anesthesia should avoid accentuation of co-existing arterial hypoxemia, systemic hypotension, and pulmonary hypertension. Nitrous oxide is not a likely choice considering the need to administer high concentrations of oxygen and the potential for this drug to increase pulmonary vascular resistance (same consideration for ketamine).

   2. Removal of embolic fragments from the distal pulmonary artery may be facilitated by applying positive-pressure ventilation to the patient's lungs when the surgeon applies suction through the arteriotomy placed in the pulmonary artery.

III. FAT EMBOLISM

   A. Fat embolism to the lungs typically appears 12 to 72 hours (lucid interval) after long bone fractures, especially of the

---

≡ Table 12–7 • Treatment of Pulmonary Embolism

Heparin bolus followed by continuous intravenous infusion

Warfarin initiated when therapeutic activated partial thromboplastin time is achieved (goal is INR of 3.0)

Inotrope to support cardiac output (isoproterenol, dopamine, dobutamine)

Tracheal intubation and positive end-expiratory pressure

Analgesia

Pulmonary artery embolectomy utilizing cardiopulmonary bypass

---

femur or tibia. The triad of arterial hypoxemia, mental confusion, and petechiae, especially over the anterior neck, shoulders, and chest (caused by embolic fat) in young adults with closed tibia or femur fractures, should arouse suspicion of fat embolism. Temperature increases and tachycardia are often present.

B. Treatment of fat embolism syndrome includes management of acute respiratory distress syndrome and immobilization of long bone fractures. The efficacy of corticosteroids has not been confirmed.

13

Chronic Obstructive Pulmonary Disease

Chronic obstructive pulmonary disease (COPD) is character-ized by the progressive development of airflow limitation that is not fully reversible (Stoelting RK, Dierdorf SF. Chronic obstructive pulmonary disease. In: Anesthesia and Co-Existing Disease, 4th ed. New York, Churchill Livingstone, 2002;177–191). The term COPD encompasses chronic obstructive bronchitis (obstruction of small airways) and emphysema (enlargement of air spaces and destruction of lung parenchyma, loss of lung elasticity, closure of small airways). Chronic bronchitis, by contrast, is defined by the presence of a productive cough for more than 3 months over more than three successive years. Most patients with COPD have all three pathologic conditions, but the extent varies among individuals.

I. CHRONIC BRONCHITIS AND PULMONARY EMPHYSEMA

See Table 13-1.

  A. **Epidemiology.** Cigarette smoking is the major predisposing factor in the development of COPD. The dominant feature of the natural history of COPD is progressive airflow obstruction, as reflected by decreased forced exhaled volume in 1 second (FEV_1). Emphysema develops in some patients because of an imbalance between protease and antiprotease results in unopposed degradation of pulmonary interstitial elastin fibers in the lungs. The genetic absence of α_1-antitrypsin is associated with the development of emphysema and cirrhosis of the liver.

  B. **Clinical features and diagnosis** (Table 13–1). Chronic productive cough and exercise limitation due to dyspnea are the hallmarks of the persistent expiratory airflow obstruction characteristic of COPD. Although these symptoms are nonspecific, the diagnosis of COPD is likely if patients are also chronic cigarette smokers. Patients with predominant chronic bronchitis present with chronic productive cough, whereas

■ Table 13–1 • Comparative Features of Chronic Obstructive Pulmonary Disease

Feature	Chronic Bronchitis	Pulmonary Emphysema
Mechanism of airway obstruction	Decreased airway lumen due to mucus and inflammation	Loss of elastic recoil
Dyspnea	Moderate	Severe
Forced exhaled volume in 1 second (FEV_1)	Decreased	Decreased
PaO_2	Marked decrease ("blue bloater")	Moderate decrease ("pink puffer")
$PaCO_2$	Increased	Normal to decreased
Diffusing capacity	Normal	Decreased
Hematocrit	Increased	Normal
Cor pulmonale	Marked	Mild
Prognosis	Poor	Good

patients with predominant emphysema complain of dyspnea. Wheezing is common in the presence of mucus accumulation in the airways and may mimic asthma. The combination of chronic bronchitis and reversible bronchospasm is referred to as asthmatic bronchitis.

1. **Physical examination** in the presence of expiratory airway obstruction reveals tachypnea and a prolonged expiratory phase.
2. **Pulmonary function tests** reveal a decreased FEV_1/forced vital capacity (FVC) ratio and even greater decreases in the forced expiratory flow between 25% to 75% of vital capacity. Measurement of lung volumes reveals an increased residual volume and normal to increased functional residual capacity and total lung volume (Fig. 13–1).
3. **Chest radiography.** Hyperlucency of the lungs owing to arterial vascular deficiency in the lung periphery and hyperinflation (flattening of the diaphragm with loss of the normal domed appearance and a vertically oriented cardiac silhouette) suggest the diagnosis of emphysema.
4. **Arterial blood gases** in the presence of advanced COPD are commonly used to categorize the patient with COPD

NORMAL   **OBSTRUCTIVE**

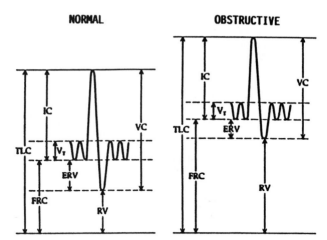

Fig. 13–1 • Lung volumes in chronic obstructive pulmonary disease compared with normal values. In the presence of obstructive lung disease, VC is normal to decreased; RV and FRC are increased; TLC is normal to increased; and the RV/TLC ratio is increased. ERV, expiratory reserve volume; FRC, functional residual capacity; IC, inspiratory capacity; RV, residual volume; TLC, total lung capacity; VC, vital capacity; V_T, tidal volume.

as a "pink puffer" ($PaO_2 > 65$ mmHg and $PaCO_2$ normal to slightly decreased) or a "blue bloater" ($PaO_2 < 65$ mmHg and $PaCO_2$ chronically increased to > 45 mmHg).

   a. Cardiovascular consequences of these two blood gas patterns manifest as pulmonary hypertension, secondary erythrocytosis, and cor pulmonale (right ventricular failure) in patients characterized as "blue bloaters."

   b. Pulmonary vasoconstriction is minimal, secondary erythrocytosis does not occur, and cor pulmonale is unlikely in patients characterized as "pink puffers."

C. Treatment. See Table 13–2.

   1. Noninvasive ventilation with a nasal mask eliminates the need for tracheal intubation and decreases the risk of mechanical ventilation during acute exacerbations of COPD.

   2. Lung volume reduction surgery may be considered in selected patients with emphysema characterized by areas of overdistended and poorly functioning emphysematous regions.

▬ Table 13–2 • Treatment of Patients with Chronic
Obstructive Pulmonary Disease

Cessation of cigarette smoking
Supplemental oxygen if PaO_2 < 55 mmHg or hematocrit > 55%
  (goal is to maintain PaO_2 at 60–80 mmHg)
β_2-Agonists (even small improvements in airway resistance to
  airflow decrease symptoms and may decrease infective
  exacerbations)
Anticholinergic drugs (most effective in patients with COPD)
Inhaled corticosteroids
Intermittent broad-spectrum antibiotics
Annual vaccinations against influenza and pneumococci
Drug-induced diuresis if right ventricular failure present

COPD, chronic obstructive pulmonary disease.

---

   a. Management of anesthesia for lung reduction surgery
      includes use of an endobronchial tube, avoidance of ni-
      trous oxide, and avoidance of excessive positive airway
      pressure (inspiratory pressure is ideally < 20 cmH$_2$O).
   b. Monitoring central venous pressure to guide fluid man-
      agement is not likely to be reliable because of gas trap-
      ping and the pulmonary tamponade effect due to large
      emphysematous bullae.
 **D. Preoperative pulmonary evaluation and risk of postopera-
    tive complications.** Postoperative cardiac and pulmonary
    (pneumonia, atelectasis, bronchospasm, acute respiratory
    failure) complications are predictable risks for surgery in
    these patients.
    1. Patient-related risk factors. See Table 13–3.
    2. Procedure-related risk factors. See Table 13–4.

▬ Table 13–3 • Patient-Related Risk Factors for the
Development of Postoperative Pulmonary
Complications in Patients with COPD

Smoking
Co-existing pulmonary disease (aggressive preoperative treatment
  of symptomatic COPD; defer elective surgery in presence of
  acute exacerbations)
Advanced age
Poor general health

Table 13–4 • Procedure-Related Risk Factors for the Development of Postoperative Pulmonary Complications in Patients with COPD

Operative site (most important predictor; risk increases as incision approaches the diaphragm and duration of surgery is > 3 hours)

Respiratory muscle function (disruption of normal coordination of respiratory muscles due to anesthetic drugs, neuromuscular blocking drugs, and surgical trauma)

E. **Preoperative clinical evaluation.** The history (exercise tolerance, chronic cough, dyspnea) and physical examination (decreased breath sounds, wheezing, prolonged expiratory phase) of patients with COPD provides a more accurate assessment of the likelihood of postoperative pulmonary complications than do pulmonary function tests and measurement of arterial blood gases.

   1. **Preoperative pulmonary function testing.** Pulmonary function tests should be viewed as a management tool to optimize preoperative function but not as a means to assess risk of postoperative pulmonary complications. Preoperative spirometry may be reserved for patients scheduled to undergo thoracic or upper abdominal surgery and who have symptoms of cough, dyspnea, or exercise intolerance. The results of preoperative pulmonary function testing should not be used to deny patients surgery.

   2. **Risk reduction strategies.** See Table 13–5.

F. **Management of anesthesia** for patients with COPD undergoing elective surgery includes efforts during the preoperative period to optimize pulmonary function, intraoperative management designed to minimize residual depressant effects of anesthetic drugs on breathing, and postoperative interventions to decrease surgical pain that could contribute to impaired oxygenation and ventilation.

   1. **Preoperative preparation** of patients with COPD includes recommendations to stop smoking, treatment of reversible processes such as bronchospasm (inhaled β-agonists), and eradication of infections.

      a. **Cessation of smoking.** Even brief periods of abstinence improve the oxygen-carrying capacity of the patient's arterial blood (12 hours is sufficient to increase the P_{50} and decrease plasma levels of carboxyhemoglobin sub-

━ **Table 13–5** • Risk Reduction Strategies to Decrease the Incidence of Postoperative Complications in Patients with COPD

Preoperative
Encourage cessation of smoking for at least 8 weeks
Treat evidence of expiratory airflow obstruction
Treat respiratory infection with antibiotics
Initiate patient education regarding lung-volume expansion maneuvers

Intraoperative
Use minimally invasive surgical (laparoscopic) techniques when possible
Consider use of regional anesthesia (?)
Avoid use of long-acting neuromuscular blocking drugs (?)
Avoid surgical procedures > 3 hours

Postoperative
Continue tracheal intubation and mechanical ventilation (likely after abdominal or intrathoracic surgery and a preoperative $PaCO_2$ > 50 mmHg and FEV_1/FVC < 0.5; maintain PaO_2 at 60–100 mmHg and $PaCO_2$ in a range that maintains the pHa at 7.35–7.45)
Institute long-volume expansion maneuvers (voluntary deep breathing, incentive spirometry, continuous positive airway pressure)
Chest physiotherapy
Maximize analgesia (neuraxial opioids, intercostal nerve blocks, patient-controlled analgesia)

FEV_1/FVC, forced expiratory volume in 1 second/forced vital capacity.
Adapted from: Smetana GW. Preoperative pulmonary evaluation. N Engl J Med 1999;340:937–44.

stantially). Likewise, the effects of nicotine on the cardiovascular system are brief, lasting only 20 to 30 minutes.

  b. Adverse effects of cigarette smoking, including mucous hypersecretion, impaired mucociliary transport, narrowed small airways, impaired immune function, and increased hepatic enzyme activity, require at least 6 weeks of abstinence to return to normal.

 2. Selection of anesthetic technique. The preoperative presence of COPD does not dictate the use of specific drugs or techniques for the management of anesthesia (incidence of postoperative pulmonary infections is not predictably influenced by the choices made). More important than the drugs or techniques selected is the realization that these patients are susceptible to the development of acute respiratory failure during the postoperative period. Continued tracheal intubation and mechanical ventilation of the patient's lungs may be necessary, particularly after upper abdominal or intrathoracic surgery. Alternatively, postoperative analgesia with neuraxial opioids that permit pain-free breathing during the postoperative period may permit early tracheal extubation.

  a. **Regional anesthesia.** The risk of pulmonary complications is often viewed as being less following surgery with epidural or spinal anesthesia then following general anesthesia, although this notion is not always supported by the literature. Regional anesthesia remains a useful choice in patients with COPD only when sedative drugs are not needed (midazolam, 1 to 2 mg IV, in increments can be administered with minimal likelihood of producing undesirable degrees of ventilatory depression, remembering that these patients, particularly elderly patients, may be extremely sensitive to depressant effects of sedatives).

  b. **General anesthesia** in patients with COPD is often provided with volatile anesthetics (prompt elimination and bronchodilation) with or without nitrous oxide (consider the risk of diffusion into bullae, diluting the delivered oxygen concentrations) using humidification of the inspired gases and mechanical ventilation of the lungs [optimizes arterial oxygenation using large tidal volumes (10 to 15 mg/kg) combined with slow breathing rates (6 to 10 breaths/min), which minimizes the likelihood of turbulent airflow and maintains optimal ventilation-to-perfusion matching].

3. **Postoperative care** of patients with COPD is intended to minimize the incidence and severity of pulmonary complications, recognizing that these patients are at increased risk for developing acute respiratory failure (Table 13–5). The likelihood of postoperative pulmonary complications is greatest following upper abdominal and intrathoracic surgery. Vital capacity and functional residual capacity decrease early postoperatively and are not restored by pain relief, suggesting that altered respiratory muscle coordination (trauma from the surgical procedure) is responsible. The incidence of postoperative pulmonary complications

is less after laparoscopic cholecystectomy than after open cholecystectomy.

II. LESS COMMON CAUSES OF EXPIRATORY AIRFLOW OBSTRUCTION

A. **Bronchiectasis** is a chronic suppurative disease of the airways that if sufficiently widespread may cause expiratory airflow obstruction similar to COPD.

1. **Pathophysiology.** Bacterial or myobacterial infection is presumed to be responsible for most cases of bronchiectasis. Once bacterial superinfection is established, it is nearly impossible to eradicate, and daily expectoration of purulent sputum persists.

2. **Diagnosis.** The history of chronic cough productive of purulent sputum is highly suggestive of bronchiectasis. Clubbing of the digits is frequent, a change not characteristic of COPD. Computed tomography confirms the presence and extent of the disease.

3. **Treatment** of bronchiectasis is administration of antibiotics and postural drainage. Massive hemoptysis may be treated by surgical resection of the involved lung or by selective bronchial arterial embolization under radiographic control.

4. **Management of anesthesia** may include use of a double-lumen endobronchial tube and avoidance of nasal instrumentation (high incidence of sinusitis).

B. **Cystic fibrosis** is the most common life-shortening autosomal recessive disorder in the United States.

1. **Pathophysiology.** Cystic fibrosis is caused by a mutation in a single gene in chromosome 7 that results in defective chloride ion transport in epithelial cells in the lungs (bronchiectasis, COPD, sinusitis), pancreas (diabetes mellitus), liver (cirrhosis), gastrointestinal tract (meconium ileus), and reproductive organs (azospermia).

2. **Diagnosis.** The presence of a sweat chloride concentration > 80 mEq/L plus characteristic clinical symptoms or a family history confirm the diagnosis of cystic fibrosis.

3. **Treatment.** See Table 13–6.

4. **Management of anesthesia** in patients with cystic fibrosis invokes the same principles as for patients with COPD and bronchiectasis. Elective operations are delayed until optimal pulmonary function can be ensured by controlling the bronchial infection and facilitating removal of secre-

Table 13–6 • Treatment of Patients with Cystic Fibrosis

Clearance of airway secretions (chest physiotherapy with postural drainage, high-frequency chest compressions with an inflatable vest)
Bronchodilator therapy
Reduction in viscoelasticity of sputum
Antibiotic therapy (treatment of exacerbations on the basis of an increase in pulmonary symptoms and airway secretions or long term in hopes of decreasing the frequency of pulmonary infections)

tions from the airways. Volatile anesthetics are helpful for decreasing the responsiveness of the hyperactive airways that is characteristic of cystic fibrosis. Frequent suctioning of the trachea is often necessary during the operative period.

C. **Primary ciliary dyskinesia** is characterized by congenital impairment of ciliary activity in respiratory tract epithelial cells (chronic sinusitis, otitis media, bronchiectasis, chronic cough) and sperm tails (infertility). The triad of chronic sinusitis, bronchiectasis, and situs inversus (dextrocardia) is known as **Kartagener syndrome.**

1. **Management of anesthesia.** Preoperative preparation is directed at treating any active pulmonary infection and determining the presence of significant organ inversion (Table 13–7).
2. Drugs that depress ventilation or ciliary activity may be avoided in the preoperative medication.
3. In view of the high incidence of sinusitis, the use of a nasopharyngeal airway is questionable.

Table 13–7 • Anesthetic Considerations in the Presence of Dextrocardia

Reverse the electrocardiogram leads
Select left internal jugular vein to avoid thoracic duct
Double-lumen endobronchial tube anatomy is reversed
Uterine displacement in parturients is to the right

D. **Bronchiolitis obliterans** is a disease of childhood and most often results from infection with respiratory syncytial virus. This process may also accompany collagen vascular diseases (especially rheumatoid arthritis) and may be a sequela of bone marrow transplantation.

E. **Tracheal stenosis** is an extreme example of COPD that typically develops after mechanical ventilation of the lungs requiring prolonged translaryngeal tracheal intubation or tracheostomy.

1. **Diagnosis.** Circumferential constricting scar formation results in symptoms (dyspnea at rest, ineffective cough) when the lumen of the adult trachea is decreased to < 5 mm. A flow-volume loop is likely to display flattened exhaled and inhaled portions. Tomograms of the trachea demonstrate tracheal narrowing.

2. **Management of anesthesia** for surgical resection of the stenotic tracheal segment requires initial placement of a translaryngeal tracheal tube. After surgical exposure the distal normal trachea is opened and a sterile cuffed tube inserted. Maintenance of anesthesia using volatile anesthetics is useful for ensuring maximum inspired concentrations of oxygen. Addition of helium to the delivered gases is a consideration.

14

Asthma

Asthma is a chronic disease characterized by chronic airway inflammation, reversible expiratory airflow obstruction due to narrowing in the airways in response to various stimuli, and airway (bronchial) hyperreactivity (Stoelting RK, Dierdorf SF. Asthma. In: Anesthesia and Co-Existing Disease, 4th ed. New York, Churchill Livingstone, 2002;193–204). The incidence of asthma in persons 5 to 34 years of age is nearly 5% (at least 10 million Americans, making it one of the most common chronic diseases in the United States) with the greatest incidence of new cases of asthma in individuals less than 5 years of age.

I. PATHOGENESIS

A. **Allergen immunologic model.** In atopic persons, repeated antigen exposure leads to synthesis and secretion of specific immunoglobulin E (IgE) antibodies. Antigens can cross-link with IgE antibodies, leading to the release of vasoactive, bronchoactive, and chemoreactive mediators (histamine, interleukins, tumor necrosis factor, leukotrienes, prostaglandins, platelet-activating factor) from mast cells.

B. **Abnormal autonomic nervous system regulation of airway function.** This hypothesis is supported by increased expiratory airflow obstruction in patients with asthma being treated with a nonselective β-antagonist (propranolol), suggesting the presence of an imbalance between excitatory (bronchoconstrictor) and inhibitory (bronchodilator) neural input.

II. CLINICAL MANIFESTATIONS

A. During periods of normal to near-normal pulmonary function, patients are likely to have no physical findings referable to their asthma.

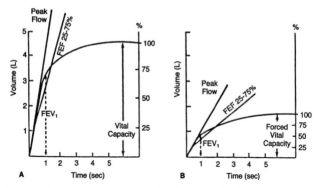

Fig. 14–1 • Spirogram changes in (A) a normal subject and (B) a patient in bronchospasm. The forced expiratory volume in 1 second (FEV_1) is typically < 80% of the vital capacity in the presence of obstructive airway disease. Peak flow and maximum midexpiratory flow rate (FEF_{25-75}) are also decreased in these patients (B). (From Kingston HGG, Hirshman CA. Perioperative management of the patient with asthma. Anesth Analg 1984;63:844–55, with permission.)

    B. As expiratory airflow obstruction increases, a number of signs and symptoms manifest and offer clues as to the severity of the asthmatic attack. Classic manifestations of asthma are wheezing, cough, and dyspnea.
        1. The forced exhaled volume in 1 second (FEV_1) and the maximum midexpiratory flow rate are direct reflections of the severity of expiratory airflow obstruction (Fig. 14–1; Table 14–1).
        2. Flow-volume loops demonstrate characteristic downward scooping of the expiratory limb (Fig. 14–2).
        3. Mild asthma is usually accompanied by normal PaO_2 and normal to decreased $PaCO_2$ values (Table 14–1). Tachypnea and hyperventilation observed during an acute asthmatic attack reflect neural reflexes in the lungs rather than arterial hypoxemia. Fatigue of the muscles necessary for breathing may contribute to the development of hypercarbia.

III. DIAGNOSIS

    A. No single laboratory test can confirm the diagnosis of asthma. In patients with baseline expiratory airflow obstruc-

Table 14–1 • Severity of Expiratory Airflow Obstruction

Severity	FEV$_1$ (% predicted)	FEF$_{25-75}$ (% predicted)	PaO$_2$* (mmHg)	PaCO$_2$* (mmHg)
Mild (asymptomatic)	65–80	60–75	> 60	< 40
Moderate	50–64	45–59	> 60	< 45
Marked	35–49	30–44	< 60	> 50
Severe (status asthmaticus)	< 35	< 30	< 60	> 50

FEV$_1$, forced exhaled volume in 1 second; FEF$_{25-75}$, forced expiratory flow at 25–75% forced vital capacity.
* Values are estimates.
Data from Kingston HGG, Hirshman CA. Perioperative management of the patient with asthma. Anesth Analg 1984;63:844–55.

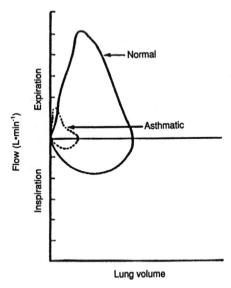

Fig. 14–2 • Flow–volume curve of a normal person and an asthmatic patient. (From Kingston HGG, Hirshman CA. Perioperative management of the patient with asthma. Anesth Analg 1984;63:844–55, with permission.)

tion, an increase (> 15%) in airflow after inhalation of a bronchodilator suggests asthma.

B. The differential diagnosis of asthma includes viral tracheobronchitis, restrictive pulmonary disease (sarcoidosis), rheumatoid arthritis, and extrinsic (thoracic aneurysm, mediastinal neoplasm) or intrinsic (epiglottitis, croup) compression causing upper airway obstruction. Congestive heart failure and pulmonary embolism may cause dyspnea.

IV. ETIOLOGIC FORMS OF ASTHMA

See Table 14–2.

V. PHARMACOLOGIC THERAPY

See Table 14–3.

A. Recognition of the consistent presence of airway inflammation in patients with asthma has resulted in a change in the

≡ Table 14–2 • Etiologic Forms of Asthma

Allergen-induced (immunologic) asthma (most common form of reversible expiratory airflow obstruction)

Exercise-induced asthma

Nocturnal asthma

Aspirin-induced asthma (includes nonsteroidal antiinflammatory drugs; patients with asthma may be sensitive to bisulfite and metabisulfite as used for preservatives and antioxidants for food-processing and certain drugs)

Occupational asthma (latex sensitivity in health care personnel may manifest as increasing expiratory obstruction to airflow during the normal workday in the operating room)

Infectious asthma

routine pharmacologic therapy of asthma with emphasis on the use of corticosteroids to prevent and control bronchial inflammation.

  B. Bronchodilator therapy with β_2-agonists is recommended only for pretreatment of exercise-induced asthma and for

≡ Table 14–3 • Pharmacologic Treatment of Asthma

Antiinflammatory Drugs

Corticosteroids [preferentially administered by inhalation; decrease airway responsiveness by decreasing airway inflammation; side effects include dysphonia, glossitis, and oropharyngeal candidiasis; systemic (suppression of the hypothalamic-pituitary-adrenal axis) whereas metabolic effects from inhalation do not occur]

Cromolyn (inhibits inflammation by preventing release of chemical mediators; administered by inhalation about 7 days before allergen exposure; not effective once bronchospasm is established and 10 to 20 minutes before exercise)

Leukotriene inhibitors

Bronchodilator Drugs

β-Adrenergic agonists [albuterol administered by metered-dose inhaler; side effects reflect sympathetic nervous system stimulation (tachycardia, cardiac dysrhythmias) and intracellular shifts of potassium]

Anticholinergic drugs (ipratropium administered by metered-dose inhaler for treatment of bronchoconstriction in patients with chronic obstructive pulmonary disease)

the symptomatic relief of acute exacerbations of asthma when antiinflammatory therapy is insufficient.

VI. TREATMENT OF STATUS ASTHMATICUS

See Table 14–4.

A. Status asthmaticus is defined as unresolving bronchospasm that, despite initial treatment, is considered life-threatening.

B. Measurement of lung function [forced expiratory volume in 1 second (FEV_1) or peak expiratory flow rate decreased to 25% of normal introduces the risk of hypercarbia] may be helpful for assessing the severity of the asthmatic attack and the response to treatment.

   1. The presence of hypercarbia ($PaCO_2 > 50$ mmHg) despite aggressive antiinflammatory and bronchodilator therapy may be a sign of impending respiratory fatigue that ultimately requires tracheal intubation and mechanical support of ventilation.

   2. When the FEV_1 or peak expiratory flow rate reaches 50% of normal or more, patients usually have minimal to no symptoms. At this point the frequency and intensity of bronchodilator therapy can be decreased.

VII. MANAGEMENT OF ANESTHESIA

A. **Preoperative evaluation** begins with a clinical history to elicit the severity and characteristics of the patient's asthma

---

≡ Table 14–4 • Treatment of Status Asthmaticus

β_2-Agonist by metered-dose inhaled every 15–20 minutes (most effective emergency treatment)

Corticosteroids administered intravenously (cortisol 2 mg/kg IV followed by 0.5 mg/kg/hr or methylprednisolone 60–125 mg IV every 6 hours; may take up to 12 hours to work)

Supplemental oxygen

Tracheal intubation and mechanical ventilation (consider when $PaCO_2 > 50$ mmHg)

Antibiotic therapy

General anesthesia with volatile anesthetics (only when bronchospasm persists despite aggressive pharmacologic therapy)

(Table 14–5). The preoperative absence of wheezing during auscultation of the chest or complaints of dyspnea suggest that the patient is not experiencing an acute exacerbation of asthma. Chest physiotherapy, systemic hydration, appropriate antibiotics, and bronchodilator therapy during the preoperative period often help with the reversible components of asthma, as evidenced by pulmonary function tests (especially FEV_1). Measurement of arterial blood gases before undertaking elective surgery is indicated if there are any questions about the adequacy of ventilation or arterial oxygenation.

B. **Preoperative medication.** A preferred drug or combination of drugs for use as preoperative medication in patients with asthma has not been established (opioids, anticholinergics, and H_2-receptor antagonists may be avoided). Bronchodilators and drugs (cromolyn) used in the treatment of asthma should be continued. When the preoperative FEV_1 is $< 80\%$, a preoperative course of oral corticosteroids may be useful.

C. **Induction and maintenance of anesthesia.** The goal during induction and maintenance of anesthesia in patients with asthma is to depress airway reflexes with anesthetic drugs, thereby avoiding bronchoconstriction of the patient's hyperreactive airways in response to mechanical stimulation.

   1. **Regional anesthesia,** avoiding instrumentation of the airway and tracheal intubation, is an attractive option when the operative site is superficial or on the extremities.

☰ **Table 14–5 • Characteristics of the Asthma to be Evaluated Preoperatively**

Age of onset
Known triggering events
Hospitalization for asthma
Known allergies
Cough
Sputum (changes in color and characteristics)
Previous anesthetic history
Current medications

2. **General anesthesia.** When general anesthesia is selected, induction of anesthesia is most often accomplished with intravenous injection of short-acting drugs such as propofol (Fig. 14–3). Ketamine is an alternative based on its sympathomimetic effects.

   a. After unconsciousness is produced by intravenous induction drugs, the patient's lungs are ventilated with a gas mixture containing a volatile anesthetic to

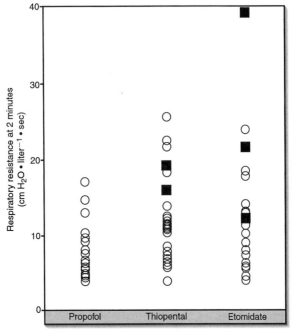

Fig. 14–3 • Respiratory resistance following tracheal intubation was lowest in healthy patients receiving propofol. *Solid squares* represent patients in whom audible wheezing was present. (From Eames WO, Rooke GA, Wu RS-C, et al. Comparison of the effects of etomidate, propofol, and thiopental on respiratory resistance after tracheal intubation. Anesthesiology 1996;84:1307–11. © 1996, Lippincott Williams & Wilkins, with permission.)

establish a depth of anesthesia that depresses hyper-reactive airway reflexes sufficiently to permit tracheal intubation without precipitating bronchospasm. An alternative to the administration of volatile anesthetics to suppress airway reflexes before tracheal intubation is intravenous injection of lidocaine 1.5 mg/kg.

b. After tracheal intubation, it may be difficult to differentiate light anesthesia from bronchospasm as the cause of decreased compliance (neuromuscular blocking drugs relieve difficulty ventilating due to light anesthesia but have no effect on bronchospasm).

c. Theoretically, antagonism of nondepolarizing neuromuscular blockade with anticholinesterase drugs could precipitate bronchospasm secondary to stimulation of postganglionic cholinergic receptors in airway smooth muscle. Nevertheless, bronchospasm does not predictably occur after administration of anticholinesterase drugs, perhaps reflecting protective effects of simultaneously administered anticholinergic drugs.

d. Intraoperatively, the desirable level of arterial oxygenation and ventilation are best provided by mechanical ventilation of the lungs. A slow inspiratory flow rate provides optimal distribution of ventilation-to-perfusion. Sufficient time for passive exhalation to occur is necessary to prevent air trapping in the presence of expiratory airflow obstruction characteristic of asthma.

e. Liberal intravenous administration of crystalloid solutions during the perioperative period is important for maintaining adequate hydration and ensuring the presence of less viscous secretions.

f. At the conclusion of anesthesia for elective surgery, it is prudent to remove the tracheal tube while anesthesia is sufficient to suppress hyperreactive airway reflexes. If it is not deemed acceptable to remove the tracheal tube, it may be helpful to minimize the likelihood of airway stimulation due to the tracheal tube by the continuous intravenous infusion of lidocaine, 1 to 3 mg/kg/hr.

3. Intraoperative bronchospasm is usually due to factors other than an acute asthma attack (Table 14–6).

■ **Table 14–6** • Differential Diagnosis of Intraoperative
Bronchospasm and Wheezing

Mechanical obstruction of tracheal tube (rule out with fiberoptic
  bronchoscopy)
  Kinking
  Secretions
  Overinflation of the tracheal tube cuff
Inadequate depth of anesthesia
  Active expiratory efforts
  Decreased function residual capacity
Endobronchial intubation
Pulmonary aspiration
Pulmonary edema
Pulmonary embolus
Pneumothorax
Acute asthmatic attack (improved with deepening of anesthesia
  but not skeletal muscle paralysis; if bronchospasm persists,
  treat with metered-dose albuterol delivered to the anesthesia
  system with a T-connector or via a catheter placed near the
  distal end of the tracheal tube)

    D. Emergency surgery. The combination of emergency surgery
    and asthma introduces a conflict between protecting the
    airway in patients at risk for aspiration and the risk of
    triggering bronchospasm in the presence of light anesthesia.
    Awake tracheal intubation may stimulate laryngeal and
    tracheal reflexes, which may induce bronchospasm.

15

Restrictive Lung Disease

Restrictive lung disease is characterized by decreases in total lung capacity, most often reflecting an intrinsic disease process that alters the elastic properties of the lungs, causing the lungs to stiffen (Figs. 15–1, 15–2; Table 15–1) (Stoelting RK, Dierdorf SF. Restrictive lung disease. In: Anesthesia and Co-Existing Disease, 4th ed. New York, Churchill Livingstone, 2002;205–216). The classic manifestation of restrictive lung disease is decreased vital capacity (normal > 70 ml/kg); but in contrast to obstructive airway disease, expiratory flow rates and the ratio of the forced exhaled volume in 1 second to the forced vital capacity (FEV_1/FVC) remain normal. Patients with restrictive lung disease complain of dyspnea, reflecting the increased work of breathing necessary to expand the poorly compliant lungs. Despite compensatory increases in breathing frequency (rapid shallow breathing pattern minimizes the work of breathing), there are subsequent decreases in alveolar ventilation that produce proportional increases in $PaCO_2$. Hypercarbia and associated arterial hypoxemia cause pulmonary hypertension and cor pulmonale.

I. ACUTE INTRINSIC RESTRICTIVE LUNG DISEASE

Acute intrinsic restrictive lung disease is most often due to leakage of intravascular fluid into the interstitium of the lungs and into the alveoli (pulmonary edema).

A. Clinical manifestations. Acute pulmonary edema can be categorized as pulmonary edema caused by increased capillary pressure (hydrostatic or cardiogenic edema) or pulmonary edema caused by increased capillary permeability (Table 15–2).

1. Acute respiratory distress syndrome (ARDS) is characterized by diffuse pulmonary endothelial injury leading to pulmonary edema due to a marked increase in pulmonary capillary permeability to water, solutes, and macromolecules. Most ARDS-related deaths are not caused by

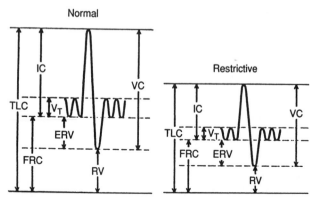

Fig. 15–1 • Lung volumes in restrictive lung disease compared with normal values. In the presence of restrictive lung disease total lung capacity (TLC), functional residual capacity (FRC), residual volume (RV), and vital capacity (VC) are decreased. ERV, expiratory reserve volume; IC, inspiratory capacity; V_T, tidal volume.

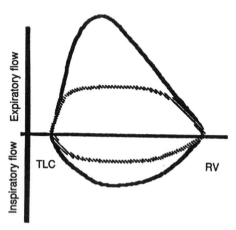

Fig. 15–2 • Flow–volume loop in a normal patient (*solid line*) and in the presence of an intrathoracic (mediastinal) mass (*hatched line*). (From Pullerits J, Holzman R. Anaesthesia for patients with mediastinal masses. Can J Anaesth 1989;36:681–8, with permission.)

≡ Table 15–1 • Causes of Restrictive Lung Disease

Acute Intrinsic Restrictive Lung Disease (Pulmonary Edema)
Acute respiratory distress syndrome
Aspiration
Neurogenic disorder
Opioid overdose
Altitude
Reexpansion of collapsed lung
Upper airway obstruction (negative pressure)
Congestive heart failure
Chronic Intrinsic Restrictive Lung Disease
Sarcoidosis
Hypersensitivity pneumonitis
Eosinophilic granuloma
Alveolar proteinosis
Lymphangiomyomatosis
Drug-induced pulmonary fibrosis
Chronic Extrinsic Restrictive Lung Disease
Obesity
Ascites
Pregnancy
Deformities of the costovertebral skeletal structures
   Kyphoscoliosis
   Ankylosing spondylitis
Deformities of the sternum
Flail chest
Neuromuscular disorders
   Spinal cord transection
   Guillain-Barré syndrome
   Myasthenia gravis
   Eaton-Lambert syndrome
   Muscular dystrophies
Disorders of the Pleura and Mediastinum
Pleural effusion
Pneumothorax
Mediastinal mass
Pneumomediastinum

gas exchange failure but, rather, by sepsis and multiorgan failure.

  a. **Posttraumatic multiple organ system failure** is characterized initially by hyperdynamic and hypermetabolic states similar to sepsis occurring in critically ill or injured patients (Table 15–3).

≡ **Table 15–2** • Clinical Manifestations of Pulmonary Edema

Increased Capillary Pressure Pulmonary Edema
Perihilar distribution ("butterfly") of a lung opacity on chest radiography
Dyspnea
Tachypnea
Sympathetic nervous system stimulation (systemic hypertension, tachycardia, diaphoresis)
Increased Capillary Permeability Pulmonary Edema
Air bronchograms on chest radiography
Less pronounced sympathetic nervous system stimulation
High concentrations of protein in pulmonary edema fluid
Diffuse alveolar damage

    b. Mortality approaches 100% if three or more organ systems become involved.

  2. Aspiration pneumonitis. Inhaled gastric fluid is rapidly distributed throughout the lungs (chest radiograph may not reveal evidence of pneumonitis for 6 to 12 hours) resulting in atelectasis, intravascular fluid leak into the lungs, tachypnea, bronchospasm, pulmonary vascular vasoconstriction, and arterial hypoxemia.

    a. Treatment. See Table 15–4.

    b. The most effective treatment of aspiration pneumonitis is delivery of supplemental oxygen and institution of positive end-expiratory pressure.

  3. Neurogenic pulmonary edema develops in a small proportion of patients experiencing acute brain injury (mas-

≡ **Table 15–3** • Posttraumatic Multisystem Organ Failure

Failure of the gastrointestinal tract to act as a barrier to systemic access of luminal bacteria
Cardiac dysfunction (wall motion abnormalities on transesophageal echocardiography)
Paradoxical increase in cardiac output
Central nervous system dysfunction (accumulation of catabolic products)

▤ Table 15–4 • Treatment of Aspiration Pneumonitis

Tracheal intubation (supplemental oxygen and institute positive end-expiratory pressure)

Inject small volumes of saline (5 ml) through the tracheal tube (large volume lavage could exaggerate spread of gastric fluid to periphery of lungs)

Measure gastric fluid pH

Fiberoptic bronchoscopy if aspiration of solid materials is a possibility

β_2-Agonist (albuterol) by metered-dose inhaler if bronchospasm is present

Prophylactic antibiotics (no evidence effective)

Corticosteroids (empirical)

Albumin if hypoalbuminemia is present due to extravasation of protein-containing fluids into the alveoli (could also leak into alveoli and exacerbate fluid injury)

---

sive outpouring of sympathetic nervous system impulses from the injured brain, resulting in generalized vasoconstriction and a shift of blood volume into the pulmonary circulation).

    a. Diagnosis. The association of pulmonary edema with a recent central nervous system injury suggests the diagnosis of neurogenic pulmonary edema (difficult to differentiate from aspiration pneumonitis).

    b. Treatment of neurogenic pulmonary edema is directed at decreasing intracranial pressure and support of oxygenation and ventilation. Digitalis and diuretics are not recommended.

4. Drug-induced pulmonary edema may occur after administration of heroin and cocaine (high-permeability pulmonary edema is suggested by high protein concentrations in the pulmonary edema fluid).

5. High-altitude pulmonary edema is presumed to reflect hypoxic pulmonary vasoconstriction, which increases pulmonary vascular resistance. Treatment of this high permeability pulmonary edema includes prompt descent from high altitude.

6. Reexpansion of collapsed lung (evacuation of a pneumothorax or pleural effusion) may result in high permeability pulmonary edema.

7. Negative-pressure pulmonary edema may follow relief of acute upper airway obstruction (postextubation laryngospasm, epiglottitis, tumors, obesity, obstructive sleep apnea). Tachypnea, cough, and failure to maintain arterial oxygen saturations at > 95% are common presenting symptoms and may be confused with pulmonary aspiration or pulmonary embolism. It is possible that some cases of postoperative arterial hypoxemia are due to unrecognized negative-pressure pulmonary edema.

    a. Pathogenesis. It is likely that development of highly negative intrapleural pressures due to vigorous inspiratory efforts against an obstructed airway results in pulmonary edema. In addition, such negative pressures may lead to intense sympathetic nervous system activation, systemic hypertension, and central pooling of blood.

    b. Treatment. Maintenance of a patent upper airway and administration of supplemental oxygen is usually sufficient treatment, as this form of pulmonary edema is transient and self-limited.

II. CHRONIC INTRINSIC RESTRICTIVE LUNG DISEASE

Chronic intrinsic restrictive lung disease is characterized by pulmonary fibrosis and loss of pulmonary vasculature leading to dyspnea, pulmonary hypertension, and cor pulmonale (Table 15–1). Pneumothorax is common when pulmonary fibrosis is far advanced.

A. Sarcoidosis is a systemic granulomatous disorder that involves many tissues (liver, spleen, heart), but it has a marked predilection for the thoracic lymph nodes and lungs (fibrosis). Laryngeal sarcoid may occur and interfere with passage of an adult-sized tracheal tube. Hypercalcemia is a rare but classic manifestation of sarcoidosis.

    1. Mediastinoscopy is used to provide thoracic lymph node tissue for diagnosis of sarcoidosis.

    2. Corticosteroids are frequently used to treat sarcoidosis associated with restrictive lung disease.

B. Hypersensitivity pneumonitis is characterized by diffuse interstitial granulomatous reactions in the lungs after inhalation of dust containing fungi, spores, or animal or vegetable material. Repeated episodes of hypersensitivity pneumonitis may lead to pulmonary fibrosis.

C. Pulmonary alveolar proteinosis, a disease of unknown etiology, is characterized by deposition of lipid-rich proteinaceous material in the alveoli. Dyspnea and arterial hypoxemia are typical clinical manifestations.

D. **Lymphangiomyomatosis** is the proliferation of smooth muscle in abdominal and thoracic lymphatics, veins, and bronchioles that occurs in females of reproductive age. Clinical presentation is as progressive dyspnea, hemoptysis, recurrent pneumothoraces, and ascites.

III. CHRONIC EXTRINSIC RESTRICTIVE LUNG DISEASE

Chronic extrinsic restrictive lung disease is most often due to disorders of the thoracic cage that interfere with lung expansion (Table 15–1). The lungs become compressed, and lung volumes are decreased.

A. **Obesity** imposes a restrictive load on the thoracic cage directly by the weight that has been added to the rib cage and indirectly by the large abdominal panniculus, which impedes movement of the diaphragm when the individual is in the supine position. Functional residual capacity is decreased, and the likelihood of ventilation-to-perfusion mismatching with associated arterial hypoxemia is increased.

B. **Deformities of the costovertebral skeletal structures** are represented by scoliosis (lateral curvature with rotation of the vertebral column) and kyphosis (anterior flexion of the vertebral column) which often occur in combination (kyphoscoliosis). Severe deformities may lead to chronic alveolar hypoventilation, arterial hypoxemia, secondary erythrocytosis, pulmonary hypertension, and cor pulmonale. Patients with severe kyphoscoliosis are at increased risk for the development of pneumonia and hypoventilation induced by central nervous system depressant drugs.

C. **Deformities of the sternum** and costochondral articulations are characterized by pectus excavatum (inward concavity) and pectus carinatum (outward protuberance). Surgical correction is indicated when the sternal deformity is accompanied by evidence of pulmonary restriction or cardiovascular dysfunction.

D. **Flail chest.** Multiple rib fractures, especially when they occur in a parallel vertical orientation, can produce a flail chest characterized by paradoxical inward movement of the unstable portion of the thoracic cage as the remainder of the thoracic cage moves outward during inspiration. The pathophysiologic disturbances of a flail chest may also result from dehiscence of a median sternotomy, as following cardiac surgery.

1. Progressive arterial hypoxemia and alveolar hypoventilation with associated increases in $PaCO_2$ occur.
2. Treatment of flail chest is positive pressure ventilation of the patient's lungs until definitive stabilization procedures can be accomplished or rib fractures stabilize.

E. **Neuromuscular disorders** that interfere with transfer of central nervous system output to skeletal muscles necessary for inspiration and exhalation can result in restrictive lung disease (Table 15–1). Measurement of vital capacity is an important indicator of the total impact of neuromuscular disorders on ventilation.

1. **Diaphragmatic paralysis.** In the absence of associated pleuropulmonary disease, most adult patients with unilateral diaphragmatic paralysis remain asymptomatic.
   a. **Postoperative diaphragmatic dysfunction** is a transient form of diaphragmatic dysfunction that may follow abdominal surgery.
   b. As a result of postoperative diaphragmatic dysfunction, atelectasis and arterial hypoxemia may occur. Incentive spirometry may alleviate these abnormalities.

2. **Spinal cord transection.** Breathing is maintained solely or predominantly by the diaphragm in quadriplegic patients (transection above C4 results in paralysis of the diaphragm). Because the diaphragm is active only during inspiration, cough, which requires activity by expiratory muscles, including those of the abdominal wall, is almost totally absent. Respiratory failure almost never occurs in quadriplegic patients in the absence of complications such as pneumonia.

3. **Guillain-Barré syndrome** may result in respiratory insufficiency requiring prolonged mechanical support of ventilation.

4. **Disorders of neuromuscular transmission.** Myasthenia gravis is the most common of the disorders that affect neuromuscular transmission resulting in respiratory failure (may be confused with Eaton-Lambert syndrome or other paraneoplastic syndromes). Skeletal muscle paralysis or weakness may follow prolonged administration of nondepolarizing neuromuscular blocking drugs, as administered to facilitate mechanical ventilation of the lungs.

5. **Muscular dystrophy** predisposes patients to pulmonary complications and respiratory failure. Chronic alveolar

hypoventilation caused by inspiratory muscle weakness may develop. Expiratory muscle weakness impairs cough, and accompanying weakness of the muscles of deglutition often leads to pulmonary aspiration. Central nervous system depressant drugs should be avoided or administered in minimal doses when necessary.

IV. DISORDERS OF THE PLEURA AND MEDIASTINUM

Disorders of the pleura and mediastinum may contribute to mechanical changes that interfere with optimal expansion of the lungs (Table 15–5).

V. PREOPERATIVE PREPARATION

Preoperative preparation of patients with restrictive lung disease includes an assessment of the severity of the lung disease and treatment of reversible components.

A. A preoperative history of dyspnea that limits activity and can be attributed to restrictive lung disease may be viewed as an indication for pulmonary function studies and arterial blood gas determinations. The most detailed assessment of flow-resistive properties of the airways is obtained by analysis of flow-volume loops (Fig. 15–2).

1. Decreases in the vital capacity to 15 ml/kg (normal > 70 ml/kg) or the presence of resting increases in the $PaCO_2$ suggests that these patients are at increased risk for the development of exaggerated pulmonary dysfunction during the postoperative period.

≡ Table 15–5 • Disorders of the Pleura and Mediastinum

Pleural effusion

Pneumothorax (severe chest pain and dyspnea; arterial hypoxemia and hypotension likely if tension pneumothorax develops)

Mediastinal mass (superior vena cava syndrome is most often due to cancer; may be evidence of increased intracranial pressure)

Acute mediastinitis

Pneumomediastinum (may follow tracheostomy; treatment rarely necessary)

Bronchogenic cysts (avoid nitrous oxide and positive-pressure ventilation)

---

2. Eradication of acute pulmonary infections, improvement of sputum clearance, and treatment of cardiac dysfunction are part of the preoperative preparation.

B. **Preoperative evaluation in the presence of mediastinal tumors.** Preoperative evaluation of patients with mediastinal tumors includes chest radiography, flow–volume loops, computed tomography (evidence of tracheal compression is a predictor of airway difficulty during anesthesia), and clinical evaluation of evidence of tracheobronchial compression. Flexible fiberoptic bronchoscopy under topical anesthesia is an alternative method for evaluating airway obstruction. Nevertheless, the severity of pulmonary symptoms may bear no relation to the degree of respiratory compromise encountered during anesthesia (supine position may accentuate airway or vascular obstruction, or both). Preoperative irradiation should be considered for patients whose mediastinal tumors are radiation-sensitive.

VI. MANAGEMENT OF ANESTHESIA

A. Restrictive lung disease unrelated to the presence of mediastinal tumors does not influence the choice of drugs used for induction or maintenance of general anesthesia. A high index of suspicion for the presence of a pneumothorax and the need to avoid or discontinue nitrous oxide must be maintained.

1. Regional anesthesia can be considered for peripheral operations, but it must be appreciated that sensory levels

---

≡ Table 15–6 • Considerations in the Management of Anesthesia in the Presence of a Mediastinal Mass

---

External edema associated with superior vena cava syndrome (may be accompanied by intraoral edema; consider establishing intravenous access in the legs)

Awake fiberoptic laryngoscopy (especially in patients who must remain sitting)

Place patients in lateral or prone position should unexpected airway obstruction develop

Spontaneous ventilation and avoidance of skeletal muscle paralysis (may not be possible)

Increased surgical bleeding owing to increased venous pressure

Be prepared to reintubate the trachea postoperatively

≡ Table 15–7 • Diagnostic Techniques for Visualizing the Airways and Obtaining Samples

Fiberoptic bronchoscopy (pneumothorax a risk after transbronchial lung biopsies)

Pleuroscopy (alternative to thoractomy to obtain a biopsy)

Mediastinoscopy (complications include pneumothorax, hemorrhage, venous air embolism, recurrent laryngeal nerve injury, stroke due to compression of right carotid artery by mediastinoscope; monitor blood pressure in left upper extremity as compression by mediastinoscope may compress right subclavian artery)

above T10 can be associated with impairment of the respiratory muscle activity necessary for patients with restrictive lung disease to maintain acceptable ventilation.

2. Controlled ventilation of the lungs during the operative period (increased inflation pressures may be necessary to expand the poorly compliant lungs) optimizes oxygenation and ventilation. Mechanical ventilation of the lungs during the postoperative period is often required for patients with impaired pulmonary function documented preoperatively.

B. The method selected for induction of anesthesia and tracheal intubation in the presence of mediastinal tumors depends on the preoperative assessment of the airway (Table 15–6).

VII. DIAGNOSTIC TECHNIQUES

See Table 15–7.

16

Acute Respiratory Failure

Respiratory failure is the inability of the patient's lungs to provide adequate arterial oxygenation with or without acceptable elimination of carbon dioxide (From Stoelting RK Dierdorf SF. Acute respiratory failure. In: Anesthesia and Co-Existing Disease, 4th ed. New York, Churchill Livingstone, 2002;217–232). Fatigue of the muscles of breathing is an important factor in the development of acute respiratory failure. Arterial hypoxemia resulting from right-to-left intracardiac shunts or low ambient oxygen concentrations are not considered causes of acute respiratory failure, as these defects do not represent disorders of the patient's respiratory system.

I. DIAGNOSIS OF ACUTE RESPIRATORY FAILURE

See Table 16–1.

A. Significant desaturation of arterial blood occurs only when the PaO_2 is < 60 mmHg, accounting for arterial hypoxemia commonly being defined by a PaO_2 level below this value.

B. Acute respiratory failure is distinguished from chronic respiratory failure on the basis of the relation of the $PaCO_2$ to the arterial pH (normal pHa despite an increased $PaCO_2$ reflects compensation by virtue of renal tubular reabsorption of bicarbonate).

C. **Acute respiratory distress syndrome.** Arterial hypoxemia associated with acute lung injury (aspiration, sepsis, trauma with multiple blood transfusions) characterized by diffuse alveolar damage (influx of protein-rich edema fluid into the alveoli as a consequence of increased permeability of alveolar-capillary membranes) and noncardiogenic pulmonary edema is designated the acute respiratory distress syndrome (ARDS).

1. **Signs and symptoms.** Arterial hypoxemia resistant to treatment with supplemental oxygen is a feature of

---

▬ Table 16–1 • Diagnosis of Acute Respiratory Failure

$PaO_2 < 60$ mmHg despite supplemental oxygen and in the absence of a right-to-left intracardiac shunt
$PaCO_2 > 50$ mmHg in the absence of respiratory compensation for metabolic alkalosis
Decreased functional residual capacity
Decreased lung compliance
Bilateral diffuse opacification of the lungs on chest radiographs
Pulmonary artery occlusion pressure < 15 mmHg despite frequent presence of pulmonary edema

---

ARDS. Radiographically, the findings are indistinguishable from those of cardiogenic pulmonary edema. Pulmonary hypertension may lead to right heart failure. Pneumothorax is a possible complication.

2. Recovery from ARDS is characterized by the gradual resolution of arterial hypoxemia and improved lung compliance.

II. TREATMENT OF ACUTE RESPIRATORY FAILURE

Treatment of acute respiratory failure is based on correcting arterial hypoxemia, removing excess carbon dioxide, and providing a patent upper airway (Table 16–2).

III. MANAGEMENT OF PATIENTS RECEIVING MECHANICAL VENTILATORY SUPPORT

Critically ill patients who require mechanical ventilation are often given continuous intravenous infusions of sedative drugs to treat anxiety and agitation and to facilitate coordination with ventilator-delivered breaths. Inadequate sedation can lead to life-threatening problems (self-extubation, acute deterioration of gas exchange, barotrauma).

A. **Sedation.** Benzodiazepines are the drugs most commonly selected to decrease anxiety and produce anterograde amnesia during mechanical ventilation of patients for management of acute respiratory failure. Permissive hypercapnia can cause patients substantial discomfort, necessitating high levels of sedation. Analgesia, if needed, is provided by intravenous administration of opioids.

1. Continuous intravenous infusions of propofol are useful, as rapid awakening from this drug occurs independent of the duration of administration.

≡ Table 16–2 • Treatment of Acute Respiratory Failure

Supplemental oxygen (maintain PaO_2 60–80 mmHg)
Continuous positive airway pressure when PaO_2 not maintained
    > 60 mmHg with supplemental oxygen delivered by nasal
    cannula or face mask
Tracheal intubation if cannot maintain acceptable oxygenation and
    ventilation
Mechanical support of ventilation if cannot maintain PaO_2 > 60
    mmHg breathing 50% oxygen by noninvasive means or if there
    is progressive hypoventilation (modalities of ventilation using
    volume-cycled ventilation are assist-control ventilation,
    synchronized intermittent mandatory ventilation, and auto-
    positive end-expiratory pressure)
Optimize intravascular fluid volume
Drug-induced diuresis
Inotropic support of cardiac function
Glucocorticoids (?)
Removal of secretions
Control of infection
Nutritional support
Inhaled β-adrenergic agonists (?)

    2. Daily interruption of intravenous sedative infusions and
    allowing patients to ''awaken'' may facilitate evaluation
    of the patient's mental status and ultimately shorten the
    period of mechanical ventilation.
  B. Paralysis. When sedation is inadequate or hypotension
    accompanies the administration of drugs utilized for seda-
    tion, the administration of nondepolarizing neuromuscular
    blocking drugs to produce skeletal muscle paralysis may
    be necessary to permit optimal mechanical ventilation. A
    risk of prolonged drug-induced skeletal muscle paralysis
    is accentuation of the diffuse polyneuropathy that may
    accompany critical illnesses.

IV. COMPLICATIONS OF TRACHEAL INTUBATION AND MECHANICAL VENTILATION

See Table 16–3.

V. CESSATION OF MECHANICAL SUPPORT OF VENTILATION

Mechanical ventilatory support should be withdrawn once
patients can maintain arterial oxygenation and carbon dioxide
elimination without external assistance.

Table 16–3 • Complications of Tracheal Intubation and Mechanical Ventilation

Infection ("ventilator-associated pneumonia")

Alveolar overdistension [consider utilizing more "gentle" forms of mechanical ventilation creating tidal volumes of 5–8 ml/kg and airway pressures not exceeding 30 cmH_2O; permissive hypercapnia ($PaCO_2$ as high as 80 mmHg) may occur]

Barotrauma (tension pneumothorax, arterial gas embolism)

Atelectasis (common cause of arterial hypoxemia that develops during mechanical ventilation; fiberoptic bronchoscopy needed to remove mucoid plugs responsible for persistent atelectasis)

Critical illness myopathy (neuromuscular weakness that persists long after respiratory failure has resolved; may reflect an axonal disorder that occurs in the presence of sepsis and multiorgan failure; may be accentuated by prolonged administration of nondepolarizing neuromuscular blocking drugs)

    A. When considering whether a patient can be safely weaned from mechanical ventilation and tolerate tracheal extubation, it is important that the patient be alert and cooperative and able to tolerate trials of spontaneous ventilation without excessive tachypnea, tachycardia, or obvious respiratory distress.

        1. Arbitrary guidelines have been proposed for indicating the feasibility of discontinuing mechanical support of ventilation (Table 16–4).

        2. Ultimately, the decision to attempt withdrawal of mechanical ventilation is individualized, considering not only the status of pulmonary function but also co-

Table 16–4 • Arbitrary Guidelines for Discontinuing Mechanical Support of Ventilation

Vital capacity > 15 ml/kg

$A\text{-}aDO_2$ < 350 mmHg while 100% breathing oxygen

PaO_2 > 60 mmHg breathing < 50% oxygen

Maximal inspiratory pressure more than −20 cmH_2O with airway occlusion

Maintenance of a normal pHa

Spontaneous breathing rate < 20 breaths/min

V_D/V_T ratio < 0.6

▬ Table 16–5 • Methods Utilized for Withdrawal of Mechanical Ventilation

Synchronized intermittent mandatory ventilation (allows spontaneous breathing and diminishing numbers of mandatory breaths per minute until the patient is breathing unassisted)

Intermittent trials with total removal of mechanical support while breathing through a T-piece

Decreasing levels of pressure-support ventilation

existing abnormalities (anemia, hypokalemia, hypovolemia).

B. Removing ventilator support. Correcting the conditions responsible for the need for mechanical support of ventilation seems to be more important to successful tracheal extubation than is the method of weaning (Table 16–5).

1. Deterioration of oxygenation after withdrawal of mechanical support of ventilation may reflect progressive alveolar collapse that is responsive to treatment with continuous positive airway pressure (CPAP) (1.5 to 5.0 cmH$_2$O) rather than reinstitution of mechanical ventilation.

2. Several events may interfere with successful cessation of mechanical support of ventilation (Table 16–6).

C. Tracheal extubation should be considered if patients tolerate 2 hours of spontaneous breathing during T tube weaning or a spontaneous mandatory intermittent ventilation rate of 1 to 2 breaths/min is tolerated without deterioration of arterial blood gases (PaO$_2$ remains at > 60 mmHg breathing < 50% oxygen, PaCO$_2$ remains at < 50 mmHg, and

▬ Table 16–6 • Events that May Interfere with Successful Cessation of Mechanical Ventilation

Depressed ventilatory drive due to respiratory alkalosis or persistent sedation

Inability of the patient's muscles of respiration to perform the necessary level of ventilatory work

Excessive workload on patient's respiratory muscles (excessive secretions, bronchospasm, increased lung water, increased carbon dioxide production due to fever or parenteral nutrition)

pHa remains at > 7.30), mental status, or cardiac function. These patients should be alert with active laryngeal reflexes and the ability to generate an effective cough to clear secretions from the airway. Protective glottic closure function may be impaired following tracheal extubation.

D. Supplemental oxygen is often needed after tracheal extubation reflecting persistence of ventilation-to-perfusion mismatching.

VI. ACUTE RESPIRATORY FAILURE AND CHRONIC OBSTRUCTIVE PULMONARY DISEASE

Acute deterioration is most often triggered by events such as pneumonia, congestive heart failure, or increased metabolic production of carbon dioxide, as produced by febrile states leading to increasing arterial hypoxemia and hypercarbia.

A. Treatment. Analysis of arterial blood gases is crucial for the proper treatment of acute exacerbations of chronic obstructive pulmonary disease (COPD) (Table 16–7).

B. Tracheal intubation versus noninvasive ventilation. Tracheal intubation is performed when patients demonstrate hemodynamic instability, somnolence occurs, or secretions cannot be cleared. When patients remain alert despite hypercarbia, delivery of positive-pressure ventilation via a tight-fitting face mask (''noninvasive ventilation'') is an alternative to tracheal intubation.

1. The most common method of noninvasive ventilation is delivery of a specified amount of inspiratory pressure (15 to 20 cmH$_2$O) combined with a low level of expiratory pressure (3 to 5 cmH$_2$O) to decrease the effort

---

≡ Table 16–7 • Treatment of Acute Exacerbations of Chronic Obstructive Pulmonary Disease

Supplemental oxygen (maintain PaO$_2$ 50–60 mmHg)
Accept PaCO$_2$ increases during supplemental oxygen administered so long as pHa remains > 7.2
Bronchopulmonary lavage (encourage to cough, inhaled bronchodilators, systemic administration of corticosteroids)
Antibiotics
Mechanical support of ventilation (pHa < 7.2, mental status deterioration, respiratory muscle fatigue)

---

required to trigger the ventilator. The risk of nosocomial infections is decreased.

2. When tracheal intubation is required to treat acute exacerbations of COPD, the initial settings on the ventilator are likely to include a tidal volume of 10 ml/kg and a breathing rate of 10 breaths/min. Patients with chronic hypercarbia should not have their $PaCO_2$ decreased abruptly, as respiratory alkalosis and cardiac dysrhythmias may occur.

VII. ACUTE RESPIRATORY FAILURE IN PATIENTS WITH ACUTE LUNG INJURY AND THE ACUTE RESPIRATORY DISTRESS SYNDROME

Death is most often attributed to sepsis or multiorgan failure rather than primary respiratory causes.

A. **Epidemiology and pathogenesis.** See Table 16–8. Sepsis is associated with the highest risk of progression of acute lung injury to ARDS. There is an influx of protein-rich edema fluid into the alveoli as a result of increased alveolar-capillary permeability.

≡ **Table 16–8 •** Clinical Disorders Associated with Acute Lung Injury and Acute Respiratory Distress Syndrome

Direct Lung Injury
Pneumonia
Aspiration of gastric contents
Pulmonary contusion
Fat emboli
Near-drowning
Inhalational injury
Indirect Lung Injury
Sepsis
Trauma associated with shock
Multiple blood transfusions
Cardiopulmonary bypass
Drug overdose
Acute pancreatitis

B. **Treatment.** See Table 16–9.

C. **Monitoring the treatment** includes evaluation of pulmonary gas exchange (arterial and venous blood gases, pHa) and cardiac function (cardiac output, cardiac filling pressures, intrapulmonary shunt). It is often facilitated by measurements obtained from a pulmonary artery catheter (Table 16–10).

≡ Table 16–9 • Treatment of Acute Lung Injury and Acute Respiratory Distress Syndrome

Search for any underlying cause (treatable infection such as pneumonia)

Prevention or early treatment of any nosocomial infections

Adequate nutrition (enteral feeding preferred to parenteral nutrition as it does not introduce risk of catheter-induced sepsis)

Prevention of gastrointestinal bleeding

Prevention of thromboembolism

Tracheal intubation and mechanical ventilation with a volume-cycled ventilator when cannot maintain adequate oxygenation (goal is PaO_2 60–80 mmHg and minimize risk of barotrauma by using tidal volumes of 8–10 ml/kg)

Positive end-expiratory pressure (PEEP) indicated when cannot maintain an adequate PaO_2 with < 50% oxygen (decreased cardiac output could offset beneficial effect of PEEP on oxygenation; offset with intravascular fluid replacement [guide with pulmonary artery catheter] and administration of inotropes)

Inverse-ratio ventilation (inspiratory time that exceeds time for exhalation) may improve arterial oxygenation without PEEP (risks are barotrauma and hypotension due to auto-PEEP)

Fluid and hemodynamic management (goal is to maintain intravascular fluid volume at the lowest level consistent with adequate organ perfusion as assessed by metabolic acid-base balance and renal function; pulmonary artery occlusion pressure < 15 mmHg may reflect inadequate intravascular fluid volume)

Corticosteroids (value remains unproven)

Removal of secretions (facilitated by adequate systemic hydration and humidification of inspired gases; fiberoptic bronchoscopy may be needed)

Control of infection (prophylactic antibiotics not recommended; earliest evidence of infection may be further deterioration of pulmonary function)

Nutritional support (skeletal muscle weakness may interfere with cessation of mechanical support of ventilation)

≣ **Table 16–10** • Monitoring Treatment of Acute Respiratory Failure

Adequacy of oxygen exchange and arterial oxygenation
   PaO_2 (> 60 mmHg)
   A-aDO_2
Adequacy of alveolar ventilation
   $PaCO_2$ (< 45 mmHg unless permissive hypercarbia)
   V_D/V_T (< 0.6)
Adequacy of cardiac output
   PvO_2 (> 30 mmHg)
   CaO_2-CvO_2 (< 6 ml/dl)
Arterial pH
Intrapulmonary shunt ($< 5\%$)

VIII. LUNG TRANSPLANTATION

   A. Management of anesthesia. See Table 16–11.
   B. Physiologic effects of lung transplantation. See Table 16–12.
   C. Complications of lung transplantation. See Table 16–13.
   D. Anesthetic considerations in lung transplant recipients. See Table 16–14.

≣ **Table 16–11** • Management of Anesthesia and Postoperative Period for Lung Transplantation

Strict attention to asepsis
Pulmonary artery catheter
Avoid drug-induced histamine release
Double-lumen endobronchial tube (verify placement by fiberoptic bronchoscopy)
Arterial hypoxemia may accompany one-lung ventilation (trial of PEEP when it occurs)
Pulmonary hypertension may occur when pulmonary artery is clamped (prostacyclin infusion, cardiopulmonary bypass)
Bronchospasm may occur despite denervation of transplanted lung
Maintain postoperative mechanical support of ventilation (denervated lung deprives patient of cough reflex and predisposes to pneumonia)
Principal causes of mortality are bronchial dehiscence or respiratory failure owing to infection or rejection

≡ Table 16–12 • Physiologic Effects of Lung Transplantation

Peak improvement in lung function usually achieved in 3–6 months
Arterial oxygenation rapidly returns to normal
Normalization of pulmonary vascular resistance and pulmonary vascular pressures
Increase in cardiac output
Improved exercise tolerance
Lung denervation
    Loss of cough reflex
    Inhaled β_2-agonists produce bronchodilation
    Mucociliary clearance impaired
    Blunted ventilatory response to carbon dioxide

≡ Table 16–13 • Complications of Lung Transplantation

Pulmonary edema
Dehiscence of the bronchial anastomosis
Anastomotic stenosis
Infection
Acute rejection (most likely first 100 days following transplantation)
Chronic rejection (bronchiolitis obliterans)

≡ Table 16–14 • Anesthetic Considerations for Patients Requiring Surgery after Lung Transplantation

Function of the transplanted lung
Possibility of rejection or infection in the transplanted lung
Effect of immunosuppressive therapy on other organs and the effect of organ dysfunction on the transplanted lung
Disease of the native lung
Planned surgical procedure and its effect on the lungs

1. **Preoperative evaluation** includes eliciting a history of increasing dyspnea or need for supplemental oxygen. Side effects of immunosuppressive drugs (systemic hypertension, renal dysfunction) are considerations during the preoperative evaluation.

   a. **Chronic rejection** may be difficult to differentiate from infection, including upper respiratory tract infection (fever and fatigue). If chronic rejection is occurring, the forced expiratory volume, vital capacity, and total lung capacity may decrease; and arterial hypoxemia and increased A-aDO$_2$ are present. Chronic cough may reflect obliterative bronchiolitis.

   b. **Preoperative medication** is acceptable provided pulmonary function is adequate. Hypercarbia is common during the early posttransplant period, and increased sensitivity to opioids is a theoretical consideration. Supplemental corticosteroids are considerations especially for long, stressful operations. Prophylactic antibiotics are indicated, and strict sterile technique is needed when placing intravascular catheters. Increased bronchial responsiveness causing bronchoconstriction is common.

2. **Choice of anesthetic technique.** In view of the decreased cough reflex, the potential for bronchoconstriction, and the increased risk of pulmonary infections, it may be recommended that regional anesthesia be selected in preference to general anesthesia and tracheal intubation. Fluid preloading may be a risk in patients with transplanted lungs reflecting disruption of the lymphatic drainage in the transplanted lung causing interstitial fluid accumulation (treat with diuretics and limited crystalloid infusions).

   a. The value of invasive monitoring is balanced against the risk of infection. Transesophageal echocardiography may be useful for monitoring volume status and cardiac function.

   b. An important goal of anesthetic management is the recovery of adequate respiratory function and early tracheal extubation. Immunosuppressive drugs may interact with neuromuscular blocking drugs, and impaired renal function may prolong the effects of certain muscle relaxants (routine pharmacologic antagonism recommended, as even minimal residual drug-induced weakness could compromise ventilation in these patients).

c. These patients may be at increased risk for aspiration in view of compromised upper airway protective reflexes.

d. When positioning a tracheal tube, it is best to place the cuff just beyond the vocal cords to minimize the risk of traumatizing the tracheal or bronchial anastomosis. If the surgery requires a double-lumen endobronchial tube, it is preferable to place the endobronchial lumen in the native bronchus.

17

Diseases of the Nervous System

Patients with diseases affecting the nervous system may undergo surgery as a result of this disease whereas in others the need for surgery is unrelated to the nervous system disease (Stoelting RK, Dierdorf SF. Diseases of the nervous system. In: Anesthesia and Co-Existing Disease, 4th ed. New York, Churchill Livingstone, 2002;233–298). Regardless of the reason for surgery, co-existing nervous system diseases often have important implications when selecting anesthetic drugs, techniques, and monitors. In addition, concepts of cerebral protection and resuscitation may assume unique importance in these patients.

I. INTRACRANIAL TUMORS

See Table 17–1.

  A. **Diagnosis** of a brain tumor is based on classic symptoms and findings on the neurologic examination that are substantiated by specific diagnostic imaging techniques (computed tomography, magnetic resonance imaging).

  B. **Surgery** is part of the initial management of virtually all brain tumors, as it quickly establishes the diagnosis and relieves symptoms due to the space-occupying intracranial mass. Radiation therapy is particularly useful for management of malignant brain tumors.

  C. **Signs and symptoms.** Increased intracranial pressure (ICP) is the most likely explanation for signs and symptoms caused by brain tumors (Table 17–2).

  D. **Management of anesthesia** for resection of brain tumors requires an understanding of pressure–volume compliance relations of the brain, methods available to monitor and decrease ICP, and the determinants of cerebral blood flow (CBF). Goals of perioperative anesthesia management are often based on keeping the ICP within normal ranges and recognizing that autoregulation of CBF may be impaired.

≡ **Table 17–1** • Classification of Brain Tumors

> *Primary Brain Tumor*
> Histologically benign
> > Meningioma
> > Pituitary adenoma
> > Astrocytoma
> > Acoustic neuroma
>
> Histologically malignant
> > Glioblastoma
> > Medulloblastoma
>
> *Metastatic Brain Tumor*

1. **Pressure–volume compliance curves** reflect changes produced by expanding intracranial tumors (Fig. 17–1). Eventually, a point is reached on the pressure–volume compliance curve at which even small increases in intracranial volume produced by the expanding tumor results in marked increases in ICP. At this point on the pressure–volume compliance curve anesthetic drugs and techniques that affect cere-

≡ **Table 17–2** • Signs and Symptoms of Increased Intracranial Pressure

Evidence of Increased Intracranial Pressure
Headache
Nausea and vomiting
Mental changes
Disturbances of consciousness
Systemic hypertension
Bradycardia
Midline shift (> 0.5 cm) on computed tomography

Seizures

Evidence of Brain Herniation
Dilated and unreactive pupils
Contralateral hemiplegia
Disturbances of consciousness
Apnea

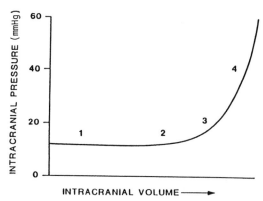

Fig. 17–1 • Pressure–volume compliance curve depicts the impact of increasing intracranial volume on intracranial pressure (ICP). As intracranial volume increases from point 1 to point 2, the ICP does not increase, as cerebrospinal fluid is shifted from the cranium into the spinal subarachnoid space. A patient with an intracranial tumor, but between points 1 and 2 on the curve, is unlikely to manifest symptoms of increased ICP. A patient on the rising portion of the curve (3) can no longer compensate for an increased intracranial volume, and the ICP begins to increase and is likely to be associated with clinical symptoms. An additional increase in intracranial volume at this point (3), as produced by increased cerebral blood flow during anesthesia, can precipitate an abrupt increase in ICP (4).

bral blood volume can adversely and abruptly increase ICP.

2. **Monitoring intracranial pressure.** The importance of monitoring ICP (epidural or subdural placement of a transducer or intraventricular via a catheter placed in a cerebral ventricle) in patients with space-occupying lesions is emphasized by the observation that alterations in ICP may not be accompanied by changes in the neurologic examination or the vital signs. The first evidence of a hazardous increase in ICP in unresponsive patients may be sudden bilateral pupillary dilatation associated with herniation of the brain stem through the foramen magnum. A normal ICP is pulsa-

---

▬ Table 17–3 • Events that May Initiate Abrupt Increases in Intracranial Pressure

Anxiety

Painful stimulation (liberal use of analgesics to avoid pain perception even in unresponsive patients)

Induction of anesthesia (establishment of an adequate depth of anesthesia before initiating direct laryngoscopy)

---

tile and varies with cardiac impulses and spontaneous breathing (mean ICP should remain < 15 mmHg) (Table 17–3).

3. **Methods to decrease intracranial pressure.** See Table 17–4.
4. **Determinants of cerebral blood flow** include the $PaCO_2$, PaO_2, arterial blood pressure and autoregulation, central venous pressure, and anesthetic drugs and techniques (Fig. 17–2).
   a. **Arterial carbon dioxide partial pressure.** Variations in $PaCO_2$ produce corresponding changes in CBF (increases 1 ml/100 g/min for every 1 mmHg increase in the $PaCO_2$ above 40 mmHg; similar decreases occur during hypocarbia). The ability of hypocapnia to decrease CBF and ICP is the basis for neuroanesthesia.

▬ Table 17–4 • Methods to Decrease Intracranial Pressure

Posture (avoid head-down position)

Hyperventilation (maintain $PaCO_2$ near 30 mmHg in adults and 20–25 mmHg in children; effect wanes after 6–12 hours)

Cerebrospinal fluid drainage

Hyperosmotic drugs (mannitol 0.25–1.00 g/kg IV over 15–30 minutes)

Diuretics (furosemide 1 mg/kg IV)

Corticosteroids (relieve localized cerebral edema that develops around an intracranial tumor)

Barbiturates (consider in presence of acute head injury)

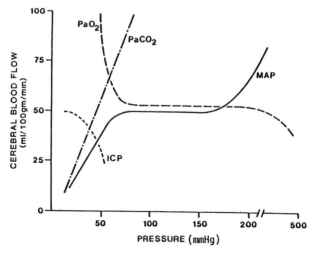

Fig. 17–2 • Effects of intracranial pressure (ICP), PaO_2, $PaCO_2$, and mean arterial pressure on cerebral blood flow.

b. **Arterial oxygen partial pressure.** Decreased PaO_2 does not lead to significantly increased CBF until a threshold value of about 50 mmHg is reached. Below this threshold there is abrupt cerebral vasodilation, and CBF increases.

c. **Arterial blood pressure and autoregulation.** Autoregulation of CBF may be lost or impaired in the presence of intracranial tumors or head trauma and the administration of volatile anesthetics. Chronic systemic hypertension shifts the autoregulation curve to the right (acute hypertension may produce signs of central nervous system dysfunction, as adaptation of cerebral vessels requires 1 to 2 months).

d. **Venous blood pressure** is usually low in supine or standing patients such that the mean arterial pressure is the predominant determinant of cerebral perfusion pressures. Increases in venous pressure are directly transmitted to intracranial veins. The impact of increased central venous pressure on cerebral perfusion pressure and ICP must be appreciated when considering the use of positive airway pressure during intracranial surgery or in patients with increased ICP.

   e. **Anesthetic drugs.** Volatile anesthetics administered during normocapnia at > 0.6 minimum alveolar concentration (MAC) are potent cerebral vasodilators that produce dose-dependent increases in CBF despite concomitant decreases in cerebral metabolic oxygen requirements. Normally, the tendency of ICP to increase in response to increases in CBF is prevented by displacement of cerebrospinal fluid from the cranium. In patients with intracranial tumors, however, this compensatory mechanism may fail, such that drug-induced increases in CBF may produce abrupt increases in ICP. In contrast to volatile anesthetics, barbiturates, etomidate, propofol, and opioids are classified as vasoconstrictors.

5. **Preoperative evaluation** of patients with intracranial tumors is directed toward establishing the presence or absence of increased ICP (Table 17–2).

6. **Preoperative medication** using drugs that may depress ventilation or the level of consciousness must be used sparingly, if at all, in patients with intracranial tumors.

7. **Induction of anesthesia.** See Table 17–5.

8. **Maintenance of anesthesia** in patients undergoing resection of supratentorial brain tumors is often achieved with combinations of drugs including nitrous oxide, volatile anesthetics (often isoflurane), opioids, and propofol. Treatment of systemic hypertension with direct vasodilators (nitroprusside, nitroglycerin) may increase CBF and ICP despite simultaneous decreases in systemic vascular resistance. Skeletal muscle paralysis is typically maintained during intracranial surgery, as unexpected movement can lead to increases in ICP.

9. **Fluid therapy** is most often with 5% glucose in lactated Ringer's solution at a rate of 1 to 3 ml/kg/hr. Glucose-in-water solutions are not recommended, as they are rapidly and equally distributed throughout the total body water.

10. **Monitoring.** See Table 17–6.

11. **Patient position** for removing supratentorial tumors is usually supine, with the head elevated 10 to 15

≡ Table 17-5 • Induction of Anesthesia in Patients with Intracranial Tumors

Intravenous induction drugs (thiopental, etomidate, propofol) producing rapid onset of unconsciousness with minimal effects on cerebral blood flow

Large doses of neuromuscular blocking drugs ($3 \times ED_{95}$) to facilitate tracheal intubation

Mechanical hyperventilation of the patient's lungs to a $PaCO_2$ near 30 mmHg

Adequate depth of anesthesia and profound skeletal muscle paralysis before initiating direct laryngoscopy for tracheal intubation (additional doses of intravenous induction drug, opioids, lidocaine)

Abrupt and sustained increases in systemic blood pressure in the absence of autoregulation in areas of intracranial pathology may be accompanied by cerebral edema and undesirable increases in cerebral blood flow and intracranial pressure

Following tracheal intubation institute mechanical hyperventilation to maintain $PaCO_2$ near 30 mmHg

degrees to facilitate cerebral venous drainage. The sitting position is often used for exploration of the posterior cranial fossa (the risk of venous air embolism may be a reason to use the lateral position).

12. **Venous air embolism** is a potential hazard whenever the operative site is above the level of the patient's

≡ Table 17-6 • Monitoring in the Presence of Intracranial Tumors

Intra-arterial blood pressure

Capnography

Intracranial pressure (not routine)

Urine output

Right atrial catheter (pulmonary artery catheter an alternative)

Peripheral nerve stimulator

Doppler transducer (placed between the second and third intercostal spaces, just to the right of the sternum)

Electrocardiogram (cardiac dysrhythmias owing to brain stem manipulation)

⊒ Table 17–7 • Detection of Venous Air Embolism

Doppler transducer (most sensitive)
Sudden decrease in end-tidal carbon dioxide concentrations
Increase in right atrial pressure and pulmonary artery pressure
Increase in end-tidal nitrogen concentration (may precede changes
  in end-tidal carbon dioxide concentration or right atrial pressure)
Sudden attempts to breath (gasp reflex)
Hypotension, cardiac dysrhythmias, and cyanosis (late signs)

heart, such that pressures in the veins are subatmospheric. In addition, veins in the skull may not collapse owing to their attachment to bone or dura.

   a. **Pathophysiology.** Presumably, when air enters the right ventricle there is interference with blood flow into the pulmonary artery. Death is usually due to acute cor pulmonale, cardiovascular collapse, and arterial hypoxemia.

   b. **Detection** of venous air embolism is important for successful treatment (Table 17–7).

   c. **Treatment.** See Table 17–8.

13. **Postoperative management.** Recognition of any adverse neurologic changes produced by the surgery may be facilitated by pharmacologic reversal of the effects of anesthetics and muscle relaxants. It is important to prevent reactions to the tracheal tube as patients awaken (consider lidocaine 0.5 to 1.5 mg/kg IV). If consciousness was depressed preoperatively or if body temperature has decreased to <34°C during sur-

⊒ Table 17–8 • Treatment of Venous Air Embolism

Occlude venous air entry site
Aspirate air via right atrial catheter
Discontinue nitrous oxide
Positive end-expiratory pressure up to 10 cmH$_2$O
Sympathomimetics and/or inotropes
β_2-Agonists

gery, it may be prudent to delay tracheal extubation until it can be confirmed that airway reflexes are present. Also, spontaneous ventilation should be sufficient to prevent carbon dioxide accumulation.

II. CEREBROVASCULAR DISORDERS

Cerebrovascular disorders ("stroke") are characterized by sudden neurologic deficits due to ischemic (80%) or hemorrhagic (intracerebral or subarachnoid) events (Table 17–9).

A. **Cerebrovascular anatomy.** Blood supply to the brain (20% of the cardiac output) is via two pairs of vessels: the internal carotid arteries and the vertebral arteries. These vessels join on the surface of the brain to form the intracranial vessels (anterior cerebral artery, middle cerebral artery, posterior cerebral artery) and the circle of Willis. Occlusion of specific arteries results in predictable clinical neurologic deficits (Table 17–10).

B. **Initial evaluation.** Patients presenting with the sudden onset of neurologic dysfunction are most likely experiencing a stroke. Early treatment to restore cerebral perfusion improves the outcome.

1. **Distinguish hemorrhage from ischemia.** Noncontrast computed tomography (CT) distinguishes acute intracerebral hemorrhage from ischemia. This is important, as treatment of hemorrhagic stroke is different from that of ischemic stroke.

2. **Define vascular lesion.** Conventional angiography demonstrates acute occlusion or an embolus lodged at a vascular bifurcation.

C. **Acute ischemic stroke** most likely reflects cardioembolism (atrial fibrillation), atherothromboembolism (carotid artery disease), and small vessel occlusive disease.

1. **Risk factors.** Systemic hypertension is the greatest risk factor for the occurrence of acute ischemic stroke. Cigarette smoking substantially increases the risk of acute ischemic stroke.

2. **Carotid endarterectomy.** Surgical treatment of symptomatic or asymptomatic carotid artery stenosis decreases the risk of stroke. Angioplasty and stenting may become alternatives to carotid endartectomy.

   a. **Preoperative evaluation.** See Table 17–11.

   b. **Management of anesthesia.** No clear advantage has been demonstrated for performing carotid end-

Table 17-9 • Characteristics of Stroke Subtypes

Characteristic	Systemic Hypoperfusion	Embolism	Thrombosis	Subarachnoid Hemorrhage	Intracerebral Hemorrhage
Risk factors	Hypotension Hemorrhage Cardiac arrest	Smoking Ischemic heart disease Peripheral vascular disease Diabetes mellitus White male	Smoking Ischemic heart disease Peripheral vascular disease Diabetes mellitus White male	Often absent Hypertension Coagulopathy Drugs Trauma	Hypertension Coagulopathy Drugs Trauma
Onset	Parallels risk factors	Sudden	Often preceded by a TIA	Sudden, often during exertion	Gradually progressive
Signs and symptoms	Pallor Diaphoresis Hypotension	Headache	Headache	Headache Vomiting Transient loss of consciousness	Headache Vomiting Decreased level of consciousness Seizures
Imaging	CT (black) MRI	CT (black) MRI	CT (black) MRI	CT (white) MRI	CT (white) MRI

CT, computed tomography; MRI, magnetic resonance imaging; TIA, transient ischemic attack.
Adapted from: Caplan LR. Diagnosis and treatment of ischemic stroke. JAMA 1991;266:2413–8.

≡ Table 17–10 • Clinical Features of Cerebrovascular Occlusive Syndromes

Occluded Artery	Clinical Features
Anterior cerebral artery	Contralateral leg weakness
Middle cerebral artery	Contralateral hemiparesis and hemisensory deficit (face and arm greater than leg)
	Aphasia (dominant hemisphere)
	Contralateral visual field defects
Posterior cerebral artery	Contralateral visual field defects
	Contralateral hemiparesis
Penetrating injuries	Contralateral hemiparesis
	Contralateral hemisensory
Basilar artery	Oculomotor deficits and/or ataxia with "crossed" sensory and motor deficits
Vertebral artery	Lower cranial nerve deficits and/or ataxia with crossed sensory deficits

Adapted from: Morgenstern LB, Kasner SE. Cerebrovascular disorders. Sci Am Med 2000:1–15.

arterectomy under regional (cervical plexus block) versus general anesthesia (Table 17–12).

    c. **Postoperative management and complications.** See Table 17–13.

3. **Medical management of acute ischemia stroke** includes consideration of the patient's airway, oxygenation, ventilation, systemic blood pressure, blood glu-

≡ Table 17–11 • Preoperative Evaluation Prior to Carotid Endarterectomy

Neurologic evaluation
Evaluate for presence of cardiovascular disease, systemic hypertension, and renal disease
Establish range of normal blood pressures as guideline for acceptable perfusion pressures during anesthesia and surgery
Determine effects of changes in head position on cerebral function (rotation, flexion, extension could compress the vertebral arteries)

≡ Table 17–12 • Management of Anesthesia for Carotid Endarterectomy

---

Cervical plexus block (early warning of cerebral dysfunction with arterial cross-clamping, yet perioperative strokes are more likely to be embolic than low flow in origin; disadvantage is the need for patient cooperation)

General anesthesia (no preferred drugs; goals are to maintain hemodynamic stability and permit prompt emergence to make rapid assessment of neurologic status possible)

Maintenance of an adequate systemic blood pressure is important, as autoregulation may be lost (phenylephrine)

Normocarbia

Monitoring during general anesthesia (electroencephalography, somatosensory evoked potentials, transcranial Doppler)

---

cose concentrations, and body temperature as well as the institution of heparin prophylaxis. Cerebral edema and increased ICP may complicate the clinical course (malignant middle cerebral artery syndrome is edematous infarcted tissue causing compression of the anterior and posterior cerebral arteries).

4. **Pharmacologic treatment of acute ischemic stroke.** Aspirin is often recommended as initial therapy for acute stroke patients and to prevent strokes or their recurrence. Intravenous recombinant tissue plasminogen activator (rt-PA) is utilized in patients who meet

---

≡ Table 17–13 • Postoperative Management and Complications Following Carotid Endarterectomy

---

Hypertension (common during immediate postoperative period, especially in patients with co-existing systemic hypertension; treat with a vasodilator)

Hypotension

Airway compression due to hematoma at the operative site

Loss of carotid body function

Myocardial infarction

Stroke

Peripheral nerve damage (facial nerve, recurrent laryngeal nerve)

---

specific eligibility requirements if treatment can be initiated within 3 hours of the onset of acute symptoms.

5. **Man-in-the barrel syndrome** is characterized by bilateral upper extremity paresis with intact motor function in the lower extremities that most often follows an episode of hypotension, causing global cerebral hypoperfusion (watershed ischemia; may be associated with cortical blindness).

D. Acute hemorrhagic stroke

1. **Intracerebral hemorrhage** cannot be distinguished from ischemic stroke by clinical criteria alone (noncontrast CT is needed to detect the presence of blood). Cerebral edema worsens during the 24 to 48 hours following the acute bleed. An ICP monitor may be utilized in patients who are obtunded.

2. **Subarachnoid hemorrhage** most commonly results from aneurysms of the circle of Willis (systemic hypertension and cigarette smoking are risk factors for aneurysm rupture).

   a. **Diagnosis** includes clinical symptoms ("worst headache of my life") and demonstration of subarachnoid blood using CT.

   b. **Treatment** of subarachnoid hemorrhage involves localizing the aneurysm with cerebral angiography and surgically excluding the aneurysmal sac from the intracranial circulation while preserving the parent artery within the first 72 hours following bleeding. Alternatively, endovascular techniques consisting of placing soft metallic coils in the lumen of the aneurysm may serve as an alternative to surgical therapy. Following aneurysm clipping, the goal is to prevent vasospasm (occurs 3 to 15 days after subarachnoid hemorrhage). "Triple H" therapy (hypertension, hypervolemic, hemodilution) is initiated at the first sign of vasospasm. Nimodipine, a calcium channel blocker, has been shown to improve outcome when initiated on the first day and continued for 21 days, presumably reflecting protective effects against the development of vasospasm.

   c. **Management of anesthesia.** The goals of anesthesia during intracranial aneurysm surgery are to limit the risks of aneurysm rupture, prevent cere-

---

Table 17–14 • Management of Anesthesia for Resection of an Intracranial Aneurysm

---

Induction of Anesthesia

Produce loss of consciousness with thiopental, etomidate, or propofol

Prevent increases in the transmural pressure of the aneurysmal sac (nitroprusside, opioids)

Patients with increased intracranial pressure prior to surgery may not tolerate decreases in mean arterial pressure to protect against aneurysm sac rupture

Monitor intra-arterial blood pressure

Place central venous pressure catheter (likely to be hypovolemic preoperatively and may experience massive blood loss intraoperatively)

Maintenance of Anesthesia

Depth of anesthesia appropriate for the level of surgical stimulation [volatile anesthetics supplemented with intermittent (fentanyl) or continuous (remifentanil) infusions of an opioid]

Facilitation of surgical exposure through optimal brain relaxation (lumbar cerebrospinal fluid drainage, mild hyperventilation, diuretics, proper patient positioning to facilitate cerebral venous drainage)

Maintenance of cerebral perfusion pressures

Normovolemia or modest hypervolemia utilizing balanced salt solutions (avoid glucose-containing solutions)

Reduction of transmural pressure in the aneurysm during clipping of the aneurysm

Prompt awakening after surgery to permit neurologic assessment

Controlled Hypotension

Regional controlled hypotension produced by placing a vascular clamp on the parent artery supplying the aneurysm

Limit temporary occlusion of the parent artery to 10 minutes [if need longer consider metabolic suppressants (thiopental) or mild hypothermia]

Level of Drug-Induced Controlled Hypotension

Mean arterial pressure about 50 mmHg (systolic blood pressure 60–70 mmHg, $PaCO_2$ about 35 mmHg and central venous pressure or intracranial pressure 10 mmHg or less)

Recognize likely rightward shift of the curve for autoregulation of cerebral blood flow in chronically hypertensive patients

Monitoring Systemic Blood Pressure During Drug-Induced Controlled Hypotension

Place transducer at the same height as the circle of Willis (level of the patient's external auditory canal)

Emergence from Anesthesia

Prompt awakening needed for neurologic evaluation

Treat systemic hypertension with labetalol or esmolol

Computed tomography or angiography if prompt awakening does not occur

---

bral ischemia, and facilitate surgical exposure (Table 17–14).

III. TRAUMATIC BRAIN INJURY

Traumatic brain injury most often follows motor vehicle accidents (closed head injury due to rapid acceleration or deceleration that causes the brain to strike the interior of the skull; associated cervical spine injuries) and is the leading cause of death in young adults in the United States.

A. **Treatment.** Initial management of acute head injury patients includes immobilizing the cervical spine, establishing a patent upper airway, and protecting the patient's lungs from aspiration of gastric contents. CT is performed as soon as possible (identify epidural or subdural hematoma). The Glasgow Coma Scale score provides a reproducible method for assessing the seriousness of the brain injury (score < 8 points is severe injury) and for following the patient's neurologic status (Table 17–15).

B. **Perioperative management** of patients with acute head trauma must consider the risks of secondary injury in

≡ Table 17–15 • Glasgow Coma Scale

Response	Score
Eye Opening	
Spontaneous	4
To speech	3
To pain	2
Nil	1
Best Motor Response	
Obeys	6
Localizes	5
Withdraws (flexion)	4
Abnormal flexion	3
Extensor response	2
Nil	1
Verbal Response	
Oriented	5
Confused conversation	4
Inappropriate words	3
Incomprehensible sounds	2
Nil	1

these patients due to cerebral ischemia (treat increased ICP).

1. **Management of anesthesia** includes efforts to optimize cerebral perfusion pressures (maintain > 70 mmHg if possible), minimize the occurrence of cerebral ischemia, and avoid drugs or techniques that could increase the ICP.

   a. **Induction and maintenance of anesthesia** is often with intravenous drugs, keeping in mind the goal to optimize cerebral perfusion pressures and prevent increases in ICP (low doses of volatile drugs may be added).

   b. **Postoperative period.** It is common to maintain skeletal muscle paralysis to facilitate mechanical ventilation of the patient's lungs.

C. **Epidural hematoma** is bleeding into the space between the skull and dura (usually rupture of a meningeal artery) in association with a skull fracture (loss of consciousness followed by a return of consciousness and a variable lucid period). If an epidural hematoma is suspected on CT, treatment is prompt placement of burr holes at the site of the skull fracture.

D. **Subdural hematoma** results from lacerated or torn bridging veins that bleed into the space between the dura and arachnoid; it is often associated with "trivial" head injury, especially in elderly patients. Diagnosis of subdural hematoma is confirmed by CT.

   1. **Signs and symptoms.** See Table 17–16.

   2. **Treatment** is most likely surgical evacuation of the clot as the prognosis is poor if coma develops.

Table 17–16 • Signs and Symptoms of Subdural Hematoma

Evolve gradually over several days (in contrast to epidural hematoma)
Headache
Drowsiness and obtundation (may fluctuate)
Lateralizing neurologic signs (hemiparesis, hemianopsia)
Unexplained progressive dementia (elderly patients)

IV. DEGENERATIVE DISEASES OF THE NERVOUS SYSTEM

See Table 17–17.

A. **Aqueductal stenosis** is caused by congenital narrowing of the cerebral aqueduct that connects the third and fourth ventricles. It leads eventually to obstructive hydrocephalus and symptoms of increased ICP. Treatment is placement of a ventricular shunt.

B. **Arnold-Chiari malformation** is herniation of the cerebellum into the cervical spinal canal requiring surgical decompression.

C. **Syringomyelia** is progressive degeneration of the spinal cord (cavitation), leading to sensory and motor (thoracic scoliosis) deficits. The possible absence of protective upper airway reflexes and a hyperkalemic response to succinylcholine are considerations in the management of anesthesia.

D. **Amyotrophic lateral sclerosis** is a degenerative disease of motor cells throughout the central nervous system and spinal cord, leading to weakness and fasciculations of skeletal muscles. Dysphagia (bulbar involvement) leading to pulmonary aspiration and a hyperkalemic response to succinylcholine are considerations in the management of anesthesia.

E. **Friedreich's ataxia** is characterized by degeneration of the spinocerebellar tracts, often in association with cardiomyopathy and kyphoscoliosis.

F. **Parkinson's disease** is a degenerative disease of the central nervous system characterized by loss of dopaminergic fibers (dopamine is an inhibitory neurotransmitter acting on the extrapyramidal motor system) in the basal ganglia of the brain (Table 17–18).

G. **Hallervorden-Spatz disease** is a disorder of basal ganglia characterized by dystonic posturing and scoliosis.

H. **Huntington's chorea** is a premature degenerative disease of the central nervous system characterized by progressive dementia, pulmonary aspiration, and involuntary skeletal muscle movements.

I. **Olivopontocerebellar degeneration** is a diverse group of diseases characterized by cerebellar disturbances (ataxic gait and kinetic motion disorders) and dysphagia.

J. **Strumpell's disease** is a neurodegenerative disorder that manifests as spastic paresis and sensory deficits predominantly of the lower limbs.

Table 17–17 • Degenerative Diseases of the Nervous System

Aqueductal stenosis
Arnold-Chiari malformation
Syringomyelia
Amyotrophic lateral sclerosis
Tuberous sclerosis
Friedreich's ataxia
Parkinson's disease
Hallervorden-Spatz disease
Polyglucosan body disease
Huntington's chorea
Olivopontocerebellar degeneration
Strumpell's disease
Isaac's disease
Spasmodic torticollis
Shy-Drager syndrome
Orthostatic intolerance syndrome
Harlequin syndrome
Congenital insensitivity to pain
Progressive blindness
    Leber's optic atrophy
    Retinitis pigmentosa
    Kearns-Sayer syndrome
    Ischemic optic neuropathy (anterior and posterior optic
      neuropathy)
    Cortical blindness
    Retinal artery occlusion
    Ophthalmic venous obstruction
Transmissible spongiform encephalopathies
    Creutzfeldt-Jakob disease
    Adrenoleukodystrophies
Leigh syndrome
Rett syndrome
Sotos syndrome
Fragile X syndrome
Menkes syndrome
Stiff-person syndrome
Von Hippel-Lindau syndrome
Painful legs and moving toes syndrome
Kallman syndrome
Multiple sclerosis
Postpolio sequelae

≡ Table 17-18 • Characteristics of Parkinson's Disease

Signs and Symptoms
Skeletal muscle rigidity
Resting tremor
Diaphragmatic spasms
Mental depression
Treatment (designed to increase the concentration of dopamine in the basal ganglia or decrease the neuronal effects of acetylcholine)
Levodopa (combine with a decarboxylase inhibitor; side effects reflect dopamine effects on the central nervous system, heart, and gastrointestinal tract)
Anticholinergic drugs
Antihistamine drugs
Management of Anesthesia
Continue levodopa therapy
Possibility of systemic blood pressure lability and cardiac dysrhythmias
Avoid drugs with antidopaminergic effects (droperidol, possibly opioids)

K. **Spasmodic torticollis** most frequently presents as spasmodic contractions of nuchal muscles that may interfere with maintenance of a patent upper airway in anesthetized but nonparalyzed patients.

L. **Shy-Drager syndrome** is characterized by autonomic nervous system dysfunction (orthostatic hypotension) and degeneration of the central nervous system and spinal cord. Management of anesthesia includes continuous monitoring of systemic blood pressure and prompt correction of hypotension with infusions of fluids and/or administration of vasopressors (possible enhanced response to drugs that act by evoking the release of norepinephrine).

M. **Orthostatic intolerance syndrome** is a chronic idiopathic disorder of primary autonomic nervous system failure characterized by postural tachycardia that occurs independent of alterations in systemic blood pressure. Medical treatment includes attempts to increase the intravascular fluid volume and consideration of long-term administration of α_1-adrenergic agonists (phenylephrine).

N. **Chronic fatigue syndrome** may be a manifestation of autonomic nervous system dysfunction.

O. **Harlequin syndrome** is characterized by unilateral cutaneous color changes, flushing, and diaphoresis that seem to be due to dysfunction of the autonomic nervous system.

P. **Ischemic optic neuropathy** due to infarction of the anterior or posterior portions of the optic nerve should be suspected in patients who complain of visual loss during the first postoperative week. The etiology of postoperative ischemic optic neuropathy appears to be multifactorial including hypotension, anemia, congenital absence of the central retinal artery, venous obstruction, and infection. Postoperative ischemic optic neuropathy has been described following prolonged spine surgery performed in the prone position, cardiac surgery, radical neck dissection, and hip arthroplasty. Nonsurgical events associated with posterior ischemic optic neuropathy include cardiac arrest, treatment of malignant hypertension, blunt trauma, and severe anemia, as due to gastrointestinal hemorrhage.

Q. **Creutzfeldt-Jakob disease** is a progressively fatal encephalopathy transmitted by an infectious pathogen (prions) that is reliably inactivated by steam, ethylene oxide, and sodium hypochlorite. Alzheimer's disease poses the most difficult differential diagnosis.

R. **Adrenoleukodystrophies** are genetic disorders caused by defective degradation of peroxisomes that lead to central nervous system demyelination and primary adrenal insufficiency.

S. **Leigh syndrome** is a necrotizing encephalomyelopathy manifesting as hypotonia, seizures, and aspiration in children.

T. **Rett syndrome** manifests exclusively in females as dementia, autistic behavior, and breathing abnormalities leading to apnea and arterial hypoxemia.

U. **Sotos syndrome** is characterized by mental retardation and macrocephaly (airway management difficult), often in association with scoliosis and the likely need for corrective surgery.

V. **Fragile X syndrome** is a common cause of mental retardation and developmental delay. It is inherited as an X-linked dominant disorder.

W. **Stiff-person syndrome** is a rare central nervous system disease characterized by persistent, painful skeletal muscle contractions resembling tetanus. Skeletal muscle rigidity may interfere with adequate ventilation.

X. **Von Hippel-Lindau syndrome** is a familial disease transmitted by an autosomal dominant gene. It is characterized by retinal angiomas, hemangioblastomas, and central nervous system (cerebellar) and visceral tumors. The incidence of pheochromocytoma is increased in these patients. The possibility of spinal cord hemangioblastomas may limit the use of spinal anesthesia.

Y. **Multiple sclerosis** is characterized by random, multiple sites of demyelination of corticospinal tract neurons in the brain and spinal cord, exclusive of the peripheral nervous system (Table 17–19).

▬ Table 17–19 • Characteristics of Multiple Sclerosis

Signs and Symptoms (reflect effects of demyelination)
Visual disturbances
Ataxia
Limb paresthesias and weakness
Spastic paresis of skeletal muscles
Exacerbations and remissions
Diagnosis
Somatosensory evoked potentials
Magnetic resonance imaging
Immersion in hot water
Examination of cerebrospinal fluid
Treatment (none curative)
Corticosteroids
Interferon
Glatiramer acetate
Azathioprine
Methotrexate
Management of Anesthesia
Regardless of the anesthetic technique or drugs selected, the symptoms are usually exacerbated during the postoperative period
Increase in body temperature (1°C) is more likely than drugs to be responsible for exacerbation of symptoms postoperatively
Regional anesthesia has been utilized, but unpredictable progression of disease must be considered
Unpredictable responses to nondepolarizing muscle relaxants and risk of potassium release in response to administration of succinylcholine
Corticosteroid supplementation

≡ Table 17–20 • Postpolio Sequelae

Exquisite sensitivity to sedatives and delayed awakening from anesthesia (may reflect damage to the reticular activating system from the original infection)
Sensitivity to muscle relaxants
Severe back pain following surgery
Postoperative shivering
Increased postoperative pain sensitivity
Outpatient surgery may not be appropriate

    Z. Postpolio sequelae manifest as fatigue, skeletal muscle weakness, joint pain, cold intolerance and swallowing, sleep, and breathing problems that presumably reflect neurologic damage from the original polio virus infection (Table 17–20).

V. CRANIAL NEUROPATHIES

    See Table 17–21.

    A. Idiopathic facial paralysis (Bell's palsy) is characterized by the rapid onset of motor weakness or paralysis (no sensory loss) of all the facial muscles innervated by the facial nerve (presumed to reflect inflammation and edema of the facial nerve). Prednisone dramatically relieves pain. Surgical decompression of the facial nerve may be needed for persistent or severe cases. Trauma to the facial nerve can reflect stretch injury produced by excessive traction on the angle of the mandible during maintenance of the upper airway in unconscious patients.

≡ Table 17–21 • Cranial Mononeuropathies

    Idiopathic facial paralysis (Bell's palsy)
    Melkersson-Rosenthal syndrome
    Trigeminal neuralgia (tic douloureux)
    Myofascial pain dysfunction syndrome
    Glossopharyngeal neuralgia
    Vestibular neuronitis
    Metastatic cancer
    Möbius syndrome

≡ Table 17–22 • Management of Anesthesia in Patients with Glossopharyngeal Neuralgia

Anticipate hypovolemia
Consider placement of an artificial transvenous cardiac pacemaker
Topical anesthesia of the oropharynx
Anticholinergic drugs promptly available
Postoperative systemic hypertension
Vocal cord paralysis

B. **Trigeminal neuralgia (tic douloureux)** is characterized by the sudden onset of brief but intense unilateral facial pain triggered by local sensory stimuli to the affected side of the face (most often the mandibular division of the trigeminal nerve).

1. **Treatment.** Medical management is with the anticonvulsant drug, carbamazepine. Surgical treatment consists of selective radiofrequency destruction of the trigeminal nerve fibers, transection of the sensory root of the trigeminal nerve fibers, or microsurgical decompression of the trigeminal nerve.

2. **Management of anesthesia.** Patients undergoing surgical therapy for trigeminal neuralgia may experience significant increases in systemic blood pressure during destruction of nerve fibers, necessitating treatment with nitroprusside. Carbamazepine can cause altered hepatic function, leukopenia, and thrombocytopenia.

C. **Glossopharyngeal neuralgia** is characterized by intense pain in the sensory distribution of the nerve (throat, neck, tongue, ear). It is associated with bradycardia (sudden death) and seizures.

1. **Treatment** is with topical anesthesia and administration of carbamazepine. Intracranial section of the nerve is undertaken in life-threatening situations.

2. **Management of anesthesia.** See Table 17–22.

VI. PERIPHERAL NEUROPATHIES

See Table 17–23.

A. **Inherited Peripheral Neuropathies**

1. **Charcot-Marie-Tooth disease** (peroneal muscle disease) is the most common inherited cause of chronic motor and sensory peripheral neuropathy, manifest-

---

≡ Table 17–23 • Peripheral Neuropathies

Inherited Peripheral Neuropathies
Charcot-Marie-Tooth disease
Hereditary neuropathy with liability to pressure palsies
Inflammatory-Immune Peripheral Neuropathies
Brachial plexus neuropathy
Postherpetic neuralgia
Guillain-Barré syndrome (acute idiopathic polyneuritis)
Entrapment Neuropathies
Carpal tunnel syndrome
Cubital tunnel entrapment syndrome
Meralgia paresthetica
Diseases Associated with Peripheral Neuropathies
Diabetes mellitus
Alcohol abuse
Vitamin B_{12} deficiency
Uremia
Cancer
Collagen vascular disease
Sarcoidosis
Refsum's disease

---

ing as distal skeletal muscle weakness and wasting
(peroneal muscle atrophy, quadriceps muscle wasting). Despite concerns regarding responses to neuromuscular blocking drugs, development of malignant
hyperthermia, and the possibility of postoperative respiratory failure, these patients seem to tolerate anesthesia without increased risks.

2. **Hereditary neuropathy with liability to pressure palsies** is characterized by periodic and recurrent episodes of focal demyelinating neuropathy following
minor trauma or compression of peripheral nerves
(entrapment neuropathies are common).

B. **Inflammatory-immune peripheral neuropathies**

1. **Brachial plexus neuropathy** (idiopathic brachial neuritis, Parsonage-Turner syndrome) is characterized by
the acute onset of severe pain that is maximum in
intensity at the onset of the neuropathy. As the pain
diminishes there is an appearance of patchy paresis
or paralysis of the skeletal muscles of the shoulder
girdle and arm, as innervated by the individual
branches of the brachial plexus (especially axillary,

suprascapular, and long thoracic nerves). Overall, recovery may take 24 to 36 months but is nearly always complete.

   a. **Etiology.** Autoimmune neuropathies may occur during the postoperative period independent of the site of surgery.

   b. It is possible that the stress of surgery activates an unidentified dormant virus in the nerve roots (similar to herpes zoster).

2. **Postherpetic neuralgia** is characterized by severe burning and lancinating pain (neuropathic pain) typically accompanied by allodynia (pain provoked by nonnoxious stimuli) that continues more than 1 month after the onset of herpes eruption.

   a. **Treatment** of acute herpes zoster to prevent its progression to postherpetic neuralgia or to alleviate already present postherpetic neuralgia includes tricyclic antidepressants, anticonvulsant drugs, and intrathecal administration of methylprednisolone.

   b. Corticosteroids may speed resolution of the acute neuritis, but there is no evidence that these drugs influence the likely development of postherpetic neuralgia.

3. **Guillain-Barré syndrome (acute idiopathic polyneuritis)** is characterized by the onset of skeletal muscle weakness or paralysis that typically manifests in the legs and spreads cephalad (Table 17–24). Altered function of the autonomic nervous system and the presence of lower motor neuron lesions are the two important

---

≡ Table 17–24 • Characteristics of Guillain-Barré Syndrome (Acute Idiopathic Polyneuritis)

Ascending flaccid skeletal muscle paralysis (lower motor neuron)
Bulbar involvement
Intercostal muscle weakness (monitor vital capacity and arterial blood gases as may require tracheal intubation and mechanical support of ventilation)
Pharyngeal muscle weakness (aspiration)
Sensory paresthesias and pain
Autonomic nervous system dysfunction (labile systemic blood pressure, cardiac conduction disturbances, sudden death)

considerations for management of anesthesia in these patients (Table 17–25).

C. **Entrapment neuropathies** occur at anatomic sites where peripheral nerves pass through narrow passages (median nerve and carpal tunnel, ulnar nerve and cubital tunnel) making compression a possibility. A peripheral nerve may be more susceptible to compression if the same fibers have been damaged proximally ("double crush syndrome"), as by cervical radiculopathy. Nerve conduction studies are useful for localizing the site of peripheral nerve compression. Electromyography studies are adjuncts to nerve conduction studies showing the presence of denervation impulses and ultimately reinnervation of muscle fibers.

1. **Carpal tunnel syndrome** is compression of the median nerve between the transverse carpal ligament forming the roof of the carpal tunnel and the carpal bones at the wrist. Patients (often women) describe repeated episodes of pain and paresthesias in the wrist and hand following distribution of the median nerve (may spread to arm and shoulder).

   a. **Etiology.** Afflicted individuals often have occupations that require repetitive movements of the hands and fingers. Intraoperatively, patients may accumulate significant amounts of third space fluid, and the resulting increased tissue pressure is sufficient to cause compression of the median nerve at the wrist in previously asymptomatic pa-

---

≡ **Table 17–25** • Management of Anesthesia in Patients with Guillain-Barré Syndrome (Acute Idiopathic Neuritis)

Hypotension with changes in posture, blood loss, or positive airway pressure (impaired compensatory cardiovascular responses)

Systemic hypertension with noxious stimulation (laryngoscopy)

Exaggerated responses to indirect-acting vasopressors

Possible hyperkalemic responses to succinylcholine

Anticipate need for postoperative mechanical support of ventilation

tients. Pregnancy and associated peripheral edema may be associated with the initial manifestations of carpal tunnel syndrome.

    b. Treatment is immobilization of the wrist when the etiology is presumed to be transient (pregnancy) or due to medically treatable diseases (hypothyroidism, acromegaly). Definitive treatment of carpal tunnel syndrome is decompression of the median nerve by surgical division of the transverse carpal ligament.

  2. Cubital tunnel entrapment syndrome is compression of the ulnar nerve after it passes through the condylar groove and enters the cubital tunnel. It may be difficult to differentiate clinical symptoms of ulnar nerve neuropathy due to compression in the condylar groove from symptoms that occur as a result of entrapment in the cubital tunnel. Treatment of carpal tunnel entrapment includes tunnel decompression and transposition of the ulnar nerve.

  3. Meralgia paresthetica is entrapment of the lateral femoral cutaneous nerve as it passes under the inguinal ligament, leading to burning pain over the anterolateral aspect of the thigh (obesity, tight belts contribute).

D. Diseases associated with peripheral neuropathies

  1. Diabetes mellitus is commonly associated with peripheral neuropathies with the incidence increasing with the duration of the disease. The most common neuropathy is a distal, symmetrical, predominantly sensory neuropathy (tingling, numbness, burning, and aching in the lower extremities especially at night).

    a. Signs of autonomic nervous system dysfunction (orthostatic hypotension, resting tachycardia, impotence, gastroparesis) are commonly associated with peripheral neuropathies.

    b. For reasons that are not understood, peripheral nerves of patients with diabetes mellitus are more vulnerable to ischemia from compression or stretch injury, as may occur during intraoperative and postoperative positioning despite padding and positioning during these periods.

  2. Alcohol abuse is associated with nutritional deficiencies resulting in polyneuropathy.

3. **Uremia.** Distal polyneuropathy with sensory and motor components often occurs in the extremities of patients with chronic renal failure.
4. **Cancer.** Peripheral sensory and/or motor neuropathies occur in patients with a variety of malignancies, especially those involving the lung, ovary, and breast.

VII. SPINAL CORD TRANSECTION

Anatomically, the spinal cord is not divided, but the effect physiologically is the same as if it were transected. The most common cause of spinal cord transection is trauma associated with motor vehicle accidents or diving accidents resulting in fracture dislocation of cervical vertebrae. The most frequent nontraumatic cause of spinal cord transection is multiple sclerosis.

A. **Management of unstable cervical spine injuries.** Mobility of the cervical spine makes it vulnerable to injury, especially hyperextension injury, during impact accidents (1.5% to 3.0% of all major trauma victims).

1. **Diagnosis.** Cervical spine radiographs are obtained in nearly all patients who present with blunt trauma for fear of missing occult cervical spine injuries. Certain clinical signs confirm that a cervical spine injury is unlikely, and routine imaging studies are not necessary (Table 17–26).

   a. **Imaging studies.** Routine CT or magnetic resonance imaging may not be practical, considering the risk of transporting unstable patients.

   b. The sensitivity of plain radiographs (antero-posterior, lateral, open mouth) is < 100%, and the likelihood of cervical spine injury must be inter-

---

≡ Table 17–26 • Clinical Signs that Rule Out the Likely Presence of Cervical Spine Injury Following Trauma

No midline cervical spine tenderness
No focal neurologic deficits
Normal sensorium
No intoxication
No painful distracting injury

preted in conjunction with other clinical symptoms and risk factors.

2. **Treatment** of cervical fracture-dislocations entails immediate immobilization to limit neck flexion and extension (halothoracic device is most effective). Manual in-line stabilization to keep the patient's head in a neutral position has been recommended for minimizing cervical spine flexion or extension during direct laryngoscopy for tracheal intubation.

3. **Direct laryngoscopy and tracheal intubation.** The key principle when performing direct laryngoscopy for tracheal intubation is to minimize neck movement during the procedure. Direct laryngoscopy produces minimal movements below C3, and cervical movement during direct laryngoscopy is likely to be concentrated at the occipitoatlantoaxial area.

   a. Direct laryngoscopy and oral tracheal intubation are acceptable, provided measures are taken to stabilize the head during the procedure and prior evaluation of the patient's airway did not suggest the likelihood of technical difficulty.

   b. Topical anesthesia and awake fiberoptic laryngoscopy for tracheal intubation is an alternative if the patient is cooperative and airway trauma does not preclude visualization with the fiberscope.

   c. In addition to mechanical deformation of the spinal cord produced by movement of the patient's neck in the presence of cervical spine injury, there is perhaps an even greater risk for compromise of the blood supply to the spinal cord produced by neck flexion that elongates the cord with resultant narrowing of the longitudinal blood vessels (maintenance of perfusion pressures may be more important than positioning).

B. **Pathophysiology of spinal cord injury.** See Table 17–27.

C. **Autonomic hyperreflexia** is a disorder that appears after resolution of spinal shock and in association with cutaneous (surgical incision) or visceral (bladder distension) stimulation below the level of the spinal cord transection.

   1. **Mechanism** See Figure 17–3.

   2. **Signs and symptoms.** See Table 17–28.

D. **Management of anesthesia** in patients with spinal cord transection is largely determined by the acute or chronic nature of the injury (Table 17–29).

■ Table 17–27 • Pathophysiology of Spinal
Cord Injury

Acute Manifestations (flaccid skeletal muscle paralysis, spinal
    shock)
Hypotension
Bradycardia
Ventricular premature beats
Alveolar hypoventilation
Aspiration
Arterial hypoxemia
Pneumonia
Pulmonary embolism
Chronic Manifestations (return of spinal reflexes)
Involuntary skeletal muscle spasms
Overactivity of the sympathetic nervous system
Chronic pulmonary and genitourinary infections
Anemia
Altered thermoregulation
Mental depression
Pain

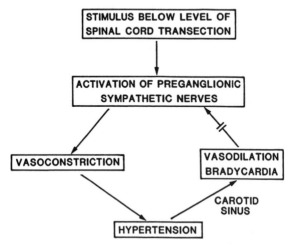

Fig. 17–3 • Sequence of events associated with clinical manifestations of autonomic hyperreflexia. Impulses that produce vasodilation cannot reach the neurologically isolated portion of the spinal
cord, such that vasoconstriction and systemic hypertension
persist.

≡ Table 17–28 • Signs and Symptoms of Autonomic Hyperreflexia

Systemic hypertension and bradycardia
Vasodilation above the level of spinal cord transection (nasal stuffiness)
Headache
Subarachnoid hemorrhage
Seizures
Cardiac dysrhythmias
Acute left ventricular failure (pulmonary edema)

VIII. SEIZURE DISORDERS

Seizure disorders are some of the most common neurologic disorders. They may occur at any age with more than 10% of the population experiencing seizures at least once in their lifetime. Transient abnormalities of brain function (hypoglycemia, hyponatremia, drug toxicity) typically result in a single seizure, and treatment of the underlying cause is curative. Epilepsy, defined as recurrent seizures resulting from congenital or acquired (cerebral scarring) factors, affects approximately 0.6% of the population (Table 17–30).

A. Treatment. See Table 17–31.
B. Side effects. See Table 17–32.

≡ Table 17–29 • Management of Anesthesia in the Presence of Spinal Cord Transection

Acute Spinal Cord Transection
Avoid extension of the head during direct laryngoscopy if cervical spine injury is present or a possibility
Absence of compensatory cardiovascular responses may manifest during posture changes, blood loss, or positive-pressure ventilation
Guard against hypothermia
Need for muscle relaxants dictated by operative site (succinylcholine safe within first 24 hours after acute injury)
Chronic Spinal Cord Transection
Prevent autonomic hyperreflexia (general versus spinal anesthesia; nitroprusside promptly available)
Exclusive use of nondepolarizing muscle relaxants

Table 17–30 • Classification of Epileptic Seizures

Partial (Focal and Local) Seizures
Simple partial seizures (consciousness not impaired)
Complex partial seizures (consciousness impaired)
Partial seizures evolving to generalized seizures (tonic, clonic, tonic-clonic)
Generalized Seizures (Convulsive or Nonconvulsive)
Absence seizures
Myoclonic seizures
Clonic seizures
Tonic seizures
Clonic-tonic seizures
Atonic seizures
Unclassified Epileptic Seizures

C. **Status epilepticus** is a life-threatening condition that manifests as continuous seizure activity or two or more seizures occurring in sequence without recovery of consciousness between the seizures.
   1. **Treatment** is prompt pharmacologic suppression of seizure activity combined with support of the patient's airway, ventilation, and circulation. Intravenous access must be established. Hypoglycemia is excluded

Table 17–31 • Treatment of Seizure Disorders

Pharmacologic Treatment (drug combinations when monotherapy fails; monitoring serum drug levels usually not necessary)
Carbamazepine (partial seizures, generalized seizure disorders)
Ethosuximide (generalized nonseizure disorders)
Gabapentin (generalized seizure disorders)
Lamotrigine (generalized seizure disorders)
Phenobarbital (generalized seizure disorders)
Phenytoin (partial seizures)
Primidone
Topiramate
Tiagabine
Valproate (partial seizures, generalized nonseizure disorders)
Surgical Treatment
Temporal lobe lobectomy

≡ Table 17–32 • Side Effects of Antiepileptic Drugs

Enzyme induction (carbamazepine, phenytoin, barbiturates)
Dose-dependent neurologic effects (sedation, ataxia, dyskinesias, sensory neuropathy)
Hepatic failure (valproate)
Anemia (aplastic anemia)
Leukopenia
Thrombocytopenia (valproate)
Rashes
Systemic lupus erythematosus, scleroderma, Sjögren syndrome
Hyponatremia (carbamazepine)
Altered thyroid function tests (phenytoin)

or corrected by intravenous administration of glucose (50 ml of 50% glucose solution).

2. Tracheal intubation as facilitated by short-acting muscle relaxants (short duration necessary to confirm that seizure activity is suppressed) may be needed to protect the patient's lungs from aspiration and to optimize delivery of oxygen and adequate removal of carbon dioxide.

D. **Management of anesthesia.** See Table 17–33.

≡ Table 17–33 • Management of Anesthesia in Patients with Seizure Disorders

Consider effects of antiepileptic therapy (sedation, enzyme induction)
Selection of drugs for anesthesia may be influenced by effects on central nervous system electrical activity
    Methohexital (may activate epileptic foci)
    Ketamine (unpredictable)
    Propofol
    Atracurium and cisatracurium (laudanosine)
    Enflurane (unique among inhaled anesthetics in evoking seizure activity)
Drugs that do not lower the seizure threshold
    Thiobarbiturates
    Opioids
    Benzodiazepines
    Isoflurane, desflurane, sevoflurane

≡ Table 17–34 • Characteristics of Headaches Encountered During the Perioperative Period

---

Migraine Headaches
Visual blurring
Nausea and vomiting
Traditional explanation is cerebral vasoconstriction followed by vasodilation (abnormal serotonergic transmission may be more likely)
Treatment is with β-adrenergic antagonists as prophylaxis; selective antagonists of serotoninic receptors (sumatriptan) are effective
No known anesthetic risks
Cluster Headaches
Excruciating unilateral temple or molar pain (visual disturbances, ptosis, and miosis may occur)
Headaches Associated with Increased Intracranial Pressure
See Table 17–2
Headaches Associated with Benign Intracranial Hypertension
Intracranial pressure > 20 mmHg in absence of focal intracranial lesions
Often obese women
Treatment is daily lumbar puncture to remove 20–40 ml of cerebrospinal fluid (may add acetazolamide and dexamethasone; lumboperitoneal shunt in resistant patients)
Management of anesthesia as if an intracranial tumor is present (spinal anesthesia may be therapeutic; but if shunt is present it may be ineffective as local anesthetic is lost)

IX. HEADACHES

Headaches are usually benign. During the postoperative period, headaches may reflect perioperative caffeine withdrawal (Table 17–34).

X. INTERVERTEBRAL DISC HERNIATION

Intervertebral disc herniation is confirmed by CT (Table 17–35).

XI. SLEEP DISORDERS

Sleep disorders include excessive daytime somnolence (obstructive sleep apnea, narcolepsy), insomnia (idiopathic or associated with psychiatric disorders including alcohol abuse), and abnormal movements ("restless leg syndrome").

≡ Table 17–35 • Intervertebral Disc Herniation

Cervical Disc Disease

Lateral protrusion of a cervical disc occurs at C5-6 (neck pain radiates down arm to thumbs) or C6-7 (pain in scapula to middle and index fingers)

Treatment is traction followed by surgical decompression if necessary

Lumbar Disc Disease

Lumbar disc protrusion is usually at the L4-5 or L5-S1 intervertebral spaces [produces low back pain, which radiates down the posterior and lateral aspects of the thigh and calf ("sciatica")]

Treatment has historically included bed rest and use of centrally acting muscle relaxants (continuing ordinary activities within limits permitted by pain equally acceptable); surgical laminectomy or microdiscectomy to decompress compressed nerve roots if symptoms persist; epidural corticosteroids may decrease inflammation and edema but do not decrease the need for surgery and may suppress the hypothalamic-pituitary-adrenal axis

Degenerative Vertebral Column Disease (Cervical Spondylosis)

Narrowing of the spinal canal and compression of the spinal cord by osteophytes

Neck and shoulder pain accompanied by sensory loss and skeletal muscle wasting

Spina Bifida Occulta

Spinal cord may end below the L2-3 interspace ("tethered spinal cord") in association with cutaneous manifestations (tufts of hair, hyperpigmented areas, cutaneous lipomas, skin dimples)

Performance of spinal anesthesia may be associated with an increased risk of lacerating vessels on the surface of the spinal cord (spinal hematomas)

Treatment of transient insomnia is with intermediate-acting benzodiazepines (temazepam), whereas insomnia due to depression is most often treated with sedative-antidepressants (trazodone).

A. **Narcolepsy** is a distinct neurologic disorder with a genetic predisposition. It is characterized by an uncontrollable urge to sleep and by abnormal rapid eye movement sleep.

    1. **Treatment** is with central nervous system stimulants (methylphenidate, dextroamphetamine, pemoline).

    2. **Management of anesthesia.** Anesthetic implications in patients with narcolepsy include possible increased

sensitivity to anesthetic drugs, increased risk of postoperative apnea (avoid intraoperative opioids), and interactions with treatment medications (vasodilation and hypotension).

B. **Postoperative sleep disturbances** may contribute to altered mental (cognitive) function, postoperative episodic arterial hypoxemia, and hemodynamic instability, especially in elderly patients.

1. **Treatment.** The magnitude and duration of the surgical procedure determines the degree of postoperative sleep disturbances, suggesting that a decrease in the surgical stress response, as associated with minimally invasive surgical techniques, may be helpful.

2. Postoperative pain is the most common cause for nighttime awakening. Provision of analgesia (continuous neural blockade using local anesthetics, as morphine may disrupt sleep patterns, and use of nonsteroidal antiinflammatory drugs to maximize opioid sparing effects) is the most effective intervention to improve sleep. Noise, nocturnal nursing procedures, and calorie deprivation are known factors that disrupt normal sleep patterns.

3. **Factitious disorder as a cause for failure to awaken.** Patient unwillingness to awaken ("hysteria") following general anesthesia is a rare but recognized phenomenon. It is, by necessity, a diagnosis of exclusion (rule out physiologic causes including residual effects of anesthetic drugs, inadequate antagonism of neuromuscular blocking drugs, hypoglycemia, electrolyte abnormalities, impaired oxygenation, impaired ventilation, hypothermia, organic cerebral insult).

4. **Circadian rhythm and sleep.** Disturbances in circadian rhythms (jet lag, changes in work hours, blindness) often result in sleep disturbances (melatonin secretion is based on light-dark cycles). Claims of effectiveness of melatonin for managing jet lag were exaggerated.

XII. ABNORMAL BREATHING PATTERNS

See Table 17–36.

XIII. ACUTE MOUNTAIN SICKNESS

Acute mountain sickness is most likely due to cerebral edema with ascent to altitudes > 3600 meters. Prompt descent from altitude and oxygen therapy are the principal treatments.

☰ Table 17–36 • Abnormal Breathing Patterns

Breathing Pattern	Description	Site of Lesion
Ataxic (Biot's breathing)	Unpredictable sequence of breaths varying in rate and tidal volume	Medulla
Apneustic breathing	Repetitive gasps and prolonged pauses at full inspiration	Pons
Cheyne-Stokes breathing	Cyclic crescendo-decrescendo tidal volume pattern interrupted by apnea	Cerebral hemispheres Congestive heart failure
Central neurogenic hypoventilation	Hypocarbia	Cerebral thrombosis or embolism
Posthyperventilation apnea	Awake apnea following moderately decreased $PaCO_2$	Frontal lobes

XIV. DISORDERS INVOLVING THE AUDITORY PROCESSES

Vertigo is the cardinal symptom of vestibular dysfunction and may be accompanied by nausea, vomiting, nystagmus, postural instability, and autonomic nervous system stimulation.

A. Meniere's disease (endolymphatic hydrops) is a disorder of the membranous labyrinth of the inner ear characterized by the triad of hearing loss, tinnitus, and vertigo.

B. Nitrous oxide and middle ear dynamics

1. The middle ear is an air-filled cavity bounded by the tympanic membrane and the inner ear. During inhalation of nitrous oxide middle ear pressures may increase, reflecting passage of nitrous oxide into the noncompliant confines of the middle ear. Under normal conditions, this pressure buildup is passively vented through the eustachian tubes into the nasopharynx.

2. Narrowing of the eustachian tubes by acute inflammation or the presence of scar tissue (as follows ade-

noidectomy) impairs the ability of the middle ear to vent passively pressure increases produced by nitrous oxide. Tympanic membrane rupture (bright red blood in the external auditory canal) and disruption of previous middle ear reconstructive surgery (postoperative hearing loss) may occur (highly unlikely) when nitrous oxide is administered under these conditions.

3. Absorption of nitrous oxide after discontinuing inhalation of this drug can result in negative pressure in the middle ear resulting in transient postoperative hearing loss and/or serous otitis.

XV. GLOMUS TUMORS OF THE HEAD AND NECK

Glomus tumors of the head and neck arise from neuroendocrine tissues that lie along the carotid artery, aorta, glossopharyngeal nerve, and middle ear.

A. **Signs and symptoms.** Tumor location determines the signs and symptoms, which most often reflect middle ear invasion (hearing loss) and cranial nerve invasion (facial paralysis, dysphagia and recurrent aspiration, upper airway obstruction).

B. **Treatment** is irradiation or surgical excision.

C. **Management of anesthesia.** See Table 17–37.

XVI. CAROTID SINUS SYNDROME

Carotid sinus syndrome is caused by exaggeration of normal activity of baroreceptors (bradycardia, hypotension) in re-

---

Table 17–37 • Management of Anesthesia for Excision of Glomus Jugulare Tumors

Possible symptoms related to catecholamine secretion (preoperative phenoxybenzamine or prazosin) or serotonin secretion (carcinoid syndrome)
Evidence of aspiration
Evidence of increased intracranial pressure
Invasive monitoring (avoid cannulation of central veins that may be invaded by tumor)
Risk of airway obstruction
Hypothermia accompanying prolonged surgery
Controlled hypotension may be utilized
Venous air embolism a risk (sudden death)
Need to identify facial nerve may influence use of muscle relaxants

---

**≡ Table 17–38 • Signs and Symptoms
of Neurofibromatosis**

Café au lait spots
Neurofibromatosis
    Cutaneous
    Neural
    Vascular
Intracranial tumors
Spinal cord tumors
Pseudarthrosis
Kyphoscoliosis
Short stature
Cancer
Endocrine dysfunction
Learning disability
Seizures
Congenital heart disease
Pulmonic stenosis

---

sponse to mechanical stimulation. Infiltration of lidocaine around the carotid sinus may improve hemodynamic stability.

XVII. NEUROFIBROMATOSIS

A. **Signs and symptoms.** See Table 17–38.
B. **Management of anesthesia** considers the multiple clinical features of this disease (possible presence of pheochromocytoma, increased ICP, upper airway obstruction).

18

Diseases of the Liver and Biliary Tract

Diseases of the liver and biliary tract can be categorized as parenchymal liver disease (acute and chronic hepatitis, cirrhosis of the liver) or cholestasis with or without obstruction of the extrahepatic biliary pathways (Stoelting RK, Dierdorf SF. Diseases of the liver and biliary tract. In: Anesthesia and Co-Existing Disease, 4th ed. New York, Churchill Livingstone, 2002;299–324).

I. ACUTE HEPATITIS

Acute hepatitis is most often due to a virus, although drugs and toxins can also cause it. Classic acute hepatitis is caused by one of five viruses (Table 18–1).

A. Viral hepatitis. The five types of viral hepatitis are similar and cannot be distinguished reliably by clinical features or laboratory tests. The diagnostic laboratory abnormality of acute hepatitis is a markedly increased serum aminotransferase concentration.

1. **Classification.** See Table 18–2.

2. **Diagnosis** of viral hepatitis depends on the appearance of clinical signs and symptoms, laboratory findings, serologic assays, and in some patients a liver biopsy (Table 18–3).

3. **Clinical course.** Hepatitis typically produces symptoms for 7 to 14 days before the appearance of dark urine and jaundice. Chronic hepatitis does not occur after hepatitis A but develops in 1% to 5% of patients infected with hepatitis B virus and in 85% of patients infected with hepatitis C virus.

4. **Treatment** of acute viral hepatitis is symptomatic with restriction of physical activity to levels comfortable for the patient. Acute hepatitis C is usually asymptomatic, but when chronic hepatitis C is recognized administration of interferon combined with ribavirin is recommended.

≡ **Table 18–1** • Etiology of Viral Hepatitis

Hepatitis A virus (HAV)
Hepatitis B virus (HBV) (accounts for 50% of reported cases of
  acute viral hepatitis in adults)
Hepatitis C virus (HCV)
Hepatitis D virus (HDV)
Hepatitis E virus (HEV)
Viruses that cause systemic illness and also affect the liver
  Cytomegalovirus (CMV)
  Epstein-Barr virus (EBV)

    5. **Prevention** of viral hepatitis includes avoidance of exposure to the virus, passive immunization with gamma globulin, and active immunization with specific vaccines (heaptitis B vaccine, hepatitis A vaccine).

  B. Additional viruses that cause hepatitis

    1. **Cytomegalovirus,** a herpes virus, is ubiquitous and may cause liver dysfunction that mimics viral hepatitis.

    2. **Epstein-Barr virus** usually produces mild hepatitis associated with nausea and vomiting that is part of the clinical syndrome of infectious mononucleosis.

  C. Drug-induced hepatitis. Many drugs (analgesics, volatile anesthetics, antibiotics, antihypertensives, anticonvulsants, tranquilizers) can cause hepatitis that is indistinguishable histologically from acute viral hepatitis. These idiosyncratic drug reactions are rare, unpredictable, and not dose-dependent.

    1. **Acetaminophen overdose** (usually associated with suicide attempts) produces profound hepatocellular necrosis in most persons (hepatic glutathione stores are depleted, and the toxic metabolites accumulate and destroy liver cells). Oral *N*-acetylcysteine administered within 8 hours of acetaminophen overdose decreases the hepatotoxicity.

    2. **Volatile anesthetics** may produce mild, self-limiting postoperative liver dysfunction (increased serum α-glutathione S-transferase concentrations) that likely reflects anesthetic-induced alterations in hepatic oxygen delivery relative to demand resulting in inadequate hepatocyte oxygenation.

      a. **Immune-mediated hepatotoxicity** is a rare but life-threatening form of hepatic dysfunction following

Table 18–2 • Characteristic Features of Viral Hepatitis

Characteristic	Type A	Type B	Type C	Type D
Mode of transmission	Fecal-oral; sewage-contaminated shellfish	Percutaneous; sexual	Percutaneous	Percutaneous
Incubation period	20–37 days	60–110 days	35–70 days	60–110 days
Results of serum antigen and antibody tests	IgM early; IgG appears during convalescence	HbsAg and anti-HBc early; persists in carriers	Anti-HVC in 6 weeks to 9 months	Anti-HVD late; may be short-lived
Immunity	Antibodies in 45%	Antibodies in 5%–15%	Unknown	Protected if immune to type B
Course	Does not progress to chronic liver disease	Chronic liver disease develops in 1%–5% of adults and 80%–90% of children	Chronic liver disease develops in 85%	Co-infection with type B
Prevention after exposure	Pooled gamma globulin	Hepatitis B immune globulin Hepatitis B vaccine	Unknown	Unknown
Mortality	< 0.2%	0.3%–1.5%	Unknown	2–20% (acute icteric hepatitis)

IgM, IgG, immunoglobulin M and G; HBsAg, hepatitis B surface antigen; HBc, hepatitis B core; HVC, hepatitis virus C; HVD, hepatitis virus D. Adapted from: Keefe EB. Acute hepatitis. Sci Am Med 1999;1–9.

≡ Table 18–3 • Diagnosis of Viral Hepatitis

Signs and Symptoms
Dark urine
Fatigue
Anorexia
Nausea
Fever
Emesis
Headache
Aminotransferase Concentration
Sensitive indicator of liver cell injury; increased 7–14 days before
   the appearance of jaundice
Laboratory Tests
Anemia
Leukocytosis
Bilirubinemia
Hypoalbuminemia
Serologic Measurements
Used to identify type of viral hepatitis
Liver Biopsy

---

administration of volatile anesthetics (most often halothane: *halothane hepatitis*). Immunoglobulin G antibodies are formed and directed against liver microsomal proteins on the surfaces of hepatocytes that have been covalently modified by reactive oxidative trifluoroacetyl halide metabolites of halothane to form neoantigens.

b. Like halothane, the fluorinated volatile anesthetics enflurane, isoflurane, and desflurane may form trifluoroacetyl halide metabolites resulting in cross-sensitivity with halothane. The incidence of hepatitis after these anesthetics, however, is lower than after halothane because the degree of anesthetic metabolism is less.

c. The chemical structure of sevoflurane is such that it does not undergo metabolism to trifluoroacetyl halide metabolites and thus would not be expected to produce immune-mediated hepatotoxicity or to cause cross-sensitivity in patients previously exposed to halothane.

d. **Differential diagnosis of postoperative hepatic dysfunction.** When postoperative hepatic dysfunction occurs, a predetermined approach, including serial liver function tests and a search for extrahepatic causes of hepatic dysfunction, facilitates the differential diagnosis (Table 18–4). The causes of postoperative hepatic dysfunction are likely multifactorial and difficult to confirm. When postoperative hepatic dysfunction occurs, it is important to determine the etiology rather than assuming that the history of an anesthetic establishes a cause-and-effect relation between hepatic dysfunction and the volatile anesthetic (Table 18–5).

II. CHRONIC HEPATITIS

Chronic hepatitis encompasses an etiologically diverse group of diseases characterized by long-term elevation (> 6 months) of liver chemistries and by hepatic inflammation seen on liver biopsy.

A. **Signs and symptoms** of chronic hepatitis range from asymptomatic disease to fulminant hepatic failure. The most common symptoms of chronic hepatitis are fatigue and mild abdominal pain.

B. **Laboratory tests.** Serum aminotransferase concentrations are increased, and in severe forms serum albumin concentrations are decreased and prothrombin times are prolonged.

C. **Autoimmune hepatitis** is characterized by hypergammaglobinemia and the presence of antinuclear antibodies. Treatment with corticosteroids prolongs survival.

D. **Chronic hepatitis B** is present in 5% of the world's population and an estimated 0.2% to 0.5% of the U.S. population are chronic carriers of hepatitis B surface antigen (HBsAg).

1. **Treatment.** The goal of treatment of chronic hepatitis B is to eradicate the hepatitis B virus and prevent the development of cirrhosis or hepatocellular cancer. No available therapy achieves these goals.

2. **Interferon** results in suppression of hepatitis B virus replication in about 40% of patients and resolution of symptoms of cirrhosis in about one-third of affected patients; it prolongs life.

Table 18–4 • Liver Function Tests and Differential Diagnosis

Hepatic Dysfunction	Bilirubin	Aminotransferase Enzymes	Alkaline Phosphatase	Causes
Prehepatic	Increased unconjugated fraction	Normal	Normal	Hemolysis Hematoma resorption Bilirubin overload from whole blood
Intrahepatic (intracellular)	Increased conjugated fraction	Markedly increased	Normal to slightly increased	Viral Drugs Sepsis Hypoxemia Cirrhosis
Posthepatic (cholestatic)	Increased conjugated fraction	Normal to slightly increased	Markedly increased	Stones Sepsis

☰ Table 18–5 • Steps to Determine the Etiology of Postoperative Hepatic Dysfunction

Review all drugs administered (analgesics, antibiotics, over-the-counter preparations)

Check for sources of sepsis

Evaluate the possibility of increased exogenous bilirubin overload (blood transfusions)

Rule out occult hematomas (resorption may produce hyperbilirubinemia)

Rule out hemolysis

Review perioperative records (hypotension, arterial hypoxemia, hypoventilation, hypovolemia)

Consider extrahepatic abnormalities (congestive heart failure, respiratory failure, pulmonary embolism, renal insufficiency)

Consider the possibility of benign postoperative intrahepatic cholestasis (associated with extensive and prolonged surgery often with hypotension, arterial hypoxemia, and massive blood transfusions)

Consider the possibility of immune-mediated hepatotoxicity (clinical history of a recent anesthetic that included a volatile anesthetic; confirm diagnosis by documentating the presence of circulating anti-trifluoroacetyl antibodies)

E. **Chronic hepatitis C** infection follows acute hepatitis C virus infection in 85% of patients. An estimated 1.8% of the population in the United States are carriers of hepatitis C virus.

   1. **Diagnosis** of hepatitis C is based on increased serum aminotransferase concentrations and the presence of antibodies to hepatitis C virus. The natural history of hepatitis C is insidious progression with the ultimate development of cirrhosis after about 30 years.

   2. **Treatment.** Interferon normalizes or decreases serum aminotransferase concentrations and decreases inflammation, as indicated by liver biopsy in about one-half of patients with chronic hepatitis C. Chronic hepatitis C with liver failure is one of the most common indications for liver transplantation.

F. **Less common causes of chronic hepatitis.** See Table 18–6.

≡ Table 18–6 • Less Common Causes of Chronic Hepatitis

Drug-induced chronic hepatitis (methyldopa, trazodone, isoniazid)
Wilson's disease (confirmed by liver biopsy and determination of hepatic copper content)
α_1-Antitrypsin deficiency
Primary biliary cirrhosis
Primary sclerosing cholangitis

III. CIRRHOSIS OF THE LIVER

Cirrhosis of the liver is the sequela of a large variety of chronic, progressive liver diseases that are most often the result of excessive alcohol ingestion and chronic viral hepatitis (hepatitis B, hepatitis C).

A. **Diagnosis** of cirrhosis of the liver is established by percutaneous liver biopsy. Computed tomography, magnetic resonance imaging, or hepatic ultrasonography with Doppler flow studies may reveal findings consistent with cirrhosis (splenomegaly, ascites, irregular liver surface). Upper gastrointestinal endoscopy often establishes the presence of esophageal varices.

B. **Signs and symptoms.** See Table 18–7.

C. **Specific forms of cirrhosis.** See Table 18–8.

D. **Complications of cirrhosis.** See Table 18–9.

E. **Management of anesthesia for patients with cirrhosis of the liver.** It is estimated that 5% to 10% of all patients with cirrhosis of the liver undergo surgery during the last 2 years of life. In patients who abuse alcohol the preoperative

≡ Table 18–7 • Signs and Symptoms of Cirrhosis of the Liver

Fatigue and malaise
Nondiagnostic physical findings (palmar erythema, spider nevi, gynecomastia, testicular atrophy, splenomegaly, ascites)
Decreased hepatic blood flow
Hepatomegaly (left lobe palpable below the xiphoid cartilage)
Decreased serum albumin concentration
Prolonged prothrombin time

▬ Table 18–8 • Specific Forms of Cirrhosis of the Liver

Alcoholic cirrhosis [directly attributable to chronic ingestion of large quantities of alcohol usually in association with malnutrition; diagnosis suggested by finding of an aspartate aminotransferase/alanine aminotransferase (AST/SLT) ratio of at least 2 : 1]

Postnecrotic cirrhosis [shrunken liver; predominates in females; cause often unknown ("crytogenic hepatitis"); primary liver cell cancer may develop]

Primary biliary cirrhosis (likely role of immune mechanisms; females; osteoporosis common; CREST syndrome may be present)

Hemochromatosis (iron deposits in the liver; males; diabetes mellitus, congestive heart failure, and liver cell cancer; treatment is phlebotomies)

Wilson's disease [autosomal disorder due to genetic defect in copper binding; neurologic and hepatic dysfunction (jaundice, ascites, splenomegaly, varices); treatment is with chelating drugs]

α_1-Antitrypsin deficiency (accompanying pulmonary emphysema)

Jejunoileal bypass (hepatic fat accumulation following surgery; operation no longer performed)

Nonalcoholic steatohepatitis (fat accumulation in liver associated with obesity, hyperlipidemia, and diabetes mellitus; females)

---

presence of ascites, sepsis, and chronic obstructive pulmonary disease are associated with increased postoperative morbidity (pneumonia, bleeding, sepsis, poor wound healing, further deterioration of liver function) and mortality.

1. **Preoperative preparation.** Preoperative criteria may correlate with the surgical risk and the postoperative outcome in patients with cirrhosis of the liver undergoing major surgery (Table 18–10). Identifying co-existing problems that could be optimally managed preoperatively (cardiorespiratory function, coagulation status, renal function, intravascular fluid volume, electrolyte balance, nutrition) may decrease morbidity and mortality associated with elective surgery in patients with severe liver disease.

   a. Parenteral vitamin K is administered if prothrombin times are prolonged. Thrombocytopenia may require treatment preoperatively.

≡ Table 18–9 • Complications of Cirrhosis of the Liver

Portal vein hypertension (hepatomegaly with or without ascites)
Gastroesophageal varices (treatment is endoscopic therapy with
    banding, ligation or sclerotherapy)
Ascites (portal vein hypertension and decreased serum albumin
    concentrations contribute to formation; treatment is drug-
    induced diuresis with an aldosterone antagonist, paracentesis is
    an alternative to diuretic therapy)
Spontaneous bacterial peritonitis (fever, leukocytosis, abdominal
    pain, decreased bowel sounds)
Hepatorenal syndrome
Malnutrition
Hyperdynamic circulation [increased cardiac output presumed to
    be due to vasodilating substances (glucagon), increased
    intravascular fluid volume, decreased blood viscosity due to
    anemia, arteriovenous communications especially in the lungs]
Cardiomyopathy (congestive heart failure)
Megaloblastic anemia (antagonism of folate by alcohol)
Thrombocytopenia
Accumulation of fibrin degradation products
Arterial hypoxemia (impaired diaphragm movement due to ascites,
    right-to-left intrapulmonary shunts in presence of portal vein
    hypertension, chronic obstructive pulmonary disease,
    pneumonia)
Hypoglycemia
Duodenal ulcer
Gallstones
Impaired immune defense mechanisms (alcohol suppresses)
Hepatic encephalopathy (mental obtundation, asterixis, fetor
    hepaticus; treatment includes dietary protein restriction and
    administration of lactulose; liver transplantation)

≡ Table 18–10 • Prediction of Surgical Risk Based on Preoperative Evaluation

Evaluation	Minimal	Modest	Marked
Bilirubin (mg/dl)	< 2	2–3	> 3
Albumin (g/dl)	> 3.5	3.0–3.5	< 3
Prothrombin time (seconds prolonged)	1–4	4–6	> 6
Encephalopathy	None	Moderate	Severe
Nutrition	Excellent	Good	Poor
Ascites	None	Moderate	Marked

Adapted from Strunin I. Preoperative assessment of the patient with liver
dysfunction. Br J Anaesth 1978;50:25–34.

b. Hypoglycemia is a possibility, and administration of glucose solutions are considerations during the perioperative period.

c. Assurance of adequate hydration with crystalloid solutions is evidenced by establishment of preoperative diuresis.

2. **Intraoperative management.** The optimal anesthetic drug or technique in the presence of liver disease is unknown. It is important to remember that a constant feature of chronic liver disease is decreased hepatic blood flow owing to increased resistance to blood flow through the portal vein (hepatic blood flow and hepatocyte oxygenation are more dependent on hepatic artery blood flow than in normal patients). It is prudent to limit the dose of volatile anesthetics (combine with nitrous oxide and/or opioids) to minimize the likelihood of persistent mean arterial pressure decreases.

a. Chronic alcohol ingestion may result in resistance to the effects of sedative drugs. In contrast to resistance to depressant drugs, alcohol-induced cardiomyopathy could make these patients unusually sensitive to the cardiac depressant effects of volatile anesthetics. There may be decreased responsiveness to catecholamines manifesting as impaired tolerance to acute surgical blood loss.

b. Regardless of the drugs selected for anesthesia, postoperative liver dysfunction is likely to be exaggerated in patients with chronic liver disease, presumably owing to the detrimental nonspecific effects of anesthetic drugs and to stress-induced activation of the sympathetic nervous system on hepatocyte oxygenation.

c. Regional anesthesia is useful in patients with advanced liver disease, assuming that coagulation status is acceptable.

d. **Muscle relaxants.** The role of the liver in the clearance of muscle relaxants is considered when selecting these drugs for administration to patients with cirrhosis of the liver (atracurium and cisatracurium are not dependent on liver clearance mechanisms).

e. **Monitoring** intraoperative arterial blood gases, pH, and urine output as well as providing exogenous glucose are important principles. Fluid administration must be carefully titrated in patients with cirrhosis of the liver (consider monitoring cardiac filling pressures).

3. **Postoperative management.** Regardless of the drugs selected for anesthesia, postoperative liver dysfunction is likely to be exaggerated in patients with chronic liver disease. Sepsis is a consideration when postoperative liver dysfunction occurs. Manifestations of alcohol withdrawal syndrome usually appear 48 to 72 hours after cessation of drinking and represents a life-threatening medical emergency.

4. **Intoxicated alcoholic patients.** In contrast to chronic but sober alcoholic patients, acutely intoxicated patients require less anesthetic, as there are additive depressant effects between alcohol and anesthetics. Intoxicated patients may be more vulnerable to regurgitation of gastric contents, as alcohol slows gastric emptying and decreases the tone of the lower esophageal sphincter. Surgical bleeding may reflect alcohol-induced interference with platelet aggregation.

IV. IDIOPATHIC HYPERBILIRUBINEMIA

See Table 18–11.

V. ACUTE HEPATIC FAILURE

Acute hepatic failure is characterized by altered mental status (hepatic encephalopathy) and impaired coagulation in the clinical setting (Table 18–12).

≡ Table 18–11 • Idiopathic Hyperbilirubinemia

Gilbert syndrome (defect is decreased bilirubin uptake by hepatocytes; present in varying degrees in 5–10% of the population)

Crigler-Najjar syndrome (decreased or absent glucuronyl transferase enzyme)

Dubin-Johnson syndrome (conjugated hyperbilirubinemia)

Alagille syndrome (intrahepatic cholestasis)

Benign postoperative intrahepatic cholestasis (prolonged surgery especially if complicated by hypotension, arterial hypoxemia, and need for blood transfusions)

Progressive familial intrahepatic cholestasis (end-stage hepatic cirrhosis develops before adulthood)

☰	**Table 18–12** • Causes of Acute Liver Failure

Viral Hepatitis
Drug-Induced
Acetaminophen
Idiosyncratic reactions
    Volatile anesthetics (especially halothane)
    Isoniazid
    Phenytoin
    Sulfonamides
    Propylthiouracil
    Amiodarone
Toxins
Carbon tetrachloride
Mushrooms
Vascular Events
Ischemia
Venoocclusive disease (Budd-Chiari syndrome)
Miscellaneous
Acute fatty liver of pregnancy
Wilson's syndrome
Reye syndrome

Adapted from: Lee WM. Acute liver failure. N Engl J Med 1993;329:1862–72.

A. **Signs and symptoms.** Typically, nonspecific symptoms, such as malaise or nausea, develop in previously healthy individuals, followed by jaundice, the rapid onset of altered mental status, and coma (rapid progression with coma developing in 2 to 10 days).

   1. **Acute fatty liver of pregnancy** is characterized by accumulation of fat within hepatocytes and often evidence of developing pregnancy-induced hypertension (laboratory results characteristic of the HEELP syndrome) during the third trimester of pregnancy.

   2. **Treatment is prompt termination of pregnancy.**

B. **Treatment.** There are no specific treatments of proven efficacy for management of acute liver failure (specific antidotes for acetaminophen poisoning, glucose for hypoglycemia). Cerebral edema may require aggressive intervention in the hope of preventing cerebral herniation. When survival seems unlikely (prothrombin time > 100 seconds), the only curative treatment is liver transplantation.

C. **Management of anesthesia.** See Table 18–13.

≡ Table 18–13 • Management of Anesthesia for Patients with Acute Liver Failure

Life-saving surgery only
Correct coagulation abnormalities (fresh frozen plasma)
Nitrous oxide may be sufficient for analgesia and amnesia
Consider clearance mechanisms when selecting muscle relaxants
(often associated renal dysfunction)
Exogenous glucose
Slow infusion of blood to minimize likelihood of citrate intoxication
Maintain urine output with crystalloids and/or colloids (mannitol if
necessary)
Invasive monitoring
Strict asepsis
Initiate lactulose therapy

VI. LIVER TRANSPLANTATION

Liver transplantation is the only curative therapy for patients with liver failure, as due to end-stage liver disease associated with cirrhosis of the liver. Hepatoma, biliary tract tumors, and genetically determined metabolic disturbances may also be treated with liver transplantation.

A. Management of anesthesia. Candidates for liver transplantation may present with severe multiple system organ dysfunction. Many of the physiologic derangements (coagulation defects) are not correctable until after successful liver transplantation. The likely presence of hepatitis A, B, or C in the recipient must be considered by the health care providers.

1. **Induction and maintenance of anesthesia.** For induction of anesthesia one may need to consider the presence of ascites and an associated slowing of gastric emptying. Maintenance of anesthesia is with drugs that preserve splanchnic circulation combined with muscle relaxants that are not dependent on hepatic clearance mechanisms. Nitrous oxide is usually avoided based on concerns regarding bowel distension and the ability of nitrous oxide to increase the size of bubbles (air emboli) that may enter the circulation.

    a. Fluid warming devices and rapid infusion systems designed to deliver prewarmed fluids or blood products at rates exceeding 1 L/min are routinely employed.

    b. Monitoring systemic blood pressure via the radial artery is preferred over infradiaphragmatic sites because the abdominal aorta may be cross-clamped during hepatic arterial anastomosis. Clamping the inferior vena cava above the liver dictates placement of venous access catheters above the diaphragm.

    2. Preanhepatic phase involves mobilization and removal of the native liver. Cardiovascular instability (hemorrhage, impaired venous return) and oliguria are common.

    3. Anhepatic phase begins when the native liver is removed, following which support of cardiac output with inotropes and relief of venous congestion (occlusion of inferior vena cava) with a venovenous bypass system may be needed.

    4. Neohepatic phase begins with reanastomosis of the major vascular structures. Subsequent unclamping can release large amounts of potassium and metabolic acids (cardiac dysrhythmias and hypotension). Postoperative support of the recipient's ventilation and oxygenation is likely to be needed.

B. Anesthetic considerations in liver transplant recipients. Potential adverse effects (systemic hypertension, anemia, thrombocytopenia) and drug interactions related to chronic immunosuppressive therapy are considered when planning management of anesthesia. Liver function tests and drug metabolizing capabilities return to normal following liver transplantation. There is no evidence of an increased risk of developing hepatitis after administration of volatile anesthetics to liver transplant recipients.

VII. DISEASES OF THE BILIARY TRACT

Cholelithiasis and inflammatory biliary tract disease constitute major health problems in the United States, with an estimated 10% of adults > 40 years of age having gallstones (prevalence higher in women).

A. Cholelithiasis and cholecystitis. Patients who have stones in the gallbladder or biliary tree manifest symptoms that range from acute disease to chronic symptomatic or silent disease.

    1. Acute cholecystitis is nearly always caused by an obstruction of the cystic duct by a gallstone.

        a. Signs and symptoms of acute cholecystitis include nausea, vomiting, fever, severe abdominal pain ("biliary colic"), and right upper quadrant tenderness.

    b. **Diagnosis.** Ultrasonography is noninvasive and is the diagnostic procedure utilized in patients with suspected gallstones and acute cholecystitis.

    c. **Differential diagnosis.** See Table 18–14.

    d. **Treatment.** Patients with a clinical diagnosis of acute cholecystitis are treated with intravenous fluids and electrolytes and administration of opioids for management of pain. Febrile patients are treated with antibiotics. Laparoscopic cholecystectomy is preferred to open cholecystectomy, as postoperative pain and pulmonary complications are less and convalescence is more rapid. Preoperative endoscopic retrograde cholangiopancreatography (ERCP) is recommended for removing common duct stones. If endoscopic removal of common duct stones is not possible, the operative procedure of choice is open cholecystectomy with common bile duct exploration and stone removal.

    e. **Complications.** Localized perforation and abscess formation are likely when symptoms persist for several days. Gallstone ileus results from obstruction of the small bowel at some point (usually the ileocecal valve) by a large gallstone.

    f. **Management of anesthesia.** See Table 18–15.

2. **Chronic cholecystitis** is associated with chronic cholelithiasis and a series of acute cholecystitis attacks. Ultrasonography is used to diagnose chronic cholecystitis; treatment is elective cholecystectomy.

3. **Alternative forms of therapy for cholelithiasis** include oral dissolution therapy (recurrence after discontinuation of ursodiol is common) and extracorporeal biliary lithotripsy.

Table 18–14 • Differential Diagnosis of Acute Cholecystitis

Acute viral hepatitis
Alcoholic hepatitis
Penetrating duodenal ulcer
Appendicitis
Pyelonephritis
Right lower lobe pneumonia
Pancreatitis
Acute myocardial infarction

☰ Table 18–15 • Management of Anesthesia for Laparoscopic Cholecystectomy

Creation of pneumoperitoneum (carbon dioxide) may interfere with spontaneous ventilation and venous return

Head-down position improves operative visualization

Mechanical ventilation of the lungs

Tracheal intubation

Capnography (facilitates recognition of venous carbon dioxide embolism)

Decompression of stomach with an orogastric tube

Vigilance for recognizing accidental injury to abdominal structures and blood vessels (prompt open laparotomy when loss of hemostasis)

No evidence that nitrous oxide expands bowel gas or interferes with surgical working conditions

Use of opioids is controversial (choledochoduodenal sphincter spasm)

B. **Choledocholithiasis** is lodgement of a stone in the common bile duct after passage from the gallbladder and the cystic duct.

   1. **Signs and symptoms** may include fever, shaking chills, jaundice, and right upper quadrant pain as evidence of cholangitis.

   2. **Diagnosis.** Ultrasonography may reveal a dilated common bile duct.

   3. **Differential diagnosis** includes ureterolithiasis (similar pain but liver function tests are normal), acute pancreatitis, acute myocardial infarction, and viral hepatitis.

   4. **Treatment** is endoscopic sphincterotomy. ERCP can be used to identify the cause of common bile duct obstruction and to remove a stone or place a stent.

19

Diseases of the Gastrointestinal System

The principal function of the gastrointestinal tract is to provide the body with continual supplies of water, nutrients, and electrolytes (Stoelting RK, Dierdorf SF. Diseases of the gastrointestinal system. In: Anesthesia and Co-Existing Disease, 4th ed. New York, Churchill Livingstone, 2002;325–340).

I. ESOPHAGEAL DISEASES

Dysphagia is the classic symptom produced at some stage in all diseases of the esophagus (evaluate by barium contrast study followed by esophagoscopy).

A. **Diffuse esophageal spasm** occurs most often in elderly patients, and the pain may mimic angina pectoris (some patients respond favorably to nitroglycerin).

B. **Chronic peptic esophagitis** is caused by reflux of acidic gastric fluid into the esophagus producing retrosternal discomfort ("heartburn") relieved by oral administration of antacids. Reflux esophagitis is a common problem (one-third of healthy adults experience symptoms at least once every 30 days). The presumed underlying defect seems to be a decrease in the resting tone of the lower esophageal sphincter. Esophagoscopy is useful for documenting inflammation.

1. **Treatment** of reflux esophagitis is initially with oral antacids and avoidance of substances (fat, chocolate, alcohol, nicotine) that decrease lower esophageal sphincter pressures. Administration of H_2-receptor antagonists may promote healing. Persistent and severe symptoms may be treated with surgical procedures designed to create a valve mechanism by wrapping a gastric pouch around the distal esophagus (Nissen fundoplication).

2. **Management of anesthesia.** See Table 19–1.

≡ Table 19-1 • Management of Anesthesia in Patients with Chronic Peptic Esophagitis

---

Exclude the preoperative presence of pneumonia

Consider known ability of anticholinergic drugs to decrease lower esophageal sphincter pressure (no evidence that incidence of silent regurgitation or aspiration is increased when these drugs are utilized in the preoperative medication)

H_2-Receptor antagonists and/or metoclopramide (not routine)

Succinylcholine increases lower esophageal sphincter pressure

---

    C. **Hiatus hernia** is protrusion of a portion of the stomach through the hiatus of the diaphragm and into the thoracic cavity (sliding type of hernia can be identified in about 30% of patients undergoing upper gastrointestinal examinations). Despite the common association with peptic esophagitis, the presence of a hiatus hernia does not predispose to esophageal reflux, emphasizing the importance of the integrity of the lower esophageal sphincter.

    D. **Esophageal diverticula** are classified, according to their location, as a Zenker's diverticulum (upper esophagus), traction diverticulum (midesophagus), or epiphrenic diverticulum (near the lower esophageal sphincter). Regurgitation of previously ingested food from a Zenker's diverticulum may predispose patients to pulmonary aspiration, even in the absence of recent food intake.

II. PEPTIC ULCER DISEASE

Peptic ulcer disease describes focal defects (ulcerations) in the gastrointestinal mucosa [most commonly the duodenal bulb and distal stomach (antrum)] associated with the presence of hydrochloric acid and pepsin in the gastric fluid.

    A. **Pathogenesis.** See Table 19-2.

    B. **Incidence.** Peptic ulcer disease in the United States affects 10% of men and 4% of women at some time in their lives. Eradication of *Helicobacter pylori* from the stomach and duodenum, especially in patients who smoke, greatly decreases the risk of recurrence of peptic ulcers.

    C. **Diagnosis** of peptic ulcer disease is suggested by clinical signs and symptoms, but ultimately the diagnosis depends on endoscopy or surgery.

☰ Table 19–2 • Risk Factors for the Development of Peptic Ulcer Disease

Presence of hydrochloric acid *and* pepsin (alone not sufficient)

Emotional stress

Infection with *Helicobacter pylori* (most important risk factor and cure of infection decreases the incidence of peptic ulcer recurrence)

Nonsteroidal antiinflammatory drugs (ulcers most often in the stomach; greatest risk of injury occurs during the first 7–30 days after initiation of treatment)

Acute stress ulcers (trauma including head injury and burn injury, septic shock, respiratory failure requiring mechanical ventilation, major surgical procedures; painless upper gastrointestinal bleeding or decreasing hematocrit may be first clinical evidence)

Gastrinoma (Zollinger-Ellison syndrome) [gastrin-secreting tumor that is often associated with other features suggesting multiple endocrine neoplasia type 1 syndrome (parathyroid adenoma, hypercalcemia, pituitary adenoma)]

1. **Signs and symptoms.** Peptic ulcers produce a variety of signs and symptoms, but none is specific for the disease. It is not possible to distinguish symptoms of duodenal ulcers from those of gastric ulcers (Table 19–3).

☰ Table 19–3 • Signs and Symptoms of Peptic Ulcer Disease

Epigastric pain [relieved by food or antacids; severe pain or a rapid increase in pain suggests perforation or another diagnosis (acute pancreatitis)]

Repeated vomiting (suggests gastric outlet obstruction; hypokalemic, hypochloremic metabolic alkalosis may develop)

Hematemesis or melena (peptic ulcers are most common cause of upper gastrointestinal bleeding; hemoglobin concentrations do not reflect initial severity of bleeding; azotemia develops from digestion and intestinal absorption of nitrogenous components)

Anemia (chronic hemorrhage)

Abdominal tenderness or rigidity and absence of bowel sounds (perforation with peritonitis, free air below diaphragm on chest radiography)

2. **Endoscopy** is the most accurate method for confirming the clinical diagnosis of peptic ulcer (biopsy for the presence of *H. pylori* and to exclude malignancy) and the presence of associated bleeding and/or intestinal obstruction. Most patients require local pharyngeal anesthesia and conscious sedation (midazolam) for endoscopy. Complications of endoscopy include depression of ventilation, perforation of the gastrointestinal tract, and bleeding.

3. **Surgery** may be needed to confirm the diagnosis of peptic ulcer disease in certain patients (acute abdomen and diagnosis at exploratory laparotomy; upper gastrointestinal bleeding makes visualization by endoscopy difficult).

D. **Treatment.** See Table 19–4.

1. **Zollinger-Ellison syndrome** is initially treated with proton-pump inhibitors. Curative surgical resection of the gastrinoma is indicated in selected patients.

   a. **Management of anesthesia** for surgical excision of a gastrinoma considers the presence of gastric acid hypersecretion and the likely presence of large gastric fluid volumes at the time of induction of anesthesia (gastric tube placed preoperatively). Depletion of intravascular fluid volume and electrolyte imbalance (hypokalemia, metabolic alkalosis) may accompany profuse watery diarrhea.

   b. **Antacid prophylaxis** with proton-pump inhibitors and H_2-receptor antagonists is maintained until surgery. Intravenous ranitidine is useful for preventing gastric acid hypersecretion during surgery.

2. **Bleeding ulcers.** The first priority in patients with suspected upper gastrointestinal bleeding is stabilization with intravascular fluid volume replacement guided by appropriate hemodynamic monitoring. Surgery is

---

═ Table 19–4 • Treatment of Peptic Ulcer Disease

Eradicate infection with *Helicobacter pylori* (bismuth subsalicylate, metronidazole, and tetracycline)
Discontinue nonsteroidal antiinflammatory drugs
Antacids, H_2-receptor antagonists, and proton-pump inhibitors (sucralfate is an alternative)

---

needed to control bleeding only if endoscopic treatment (injection of epinephrine or saline, thermal application) is not effective.

3. **Perforated ulcers.** When a perforated ulcer is confirmed or highly suspected, patients are rendered NPO with nasogastric suction, evaluated for electrolyte disturbances, and treated with intravenous fluids and broad-spectrum antibiotics. Exploratory laparotomy for closure of the perforation is performed when patients are stabilized.

4. **Obstructing ulcers.** Endoscopic diagnosis of gastrointestinal obstruction due to a peptic ulcer is followed by rendering the patient NPO and instituting nasogastric suction and treatment with intravenous fluids, electrolytes, and H_2-receptor antagonists. Gastric outlet obstruction may resolve over 5 to 14 days as edema subsides during healing of the ulcer. Gastrointestinal obstruction that occurs after endoscopic balloon dilation is an indication for surgical drainage procedures (pyloroplasty, gastroenterostomy) often combined with a vagotomy to decrease the likelihood of recurrent ulceration.

5. **Acute stress ulcers.** Treatment of bleeding acute stress ulcers includes intravascular fluid replacement and attempts to treat the underlying associated disease (endoscopic therapy is not usually curative because multiple bleeding sites are typically present). Patients at high risk for developing bleeding acute stress ulcers (multiple organ failure plus mechanical ventilation) should be treated with prophylactic intragastric or oral antacids or sucralfate or with intravenous H_2-receptor antagonists or proton-pump inhibitors (goal is gastric fluid pH > 4)

III. IRRITABLE BOWEL SYNDROME

Irritable bowel syndrome is characterized by generalized bowel discomfort usually confined to the left lower quadrant. Many patients have associated symptoms of vasomotor instability (tachycardia, hyperventilation, fatigue, headaches), and the feces are often covered with mucus ("mucous colitis"). This syndrome appears to be an intense intraabdominal response to emotional stress.

IV. INFLAMMATORY BOWEL DISEASE

Inflammatory bowel disease is the second most common chronic inflammatory disorder after rheumatoid arthritis (Table 19–5).

A. Ulcerative colitis is an inflammatory disease of the colonic mucosa (exacerbations and remissions) that primarily affects the rectum and distal colon.

1. **Complications** of ulcerative colitis are classified as colonic and extracolonic (Table 19–6).

2. **Treatment** of mild to moderately severe ulcerative colitis is most often with sulfazalazine and 5-aminosalicylic acid. Corticosteroid treatment is indicated for short-term induction of a remission of ulcerative colitis (dependence is often encountered in these patients). The only curative treatment is proctocolectomy with ileostomy. Immunomodulatory drugs (azathioprine, mercaptopurine) are appropriate for long-term treatment of some patients with ulcerative colitis (risks are pancreatitis and bone marrow suppression). Nutritional therapy in patients with ulcerative colitis may be useful to compensate for decreased caloric intake and increased colonic losses.

Table 19–5 • Comparative Features of Ulcerative Colitis and Crohn's Disease

Feature	Ulcerative Colitis	Crohn's Disease
Acute toxicity	Common	Rare
Stools	Bloody and watery	Watery
Perirectal involvement	Occurs in 10%–20% but usually self-limiting	Rectocutaneous fistulas in 50%
Extracolonic complications	Common	Common
Carcinoma of the colon	5% after 10 years	1% but unrelated to extent or duration of the disease
Treatment	Protocolectomy is curative	Recurrence is likely despite surgical resection

▤ Table 19–6 • Complications Associated with Ulcerative Colitis

Colonic Complications
Toxic megacolon (sudden onset of fever, tachycardia, dehydration, dilation of the colon)
Intestinal perforation (corticosteroids may mask symptoms)
Carcinoma of the colon
Hemorrhage
Stricture
Extracolonic Complications
Erythema nodosum
Iritis
Ankylosing spondylitis
Fatty liver infiltration
Pericholangitis
Cirrhosis of the liver

    B. Crohn's disease is characterized by ileal involvement (regional enteritis), and/or colonic involvement (granulomatous colitis), due to unknown causes.

        1. Complications often reflect chronic inflammation of all layers of the bowel (Table 19–7).

        2. Treatment of Crohn's disease is similar to that for ulcerative colitis. In contrast to patients with ulcerative colitis, total parenteral nutrition with bowel rest alleviates symptoms in patients with Crohn's disease. Surgery is necessary when drugs fail to control symptoms or complications of the disease (intra-abdominal fistulas) develop.

▤ Table 19–7 • Complications Associated with Crohn's Disease

Rectal fissures and perirectal abscesses
Intra-abdominal fistulas (often the reason for surgery)
Arthritis
Iritis
Renal stones
Gallstones
Anemia
Hypoalbuminemia (may require hyperalimentation)

C. **Pseudomembranous enterocolitis** is often associated with antibiotic therapy or intestinal ischemia, manifesting as dehydration, hypotension, and metabolic acidosis.

D. **Management of anesthesia** for surgical treatment of inflammatory bowel disease includes preoperative evaluation of intravascular fluid volume and electrolyte status as well as assessment of complications associated with these diseases (Tables 19–6, 19–7). Underlying liver disease may influence the selection of volatile anesthetics and muscle relaxants. In the presence of bowel distension, administration of nitrous oxide may be limited or avoided. The need to provide additional corticosteroids during the perioperative period may be a consideration.

V. CARCINOID TUMORS

Carcinoid tumors arise from enterochromaffin tissues and are typically found in the gastrointestinal tract (stomach, appendix, jejunum, ileum, colon, rectum) but may also occur in the bronchi and lungs. These tumors secrete a variety of amine and neuropeptide hormones, including serotonin, histamine, prostaglandins, corticotropin, and kallikrein (generates kinins including bradykinin).

A. Measurement of the serotonin metabolite 5-hydroxyindoleacetic acid in a 24-hour urine collection may be useful for confirming the diagnosis.

B. **Carcinoid syndrome** is present when systemic effects of carcinoid tumor secretions result in clinical symptoms, reflecting the presence of metastases to the liver or release of secretions from tumors in the lungs. Generally, release of secretory products from tumors in the gastrointestinal tract does not produce clinical symptoms, as the products are destroyed in the liver before reaching the systemic circulation.

1. **Signs and symptoms.** See Table 19–8.

2. **Treatment** of carcinoid syndrome is with the synthetic somatostatin analogue octreotide, which prevents the release of vasoactive products from carcinoid tumors. Surgical resection is the only definitive curative therapy. The development of right-sided heart failure in patients with carcinoid syndrome may be an indication for tricuspid and/or pulmonic valve replacement.

3. **Management of anesthesia.** See Table 19–9.

☰ Table 19–8 • Signs and Symptoms of Carcinoid Syndrome

Episodic cutaneous flushing
Diarrhea
Heart disease
   Tricuspid regurgitation and/or pulmonic stenosis
   Supraventricular tachydysrhythmias
Bronchoconstriction
Hypotension
Hypertension
Abdominal pain (small bowel obstruction)
Hepatomegaly (metastases)
Hyperglycemia
Hypoalbuminemia (pellegra-like skin lesions due to niacin
   deficiency)

☰ Table 19–9 • Management of Anesthesia in the Presence of Carcinoid Tumors

Octreotide 50–150 μg subcutaneously in the preoperative
   medication
Consider inclusion of histamine receptor antagonists in the
   preoperative medication
Octreotide 100 μg/hr IV during surgery
Continue preoperative therapy with octreotide every 8 hours
   throughout the perioperative period
Avoid drugs capable of evoking histamine release (meperidine,
   mivacurium, atracurium) or serotonin release (catecholamines,
   ketamine?)
Treat carcinoid crisis (hypotension and bronchoconstriction) with
   octreotide 100–200 μg IV
Treat systemic hypertension with labetalol or ketanserin
Intravenous induction (propofol, etomidate) plus opioids to blunt
   hypertensive response to direct laryngoscopy and tracheal
   intubation
Maintenance of anesthesia with volatile anesthetics (decreased
   anesthetic requirements and/or delayed awakening may reflect
   sedative effects of serotonin)
Regional anesthesia is controversial, as treatment of associated
   hypotension with catecholamines is not recommended

≣ Table 19–10 • Signs and Symptoms of Acute Pancreatitis

Excruciating and unrelenting midepigastric abdominal pain that radiates through to the back (sitting and leaning forward may decrease the pain)
Nausea and vomiting
Dyspnea (pleural effusion, ascites)
Fever
Obtundation and psychosis (may reflect delirium tremens)
Tetany (hypocalcemia)
Hyperglycemia (occasionally with hemorrhagic pancreatitis)

VI. ACUTE PANCREATITIS

Acute pancreatitis is characterized as an inflammatory disorder of the pancreas that is most likely due to pancreatic autodigestion. Normal pancreatic function is restored once the primary cause of the acute event is resolved.

A. Etiology. Gallstones and alcohol abuse are etiologic factors in most patients with acute pancreatitis. Acute pancreatitis is common in patients with acquired immunodeficiency syndrome (AIDS).

B. Signs and symptoms. See Table 19–10.

C. Diagnosis. The hallmark of acute pancreatitis is increased serum amylase concentrations. Morphologic changes associated with pancreatitis are evident on computed tomogra-

≣ Table 19–11 • Complications Associated with Acute Pancreatitis

Shock (sequestration of large volumes of fluid in the peripancreatic space, hemorrhage, decreased systemic vascular resistance)
Arterial hypoxemia
Acute respiratory distress syndrome
Renal failure
Gastrointestinal hemorrhage
Coagulation defects (disseminated intravascular coagulation)
Pseudocyst formation

≡ Table 19–12 • Treatment of
Acute Pancreatitis

Intravenous fluid administration (up to 10 L of crystalloid)
Colloid replacement if significant hemorrhage
Stop oral intake (rest the pancreas)
Nasogastric suction if persistent vomiting
Intravenous opioids for analgesia
Prophylactic antibiotics
Endoscopic removal of obstructing gallstones
Parenteral feeding if protracted course

---

phy. The differential diagnosis of acute pancreatitis includes perforated duodenal ulcer, acute cholecystitis, mesenteric ischemia, acute myocardial infarction (serum amylase not increased), and pneumonia (fever and epigastric pain).

D. Complications. See Table 19–11.

E. Treatment. See Table 19–12.

VII. CHRONIC PANCREATITIS

Chronic pancreatitis is characterized by chronic inflammation leading to irreversible damage to the pancreas.

A. Etiology. Chronic pancreatitis is most often due to chronic alcohol abuse. Less often, chronic pancreatitis is associated with cystic fibrosis, hyperparathyroidism, or obstruction of the pancreatic duct.

B. Signs and symptoms. Chronic pancreatitis is characterized by epigastric abdominal pain that radiates to the back and is often postprandial. Steatorrhea is present when at least 90% of the pancreas is destroyed.

C. Diagnosis of chronic pancreatitis may be based on a history of chronic alcohol abuse and demonstration of pancreatic calcifications (seen by abdominal radiography). Serum amylase concentrations are usually normal. Ultrasonography is useful for documenting the presence of an enlarged pancreas and identifying fluid-filled pseudocysts. Computed tomography demonstrates dilated pancreatic ducts and changes in the size of the pancreas.

D. Treatment. See Table 19–13.

≡ Table 19–13 • Treatment of Chronic Pancreatitis

Opioids for pain control (celiac plexus block may be considered)
Insulin for diabetes mellitus
Internal surgical drainage (pancreaticojejunostomy) or endoscopic
  placement or stents and extraction of stones
Lipase for treatment of steatorrhea
Surgical resection or cutaneous drainage of pseudocysts
Paracentesis and/or thoracentesis (ascites, pleural effusion)

VIII. MALABSORPTION AND MALDIGESTION

Malabsorption and maldigestion are reflected in impaired absorption of fat (steatorrhea), fat-soluble vitamin deficiencies (vitamins A, D, E, K), and possibly hypocalcemia and hypomagnesemia.

A. **Gluten-sensitive enteropathy** (previously termed celiac disease in children or nontropical sprue in adults) is a disease of the small intestine resulting in malabsorption (steatorrhea), weight loss, abdominal pain, and fatigue. Treatment is removal of gluten (wheat, rye, barley) from the diet.

B. **Small bowel resection** may result in malabsorption if the small intestine bowel surface area is decreased below a critical level. Clinical manifestations of the resulting "short bowel syndrome" include diarrhea, steatorrhea, trace element deficiencies, and electrolyte imbalance (hyponatremia, hypokalemia).

C. **Postgastrectomy steatorrhea** may follow extensive gastric resection surgery. Because of the small stomach, these patients cannot eat large meals; this, in combination with steatorrhea, results in weight loss.

IX. GASTROINTESTINAL BLEEDING

See Table 19–14.

A. **Upper gastrointestinal bleeding** most often originates from peptic ulcers and results in hypotension and tachycardia if blood loss exceeds 25% of the patient's total blood volume (1500 ml in adults). Most patients with evidence of acute hypovolemia (orthostatic hypotension characterized by decreases in the systolic blood pressure of 10 to

---

≡ Table 19–14 • Causes of Upper and Lower Gastrointestinal Bleeding

---

Upper Gastrointestinal Bleeding
Peptic ulcer (duodenal ulcer, gastric ulcer)
Mucosal erosive disease (gastritis, esophagitis)
Esophageal varices
Mallory-Weiss tear
Malignancy
Lower Gastrointestinal Bleeding
Colonic diverticulosis
Colorectal malignancy
Ischemic colitis
Acute colitis of unknown causes
Hemorrhoids

Adapted from: Young HS. Gastrointestinal bleeding. Sci Am Med 1998;1–10.

20 mmHg and corresponding increases in the heart rate) have a hematocrit lower than 30% (may be normal early in the course of acute hemorrhage because of insufficient time for equilibration of plasma volume).

1. Melena usually indicates that bleeding has occurred at a site above the cecum. Blood urea nitrogen (BUN) concentrations are usually > 40 mg/dl because of the absorbed nitrogen load in the small intestine.

2. **Treatment.** For patients with bleeding peptic ulcers, endoscopic coagulation (thermotherapy, injection with epinephrine or a sclerosant, ligation) is indicated when active bleeding is visible. Transient bacteremia, aspiration, pneumonia, and bacterial pneumonitis may occur in patients treated by endoscopic variceal ligation. Transjugular intrahepatic portosystemic shunt placement may be utilized in patients with esophageal variceal bleeding resistant to control by endoscopic coagulation or sclerotherapy.

B. **Lower gastrointestinal bleeding** usually occurs in elderly patients and typically presents as the abrupt passage of bright red blood and clots (most often due to diverticulosis).

1. In contrast to upper gastrointestinal bleeding, BUN concentrations are not significantly increased in patients developing lower gastrointestinal bleeding.

2. **Treatment.** Sigmoidoscopy to exclude anorectal lesions is indicated as soon as patients are hemodynamically stable. Colonoscopy can be performed only after the bowel has been purged with polyethylene glycol solutions. Unlike patients with upper gastrointestinal bleeding, a significant number of patients with lower gastrointestinal bleeding may require surgical therapy.

C. **Occult gastrointestinal bleeding** may present as unexplained iron deficiency anemia or intermittent positive tests for blood in the patient's feces. Peptic ulcer disease and colonic neoplasms are the most common causes of occult gastrointestinal bleeding as determined by endoscopic examination or colonoscopy.

D. **Gastrointestinal bleeding in critically ill patients.** Risk factors for the development of gastrointestinal bleeding in critically ill patients include head injuries, burns covering more than 30% of the patient's body surface area, respiratory failure that requires mechanical support of ventilation, and coagulopathy.

X. DIVERTICULOSIS AND DIVERTICULITIS

See Table 19–15.

☰ Table 19–15 • Signs and Symptoms of Diverticulosis and Diverticulitis

---

Diverticulosis
Multiple outpouchings of the colonic mucosa
Present in 10–20% of patients > 50 years of age
Usually involves the sigmoid colon and rarely causes symptoms
Diverticulitis
Left-sided lower abdominal pain, low grade fever, anorexia, nausea and vomiting
Right-sided diverticulitis may be indistinguishable from appendicitis
Diverticular abscess may rupture and produce purulent peritonitis
Fistula formation (most often sigmoid colon to bladder)
Computed tomography is useful for evaluation
Surgical resection of the diseased segment if fistula formation or bleeding

---

Table 19–16 • Signs and Symptoms of Appendicitis

Pain (typically referred to the periumbilical or epigastric areas that localizes to the right lower quadrant; pain exacerbated by coughing; nearness of inflammatory response to right psoas muscle results in pain when raising right leg)

Anorexia (vomiting is uncommon)

Fever (suggests perforation)

Laboratory tests are nonspecific

Atypical location of appendix results in atypical signs and symptoms (retrocecal appendix, pelvic appendix, pregnancy)

XI. APPENDICITIS

Appendicitis is generally caused by obstruction of the lumen of the appendix (lymphoid hyperplasia, fecaliths) followed by bacterial overgrowth distal to the obstruction (occurs in 7% to 9% of the population during their lifetime, with the peak incidence occurring at 10 to 20 years of age).

A. Signs and symptoms. See Table 19–16.

B. Treatment is prompt surgical (laparoscopic if possible) appendectomy (do not delay based on an absence of leukocytosis). A pregnancy test is performed in women of childbearing age. Preoperative preparation consists of intravenous fluid administration and antibiotic therapy.

XII. PERITONITIS

Peritonitis is a diffuse or localized inflammatory process affecting the peritoneal lining. It results from spontaneous bacterial hematogenous spread, or it is secondary to intra-abdominal disease such as a perforated viscus (appendicitis, peptic ulcer, diverticulitis, peritoneal dialysis).

A. Ultrasonography and computed tomography are the standard techniques for evaluating intra-abdominal abscesses.

B. Patients with spontaneous bacterial peritonitis or undergoing peritoneal dialysis are treated with antibiotics, whereas patients developing secondary peritonitis require antibiotic and surgical therapy.

XIII. ACUTE COLONIC PSEUDO-OBSTRUCTION

Acute colonic pseudo-obstruction (Ogilvie syndrome) refers to marked dilation of the colon in the absence of mechanical obstruction. It occurs most often in hospitalized patients with medical or surgical diseases.

A. It is speculated that sympathetic nervous system over-activity and/or parasympathetic nervous system suppression are responsible for the development of pseudo-obstruction.

B. Diagnosis is based on evidence of colonic distension on abdominal radiographs (diameter > 12 cm requires repeated colonoscopy to decompress or administration of neostigmine 2 mg IV).

20

Renal Diseases

Essential physiologic functions of the kidneys include excretion of end-products of metabolism (urea) with retention of nutrients (amino acids, glucose) and control of electrolytes and hydrogen ion concentrations of body fluids (Stoelting RK, Dierdorf SF. Renal diseases. In: Anesthesia and Co-Existing Disease, 4th ed. New York, Churchill Livingstone, 2002;341–372). It is estimated that 5% of the adult population of the United States have co-existing renal disease that could contribute to perioperative morbidity.

I. CLINICAL ASSESSMENT OF RENAL FUNCTION

Renal function can be evaluated preoperatively by laboratory tests that reflect the glomerular filtration rate (GFR) and renal tubular function (Table 20–1). Current laboratory tests of renal function are often nonspecific, insensitive (> 50% of nephrons destroyed before changes in tests occur) or impractical to perform on a routine clinical basis (Table 20–2). Furthermore, normal values for renal function tests as established in healthy individuals may not be applicable during anesthesia. Trends are more useful than a single laboratory measurement for evaluating renal function.

II. CHRONIC RENAL FAILURE

Chronic renal failure is progressive and irreversible deterioration of renal function that results from a wide variety of diseases (Table 20–3). Diabetes mellitus is the leading cause of end-stage renal disease followed closely by systemic hypertension.

A. **Approach to patients with chronic renal failure.** In the absence of any reversible components that may contribute to the progression of renal insufficiency, the approach to patients with chronic renal failure includes attempts to prevent progression of the disease by controling of hyper-

Table 20-1 • Tests Used for Evaluating Renal Function

Test	Normal	Factors that Influence Interpretation
Glomerular Filtration Rate		
Blood urea nitrogen	10–20 mg/dl	Dehydration
		Variable protein intake
		Gastrointestinal bleeding
		Catabolism
Serum creatinine	0.7–1.5 mg/dl (higher in males)	Advanced age
		Skeletal muscle mass
		Catabolism
Creatinine clearance	110–150 ml/min	Accurate timed urine volume measurements
Proteinuria (albumin)	> 150 mg/day	
Renal Tubular Function and/or Integrity		
Urine specific gravity	1.003–1.030	
Urine osmolality	38–1400 mOsm/L	
Urine sodium excretion	> 40 mEq/L	
Glucosuria		
Enzymuria		
N-Acetyl-β-glucoseaminidase		
α-Glutathione-S-transferase		

Table 20-2 • Stages of Chronic Renal Failure

Stage	No. of Functioning Nephrons (% of total)	Glomerular Filtration Rate (ml/min)	Signs	Laboratory Abnormalities
Normal	100	125	None	None
Decreased renal reserve	40	50–80	None	None
Renal insufficiency	10–40	12–50	Nocturia	Increased blood urea nitrogen Increased serum creatinine
Renal failure	10	< 12	Uremia	Increased blood urea nitrogen Increased serum creatinine Anemia Hyperkalemia Increased bleeding time

---

≡ Table 20–3 • Causes of Chronic Renal Failure

Glomerulopathies
Primary glomerular disease
  Focal glomerulosclerosis
  Membranous nephropathy
  Immunoglobulin A nephropathy
  Membranoproliferative glomerulonephritis
Glomerulopathies associated with systemic diseases
  Diabetes mellitus
  Amyloidosis
  Postinfectious glomerulonephritis
  Systemic lupus erythematosus
  Wegener's granulomatosis
Tubulointerstitial Diseases
Analgesic nephropathy
Reflux nephropathy with pyelonephritis
Myeloma kidney
Sarcoidosis
Hereditary Diseases
Polycystic kidney disease
Alport syndrome
Medullary cystic disease
Systemic Hypertension
Renal Vascular Disease
Obstructive Uropathy
Human Immunodeficiency Virus

Adapted from: Tolkoff-Rubin NE, Pascual M. Chronic renal failure. Sci Am Med 1998;1–12.

glycemia, managing systemic hypertension with angiotensin-converting enzyme (ACE) inhibitors, and managing the consequences of impaired renal function (Table 20–4).

1. **Uremic syndrome** is the constellation of signs and symptoms (anorexia, nausea, vomiting, pruritus, anemia, fatigue, coagulopathy) that reflect the kidney's progressive inability to perform their excretory, secretory, and regulatory functions. The blood urea nitrogen (BUN) concentration is a useful clinical indicator of the severity of the uremic syndrome and the patient's response to therapy (dietary protein restriction). Serum creatinine concentrations, although reliable measures of GFR, correlate poorly with uremic symptoms.

2. **Hyperkalemia.** Patients with chronic renal failure whose dietary intake of potassium exceeds the rate of

≡ Table 20–4 • Manifestations of Chronic Renal Failure

Electrolyte Imbalance
Hyperkalemia
Hypermagnesemia
Hypocalcemia
Metabolic Acidosis
Unpredictable Intravascular Fluid Volume Status
Anemia
Increased cardiac output
Oxyhemoglobin dissociation curve shifted to the right
Uremic Coagulopathies
Platelet dysfunction
Neurologic Changes
Encephalopathy
Cardiovascular Changes
Systemic hypertension
Congestive heart failure
Attenuated sympathetic nervous system activity due to treatment with antihypertensive drugs
Renal Osteodystrophy
Pruritus

---

excretion may become dangerously hyperkalemic. In addition, severe acidosis, acute infection with marked catabolism, acute hemolysis, marked hyperglycemia, or any superimposed complications leading to oliguria may result in rapid development of life-threatening hyperkalemia.

a. Treatment. Changes in the electrocardiogram (ECG) (peaked T waves, prolongation of the QRS complex and PR intervals, heart block, ventricular fibrillation) are the best guide for when immediate therapy of hyperkalemia must be considered (Table 20–5).

b. If the serum potassium concentration is > 6.5 mEq/L or if ECG changes are present, immediate therapy should be instituted. Initial treatment of hyperkalemia should be directed at antagonizing the effects of potassium on the heart (intravenous calcium gluconate) and rapidly shifting potassium into cells (intravenous glucose, insulin, bicarbonate).

Table 20-5 ▪ Treatment of Hyperkalemia

Treatment	Mechanism of Action	Onset of Effect	Duration of Action	Side Effects
Calcium gluconate (10–20 ml of a 10% solution IV)	Directly antagonizes effects of potassium on the heart	Immediate	Brief	Avoid if being treated with digitalis
Sodium bicarbonate (50–100 mEq IV)	Shifts potassium into cells	Prompt	Short	Possible sodium overload
Glucose (50 ml of a 50% solution) and regular insulin (10 units IV)	Shifts potassium into cells	Prompt	4–6 Hours	Hyperglycemia Hypoglycemia
Ion-exchange resins	Removes potassium from the body	1–2 Hours		Sodium overload
Dialysis	Removes potassium from the body	Prompt		Requires vascular access

Adapted from: Tolkoff-Rubin NE, Pascual M. Chronic renal failure. Sci Am Med 1998;1–12.

3. **Metabolic acidosis.** The kidneys remove acid produced by the metabolism of dietary protein, and the pH is maintained in a normal range until the GFR decreases below 50 ml/min, at which point metabolic acidosis develops (pH < 7.3 produces symptoms of fatigue and decreases catecholamine responsiveness).

   a. **Treatment** is with intravenous administration of sodium bicarbonate, taking care not to correct metabolic acidosis too rapidly, particularly if hypocalcemia is also present (seizures are a risk).

   b. When acidosis is corrected, serum levels of ionized calcium decrease as a result of increased protein binding of free calcium.

4. **Renal osteodystrophy** reflects the interaction of secondary hyperparathyroidism and decreased vitamin D production by the kidneys, manifesting as bone resorption (evidence of bone demineralization on radiographs of the clavicles, skull, phalanges; and increased serum alkaline phosphatase concentrations).

   a. **Treatment** is intended to prevent skeletal complications by restricting dietary phosphate intake (antacids bind phosphorus), administration of oral calcium supplements, and vitamin D therapy.

   b. Surgical parathyroidectomy may be recommended if medical therapies fail to control hypocalcemia and hyperparathyroidism.

5. **Anemia** that accompanies chronic renal failure is responsible for many of the symptoms (fatigue, weakness) and is presumed to be due to decreased erythropoietin production by the kidneys.

   a. **Treatment** of the anemia of chronic renal failure is with recombinant human erythropoietin (epoetin) with the goal of maintaining the hematocrit between 36% and 40%.

   b. Development of systemic hypertension or exacerbation of co-existing systemic hypertension is a risk of erythropoietin administration.

6. **Uremic bleeding** despite normal laboratory coagulation tests (bleeding time prolonged) is a major factor contributing to morbidity and mortality (gastrointestinal bleeding, subdural hematoma, hemorrhagic pericarditis).

   a. **Treatment.** See Table 20–6.

   b. Erythropoietin or blood transfusions to increase the hematocrit to > 30% tend to normalize bleeding times.

Table 20–6 • Treatment of Uremic Bleeding

Drug	Dosage	Onset of Effect	Peak Effect	Duration of Effect
Cryoprecipitate	10 units IV over 30 minutes	< 1 hour	4–12 hours	12–18 hours
DDAVP (desmopressin)	0.3 µg/kg IV or SC	< 1 hour	2–4 hours	6–8 hours
Conjugated estrogen	0.6 mg/kg/day IV for 5 days	6 hours	5–7 days	14 days

Adapted from: Tolkoff-Rubin NE, Pascual M. Chronic renal failure. Sci Am Med 1998;1–12.

7. **Neurologic changes** include impaired abstract thinking, insomnia, seizures, obtundation (uremic encephalopathy), and development of a distal, symmetrical mixed motor and sensory polyneuropathy ("restless leg syndrome").

8. **Cardiovascular changes.** Systemic hypertension is the most significant risk factor accompanying chronic renal failure and contributes to congestive heart failure, coronary artery disease, and cerebrovascular disease. The pathogenesis of systemic hypertension in these patients reflects intravascular fluid volume expansion (retention of sodium and water) and activation of the renin-angiotensin-aldosterone system.

   a. **Treatment.** Dialysis is the indicated treatment for patients who are hypertensive because of hypervolemia and for patients who develop uremic pericarditis (cardiac tamponade requires prompt percutaneous or surgical drainage).

   b. Hypertension due to activation of the renin-angiotensin-aldosterone system is treated with antihypertensive drugs (ACE inhibitors are used cautiously, as their effects can result in efferent arteriolar dilation and further decreases in GFR).

B. **Hemodialysis** is utilized for treatment of patients in whom chronic renal failure would otherwise result in the uremic syndrome. Inadequate dialysis shortens survival and leads to increased clinical symptoms of chronic renal failure (Table 20–7).

   1. **Vascular access.** Surgically created vascular access sites are necessary for effective hemodialysis (cephalic vein anastomosed to the radial artery has a longer lifespan and lower incidence of thrombosis than artificial grafts).

   2. **Complications during hemodialysis.** Hypotension is the most common adverse event during hemodialysis and most likely reflects osmolar shifts and ultrafiltration-induced volume depletion. Other complications that occur in patients on hemodialysis reflect progressive renal failure (Table 20–8).

C. **Peritoneal dialysis** is simple to perform and may be preferred to hemodialysis for patients with congestive heart failure or unstable angina pectoris who may not tolerate rapid fluid shifts or systemic blood pressure changes that may accompany hemodialysis.

≡ Table 20–7 • Findings Suggestive of Inadequate Hemodialysis

Clinical Findings
Anorexia, nausea, vomiting
Peripheral neuropathy
Poor nutritional status
Depressed sensorium
Pericarditis
Ascites
Minimal weight gain or weight loss between treatments
Fluid retention and systemic hypertension
Chemical Findings
Decrease in blood urea nitrogen (BUN) concentration during hemodialysis < 65%
Albumin concentration < 4 g/dl
Predialysis BUN concentration < 50 mg/dl
Predialysis serum creatinine concentration < 5 mg/dl
Persistent anemia (hematocrit < 30%) despite erythropoietin therapy

Adapted from: Ifudu O. Care of patients undergoing hemodialysis. N Engl J Med 1998;339:1054–62.

≡ Table 20–8 • Complications of Progressive Renal Failure in Patients on Hemodialysis

Nutrition and fluid balance (stringent dietary restriction of potassium is not necessary during hemodialysis; water-soluble vitamins must be replaced)
Cardiovascular disease (accounts for nearly 50% of deaths in patients on hemodialysis)
  Ischemic heart disease
  Congestive heart failure
  Systemic hypertension
  Pericarditis
Bleeding tendency
Infection (anergy is common; fever may not occur)
Decreased insulin requirements (reflects decreased catabolism)
Mental depression (misdiagnosed as functional impairment due to renal failure)

D. **Drug clearance in patients undergoing dialysis.** Patients undergoing dialysis may require special consideration with respect to drug dosing intervals. They may need supplemental dosing with drugs that have been cleared by dialysis.

E. **Perioperative hemodialysis.** Patients should have adequate hemodialysis before elective surgery to minimize the likelihood of uremic bleeding, pulmonary edema, and impaired arterial oxygenation.

III. RENAL EFFECTS OF ANESTHETIC DRUGS

Volatile anesthetics produce similar dose-related decreases in renal blood flow, GFR, and urine output that most likely reflect the effects of the anesthetic drugs on systemic blood pressure and cardiac output. Preoperative hydration attenuates or abolishes the increases in antidiuretic hormone concentrations produced by surgical stimulation as well as many of the changes in renal function associated with volatile anesthetics.

A. **Fluoride-induced nephrotoxicity.** Sevoflurane, but not desflurane or isoflurane, undergoes significant metabolism that results in production of inorganic fluoride. Despite the common view that fluoride-induced nephrotoxicity is a risk when serum fluoride concentrations are $> 50 \ \mu mol/L$, there is no evidence that this peak value is a valid indicator for renal dysfunction (intrarenal production of fluoride may be more important than hepatic metabolism that results in increased serum fluoride concentrations). Administration of sevoflurane is not associated with evidence of renal dysfunction as reflected by measurements of serum creatinine and BUN concentrations (renal tubular enzymes may increase, suggesting transient impairment of renal concentrating ability and renal tubular damage).

B. **Vinyl halide nephrotoxicity.** Carbon dioxide absorbents react with sevoflurane to form a degradation product (compound A), which may be nephrotoxic in animals. Recommendations to deliver sevoflurane in total gas flows of 1 L/min or more are intended to minimize the accumulation of compound A in the breathing circuit. Newer carbon dioxide absorbents with different constituents do not degrade sevoflurane to compound A.

IV. MANAGEMENT OF ANESTHESIA IN PATIENTS WITH CHRONIC RENAL DISEASE

A. **Preoperative evaluation** of patients with chronic renal disease includes consideration of concomitant drug therapy and evaluation of the changes considered characteristic of chronic renal failure (Table 20–4).

1. Blood volume status may be estimated by comparing body weight before and after hemodialysis, considering vital signs (orthostatic hypotension, tachycardia), and measuring atrial filling pressures.

2. Preoperative medication is individualized, remembering that these patients may exhibit uremia-induced slowing of gastric emptying and unexpected sensitivity to central nervous system depressant drugs.

3. Patients on hemodialysis should undergo dialysis during the 24 hours preceding elective surgery (control of systemic hypertension and serum potassium concentrations < 5.5 mEq/L on the day of surgery).

4. Preservation of renal function intraoperatively depends on maintaining an adequate intravascular fluid volume and minimizing drug-induced cardiovascular depression.

B. **Induction of anesthesia** and tracheal intubation can be safely accomplished with intravenous induction drugs (propofol, etomidate, thiopental) plus muscle relaxants that are not dependent on renal clearance mechanisms. Regardless of blood volume status, these patients often respond to induction of anesthesia as if they are hypovolemic.

C. **Maintenance of anesthesia** is often achieved with isoflurane or desflurane combined with nitrous oxide, as these drugs provide sufficient potency to suppress excessive increases in systemic blood pressure due to surgical stimulation, avoid the controversy related to fluoride nephrotoxicity, and decrease the dose of nondepolarizing muscle relaxants needed to produce skeletal muscle relaxation.

1. When systemic hypertension does not respond to adjustments in the depth of anesthesia, it may be appropriate to administer vasodilators, such as hydralazine or nitroprusside.

2. **Muscle relaxant** selection is influenced by the known clearance mechanisms of these drugs (renal failure may

also slow clearance of metabolites of these drugs including laudanosine). A diagnosis of residual neuromuscular blockade after apparent reversal of nondepolarizing neuromuscular blockade should be considered in anephric patients who manifest signs of skeletal muscle weakness during the early postoperative period (elimination of muscle relaxants and anticholinesterase drugs is prolonged in the presence of renal failure).

3. **Fluid management and urine output.** Patients with severe renal dysfunction but not requiring hemodialysis and those without renal disease undergoing operations associated with a high incidence of postoperative renal failure may benefit from preoperative hydration with balanced salt solutions 10 to 20 ml/kg. If fluid replacement does not restore intraoperative urine output, the diagnosis of congestive heart failure may be considered.

   a. Patients dependent on hemodialysis have a narrow margin of safety between insufficient and excessive fluid administration (noninvasive operations require only replacement of insensible water losses with 5% glucose in water). The small amount of urine output can be replaced with 0.45% sodium chloride.

   b. Measurement of central venous pressure may be helpful in guiding fluid replacement.

4. **Monitoring** may include a Doppler sensor to confirm continued patency of vascular shunts during the intraoperative period. Strict asepsis is mandatory for placing intravascular catheters, as for measurement of systemic blood pressure or cardiac filling pressures.

5. **Regional anesthesia,** such as brachial plexus block, is useful for placing the vascular shunts necessary for chronic hemodialysis. Adequacy of coagulation is considered before proceeding with regional anesthesia.

6. **Postoperative management.** See Table 20–9.

≡ **Table 20–9 •** Postoperative Management of Patients with Chronic Renal Failure

Recurarization
Systemic hypertension
Possible increased sensitivity to opioids
Cardiac dysrhythmias

V. ACUTE RENAL FAILURE

Acute renal failure is characterized by deterioration of renal function over a period of hours to days, resulting in failure of the kidneys to excrete nitrogenous waste products and to maintain fluid and electrolyte homeostasis (oliguric or nonoliguric).

A. Despite major advances in dialysis therapy and critical care, the mortality rate among patients with severe acute renal failure (primarily ischemic in origin) requiring dialysis remains high.

B. Etiology of acute renal failure may be classified as prerenal, renal (intrinsic), and postrenal (obstructive) azotemia (Table 20–10).

☰ Table 20–10 • Causes of Acute Renal Failure

Prerenal Azotemia (Decreased Renal Blood Flow)
Absolute decrease in blood volume
    Acute hemorrhage
    Gastrointestinal fluid loss
    Trauma
    Surgery
    Burns
Relative decrease in blood volume
    Sepsis
    Hepatic failure
    Allergic reactions
Renal Azotemia (Intrinsic)
Acute glomerulonephritis
Interstitial nephritis (drugs, sepsis)
Acute tubular necrosis (85% of cases)
    Ischemia
    Nephrotoxic drugs (antibiotics, anesthetic drugs?)
    Solvents (carbon tetrachloride, ethylene glycol)
    Radiographic contrast dyes
    Myoglobinuria
Postrenal (Obstructive) Azotemia
Upper urinary tract obstruction
Lower urinary tract obstruction (bladder outlet)

Adapted from: Klahr S, Miller SB. Acute oliguria. N Engl J Med 1998;338:671–5; Thadhani R, Pascual M, Bonventre JV. Acute renal failure. N Engl J Med 1996;334:1148–69.

1. **Prerenal azotemia** accounts for nearly half of the hospital-acquired cases of acute renal failure. Sustained prerenal azotemia is the most common factor that predisposes patients to ischemia-induced acute tubular necrosis. Prerenal azotemia is rapidly reversible if the underlying causes (hypovolemia, congestive heart failure) are corrected. Elderly patients are uniquely susceptible to prerenal azotemia because of their predisposition to hypovolemia (poor fluid intake) and high incidence or renovascular disease.

2. **Renal azotemia** due to injury to the renal tubules is most often due to ischemia or nephrotoxins. Prerenal azotemia and ischemic tubular necrosis present as a continuum with initial prerenal-induced decreases in renal blood flow leading to ischemia of the renal tubular cells.

3. **Postrenal azotemia** occurs when urinary outflow tracts are obstructed by prostatic hypertrophy or cancer of the prostate or cervix. Renal ultrasonography is the best diagnostic test for determining the presence of obstructive nephropathy.

C. **Risk factors for the development of acute renal failure** include co-existing renal disease, advanced age, congestive heart failure, symptomatic cardiovascular disease that is likely to be associated with renovascular disease, and major operative procedures (cardiopulmonary bypass, abdominal aneurysm resection). Sepsis and multiple organ system dysfunction due to trauma introduce a high risk of acute renal failure. Iatrogenic components that predispose to acute renal failure include inadequate fluid replacement (appropriate hydration and preservation of intravascular fluid volume are essential for maintaining adequate renal perfusion pressures), delayed treatment of sepsis, and administration of nephrotoxic drugs or dyes.

D. **Complications** of acute renal failure may manifest in the central nervous system, cardiovascular system, and gastrointestinal tract. There may also be an increased incidence of infection (Table 20–11).

E. **Management of acute renal failure.** See Figure 20–1.

1. **Dialysis.** When the diagnosis of intrinsic acute renal failure is established, therapeutic interventions are confined to supportive care and institution of dialysis in an effort to normalize the extracellular fluid volume and electrolyte concentrations and to control hyperkalemia and metabolic acidosis.

☰ Table 20–11 • Complications of Acute Renal Failure

Neurologic
Confusion
Asterixis
Somnolence
Seizures
Cardiovascular
Systemic hypertension
Congestive heart failure
Pulmonary edema
Cardiac dysrhythmias
Pericarditis
Anemia
Gastrointestinal
Anorexia
Nausea and vomiting
Ileus
Bleeding
Infection
Respiratory tract
Urinary tract

---

2. **Protein intake.** Nutritional therapy, often in the form of total parenteral nutrition, should be initiated early in the treatment of acute renal failure.

VI. PRIMARY DISEASES OF THE KIDNEYS

See Table 20–12.

A. **Glomerulonephritis.** Acute glomerulonephritis is usually due to deposition of antigen-antibody complexes in the glomeruli (source of antigens may be poststreptococcal infection or a collagen disease).

B. **Nephrolithiasis.** Predisposing factors for the formation of renal stones include primary hyperparathyroidism, alkaline urine (chronic bacterial infections), and gout.

1. **Treatment** of renal stones may include extracorporeal shock-wave lithotripsy (ESWL) utilizing an immersion or nonimmersion lithotriptor.

a. **Side effects of immersion lithotripsy.** See Table 20–13.

b. In patients at risk for cardiovascular problems, immersion should be achieved in graded steps, or con-

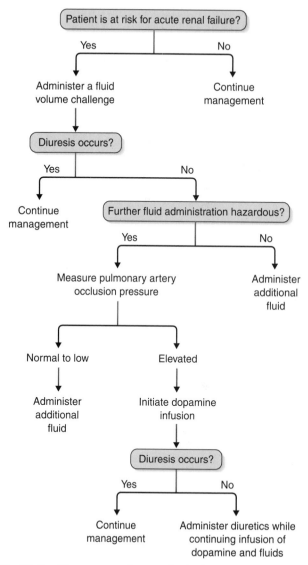

Fig. 20–1 • Management of acute oliguria during the perioperative period.

≡ Table 20–12 • Primary Diseases of the Kidneys

Glomerulonephritis (most common cause of end-stage renal failure in adults)

Nephrotic syndrome (hypoalbuminemia leads to edema and ascites; thromboembolic episodes; treatment is corticosteroids)

Goodpasture syndrome (pulmonary hemorrhage and glomerulonephritis)

Interstitial nephritis (allergic reaction to drugs)

Hereditary nephritis (accompanied by hearing loss and ocular abnormalities)

Polycystic renal disease

Fanconi syndrome (polyuria, metabolic acidosis, hypokalemia)

Bartter syndrome (hypokalemic, hypochloremic metabolic alkalosis; overproduction of prostaglandins)

Nephrolithiasis

Renal hypertension (renal disease is the most common cause of secondary systemic hypertension)

Uric acid nephropathy (most likely in patients with myeloproliferative diseases being treated with cancer chemotherapeutic drugs)

Hepatorenal syndrome (decompensated cirrhosis of the liver in association with decreased glomerular filtration rate)

≡ Table 20–13 • Side Effects of Immersion Lithotripsy

Peripheral venous compression (results in an increase in central blood volume and central venous pressure)

Hypotension (vasodilation due to warm water)

Congestive heart failure or myocardial ischemia a risk for patients with severe heart disease

Cardiac dysrhythmias (abrupt changes in right atrial pressure; shock waves are triggered from the electrocardiogram to occur 20 ms after the R wave, thus ensuring that the shock wave is delivered during the absolute refractory period of the heart)

Increased work of breathing (extrinsic pressure on the chest and abdomen results in decreases in vital capacity and functional residual capacity)

Hematuria

Pulmonary contusions

Pancreatitis

Flank pain

Sepsis

sideration should be given to utilizing a nonimmersion lithotriptor.

2. **Management of anesthesia.** The impact of shock waves at the water–cutaneous interface is painful and necessitates general or regional anesthesia; alternatively, intravenous sedation and analgesia may be used (most useful for nonimmersion lithotripsy).

    a. General anesthesia offers the advantages of controlling the patient's ventilation and avoiding the discomfort associated with immersion and exposure to the loud noise associated with operation of the lithotriptor. A disadvantage of general anesthesia is the need to position unconscious patients in the lithotriptor chair. The method for ventilating the patient's lungs during general anesthesia is a consideration, as movement of the diaphragm and abdominal contents could interfere with precise localization of the shock waves.

    b. Regional anesthesia (T6 sensory level needed) offers the advantage of an awake, cooperative patient who can help with positioning in the lithotriptor chair.

    c. Intravenous infusion techniques (propofol, fentanyl) are especially useful for nonimmersion lithotripsy.

    d. Intravenous fluid administration in intended to maintain intravascular fluid volume and systemic blood pressure and to stimulate urine output to facilitate passage of disintegrated stones. Monitors, epidural catheter insertion sites, and vascular access sites are protected with water impermeable dressings.

VII. RENAL TRANSPLANTATION

Renal transplantation is considered for selected patients with end-stage renal disease (diabetes mellitus, systemic hypertension) who are on an established chronic hemodialysis regimen. Immunosuppressive therapy is instituted during the perioperative period.

A. Management of anesthesia. See Table 20–14.

B. Postoperative complications. See Table 20–15.

C. Anesthetic considerations in renal transplant recipients. Renal transplant recipients are often elderly with co-existing cardiovascular disease and diabetes mellitus. Side effects of immunosuppressant drugs (systemic hyperten-

---

≡ Table 20–14 • Management of Anesthesia for
Renal Transplantation

Preoperative hemodialysis

Measure blood glucose concentrations if patient is diabetic

General anesthesia (isoflurane or desflurane with nitrous oxide
and/or short-acting opioids; promote renal perfusion by
maintaining a high normal systemic blood pressure; muscle
relaxant selection influenced by dependence on renal clearance
mechanisms; monitoring central venous pressure useful for
guiding fluid replacement)

Vascular unclamping may be followed by sudden hyperkalemia
(cardiac arrest) and/or hypotension

Regional anesthesia (eliminates need for tracheal intubation and
muscle relaxants; risks are hypotension from sympathetic
nervous system blockade and performance of the regional block
in the presence of abnormal coagulation)

---

sion, lowered seizure thresholds, anemia, thrombocytopenia) are considered when planning management of anesthesia. Drugs that are potentially nephrotoxic or dependent
on renal clearance are avoided, and the possibility of decreased renal blood flow or hypovolemia is minimized.

≡ Table 20–15 • Postoperative Complications
Following Renal Transplantation

Acute rejection (may manifest as soon as blood flow is
established to the transplanted kidney; only treatment is
removal of the kidney especially if disseminated intravascular
coagulation develops)

Hematoma at operative site (vascular or ureteral obstruction)

Delayed rejection (fever, local tenderness, deterioration of urine
output)

Cyclosporine toxicity

Opportunistic infections

Cancer

VIII. BENIGN PROSTATIC HYPERPLASIA

A. **Medical therapy.** The prostate gland is androgen-sensitive such that androgen deprivation decreases the size and resistance to outflow through the prostatic urethra [5α-reductase inhibitors and α-adrenergic antagonists may be effective in the symptomatic treatment of benign prostatic hyperplasia (BPH)].

B. **Minimally invasive treatments.** The most commonly utilized minimally invasive treatment of BPH is transurethral incision of the prostate (regional or general anesthesia). The advantages of laser ablation of the prostate are a brief operating time (20 minutes or less) and the absence of perioperative hemorrhage.

C. **Transurethral resection of the prostate.** Definitive treatment of BPH is transurethral resection of the prostate (TURP). The surgical procedure is accompanied by absorption of nonelectrolyte irrigating fluids (glycine, sorbitol, mannitol) used to distend the bladder and wash away blood and prostatic tissue.

    1. **TURP syndrome.** Intravascular absorption of irrigation fluid may result in acute changes in intravascular fluid volume and plasma solute concentrations, manifesting as cardiovascular and central nervous system complications known as the TURP syndrome (Table 20–16; Fig. 20–2).

        a. **Intravascular fluid volume expansion.** Rapid intravascular fluid volume expansion due to systemic absorption of irrigating fluids (absorption rates may reach 200 ml/min) can cause systemic hypertension and reflex bradycardia. The most widely used indicator of intravascular fluid volume expansion is hyponatremia or measurement of breath alcohol levels when ethanol is added as a marker to the irrigation fluids.

        b. **Hyponatremia.** Acute hyponatremia due to intravascular absorption of irrigating fluids may cause confusion, agitation, visual disturbances, pulmonary edema, cardiovascular collapse, and seizures. Changes in the ECG may accompany progressive decreases in serum sodium concentrations (widening of the QRS complex, elevated ST segment, ventricular tachycardia, ventricular fibrillation).

        c. **Hypo-osmolality** rather than hyponatremia is the crucial physiologic derangement leading to central

≡ **Table 20–16** • Signs and Symptoms of the Transurethral Resection of the Prostate Syndrome

Cardiopulmonary
Hypertension
Bradycardia
Hypotension
Cardiac dysrhythmias
Pulmonary edema
Arterial hypoxemia
Myocardial ischemia
Shock
Increased central venous pressure
Hematologic and Renal
Hyponatremia
Hypo-osmolality
Metabolic acidosis
Hyperammonemia
Hyperglycinemia
Hemolysis
Acute renal failure
Central Nervous System
Nausea and vomiting
Confusion and agitation
Seizures
Coma
Blindness

Adapted from: Gravenstein D. Transurethral resection of the prostate (TURP) syndrome: a review of the pathophysiology and management. Anesth Analg 1997;84:438–46.

Fig. 20–2 • Mechanisms and pathways that lead to transurethral resection of the prostate syndrome. The initiating event is systemic absorption of irrigating solution (A), which increases intravascular fluid volume (B) with its sequelae and decreases (C) and/or increases (D) solute concentrations. [From Gravenstein D. Transurethral resection of the prostate (TURP) syndrome: a review of the pathophysiology and management. Anesth Analg 1997;84:438–46. © 1997, Lippincott Williams & Wilkins, with permission.]

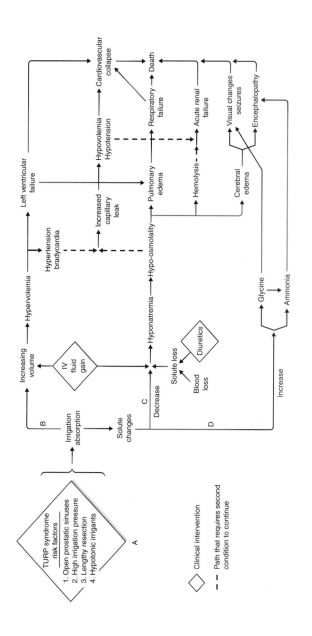

nervous system dysfunction (cerebral edema, increased intracranial pressure) during TURP. Serum osmolality should be monitored and corrected aggressively with hypertonic saline only until symptoms resolve [risk of central pontine myelinolysis (osmotic demyelination syndrome) if serum sodium concentrations are increased too rapidly].

d. **Hyperammonemia** is the result of using glycine containing irrigation solutions with subsequent systemic absorption of glycine and its oxidative deamination to glyoxylic acid and ammonia.

e. **Hyperglycinemia.** Glycine is an inhibitory neurotransmitter similar to γ-aminobutyric acid in the spinal cord and brain. Glycine is the most likely cause of visual disturbances, including transient blindness during TURP syndrome, reflecting the role of glycine as an inhibitory neurotransmitter in the retina. Glycine may also exert toxic effects on the kidneys (hyperoxaluria from metabolism of glycine to oxalate and glycolate).

2. A syndrome similar to TURP syndrome may occur in women undergoing endometrial ablation with saline, glycine, or sorbital solutions.

21

Water, Electrolyte, and Acid-Base Disturbances

Alterations of water and electrolyte content and distribution as well as acid-base disturbances can produce multiple organ system dysfunction (central nervous system, cardiac, neuro-muscular) during the perioperative period (Stoelting RK, Dierdorf SF. Water, electrolyte, and acid-base disturbances. In: Anesthesia and Co-Existing Disease, 4th ed. New York, Churchill Livingstone, 2002;374–394). Furthermore, these disorders frequently accompany events associated with the perioperative period (Table 21–1). Often the signs and symptoms of water and electrolyte disturbances are related more to the rate of change and less to absolute change.

I. TOTAL BODY WATER AND ELECTROLYTE DISTURBANCES

A. Total body water content is categorized as intracellular fluid or extracellular fluid, according to the location of water relative to cell membranes (Fig. 21–1). The distribution and concentration of electrolytes differs greatly among fluid compartments for total body water (Table 21–2). The electrophysiology of excitable cells is dependent on the intracellular and extracellular concentrations of sodium, potassium, and calcium. The unequal distribution of ions (excess potassium inside and sodium outside) produces an electrochemical difference across cell membranes.

B. **Hyponatremia** is defined as a decrease in the serum sodium concentration to < 136 mEq/L (frequent in hospitalized patients).

1. **Causes of dilutional hyponatremia.** Dilutional (hypotonic) hyponatremia is the most common form, reflecting impaired renal excretion of water and only rarely excessive water intake (Table 21–3).

a. **Hyponatremia in hospitalized patients** likely reflects a defect of water excretion due to factors that stimulate

---

≡ **Table 21–1** • Etiology of Water, Electrolyte, and Acid-Base Disturbances During the Perioperative Period

---

Disease States
Endocrinopathies
Nephropathies
Gastroenteropathies
Drug Therapy
Diuretics
Corticosteroids
Nasogastric Suction
Surgery
Transurethral resection of the prostate
Translocation of body water due to tissue trauma
Resection of portions of the gastrointestinal tract
Management of Anesthesia
Intravenous fluid administration
Alveolar ventilation
Hypothermia

---

inappropriate secretion of antidiuretic hormone (postoperative state, drugs, organ failure).

b. In infants and children, the most common causes of hyponatremia are gastrointestinal fluid loss, ingestion of dilute formula, and accidental ingestion of excess water.

2. **Signs and symptoms of dilutional hyponatremia.** Patients with serum sodium concentrations > 125 mEq/L are usually asymptomatic, whereas those with lower values may have symptoms (seizures, coma, brain stem herniation, osmotic demyelination), especially if hyponatremia has developed rapidly.

3. **Treatment of dilutional hyponatremia** balances the risk of serum hypotonicity and hypo-osmolarity with the hazards of therapy (osmotic demyelination with aggressive correction). The presence of symptoms and and their severity largely determines the speed of correction of hyponatremia.

a. **Symptomatic dilutional hyponatremia** is treated with intravenous infusions of hypertonic saline (5% sodium chloride in water) often in combination with furosemide

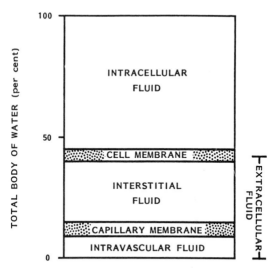

Fig. 21–1 • Total body water (constitutes about 60% of the total body weight in kilograms or about 42 L in adult men and 35 L in adult women) is designated intracellular or extracellular fluid, depending on the location of water relative to cell membranes. Water in extracellular compartments is further subdivided as interstitial or intravascular (plasma) fluid, depending on its location relative to cell membranes. About 55% of total body water is intracellular, 37% interstitial, and the remaining 8% intravascular.

≡ Table 21–2 • Approximate Composition of Extracellular and Intracellular Fluid*

Substance	Extracellular Fluid (mEq/L)		Intracellular Fluid (mEq/L)
	Intravascular	Interstitial	
Sodium	140	145	10
Potassium	5	4	150
Calcium	5	2.5	< 1
Magnesium	2	1.5	40
Chloride	103	115	4
Bicarbonate	28	30	10

* Total anion concentration consists of phosphates, sulfates, organic acids, and negatively charged sites on proteins.

≡ Table 21–3 • Causes of Dilutional Hyponatremia Reflecting Impaired Renal Water Excretion

Decreased Extracellular Fluid Volume
Renal sodium loss
  Thiazide diuretics
  Osmotic diuretics
  Adrenal insufficiency
  Ketonuria
Extrarenal sodium loss
  Vomiting
  Blood loss
  Fluid sequestration in "third spaces" (bowel obstruction, trauma, burns)
Increased Extracellular Fluid Volume
  Congestive heart failure
  Cirrhosis of the liver
  Renal failure (acute or chronic)
  Pregnancy
Normal Extracellular Fluid Volume
Syndrome of inappropriate antidiuretic hormone secretion
  Postoperative status
  Pain
  Acute respiratory failure
  Positive-pressure ventilation
  Cancer (lungs, mediastinum)
  Stroke
  Intracranial hemorrhage
  Acute brain trauma
  Drugs (desmopressin, oxytocin, tricyclic antidepressants, serotonin reuptake inhibitors, opioids, cyclophosphamide, vincristine)
  Thiazide diuretics
  Adrenal insufficiency
  Hypothyroidism

to limit treatment-induced expansion of extracellular fluid volume. Relatively small increases in serum sodium concentrations (3 to 7 mEq/L) may be sufficient to reverse cerebral edema and stop seizure activity.

  b. Most cases of osmotic demyelination occur when the rate of serum sodium concentration increase exceeds 12 mEq/L daily.

  c. **Asymptomatic dilutional hyponatremia** that accompanies edematous states or the syndrome of inappropriate secretion of antidiuretic hormone is treated with restriction of daily water intake to < 800 ml.

4. **Management of anesthesia** considers the likely presence of renal, cardiac, or liver disease as the etiology of excess total body water and dilutional hyponatremia. Decreased excitability of cells due to hyponatremia could manifest as poor myocardial contractility (unexpected hypotension) and increased sensitivity to nondepolarizing muscle relaxants.

C. **Hypernatremia** is defined as an increase in the serum sodium concentration to > 145 mEq/L.

1. **Causes** of hypernatremia are most often total body water deficits, as the kidneys closely regulate total body sodium content. Nevertheless, impairment of sodium excretion is common in the presence of congestive heart failure and cirrhosis of the liver with ascites.

2. **Signs and symptoms.** See Table 21–4.

3. **Treatment of hypernatremia due to total body water deficit** is intravenous administration of 5% glucose in water, with the volume and rate of infusion guided by changes in systemic blood pressure, central venous pressure, urine output, and repeated determinations of serum sodium concentrations. To minimize the risk of cerebral edema, it is

---

Table 21–4 • Signs and Symptoms of Hypernatremia

Total Body Water Deficit
Dehydration (decreased systemic blood pressure, venous pressure, urine output, and tachycardia)
Unchanged hematocrit (both intracellular and extracellular fluid volumes decreased)
Blood urea nitrogen and serum creatinine concentrations increased (hypovolemia results in decreased renal blood flow and glomerular filtration rate)
Increased urine specific gravity
Absent edema
Total Body Sodium Excess
Peripheral edema (interstitial fluid spaces can expand by as much as 5 L before edema is clinically detectable)
Ascites
Pleural effusions
Hypervolemia (systemic hypertension)

recommended that hypernatremia be gradually corrected at a maximum rate of 0.5 mEq/L/hr.

4. **Treatment of hypernatremia due to excess body sodium** is intravenous administration of diuretics (furosemide) to facilitate sodium excretion by the kidneys.

5. **Management of anesthesia** in the presence of hypernatremia due to total body water deficit is likely to be accompanied by hypotension, as drug-induced vasodilation unmasks hypovolemia. Measurements of cardiac filling pressures and urine output are helpful for guiding the volume and rate of intravenous fluid administration during the perioperative period.

D. **Hypokalemia** is defined as a decrease in the serum potassium concentrations to < 3.5 mEq/L (based on this definition, hypokalemia is the most common electrolyte disturbance seen clinically).

1. **Diagnosis** of hypokalemia is rarely suspected on the basis of clinical presentation; rather, the diagnosis is made by measuring the serum potassium concentration. Because 98% of potassium is intracellular, enormous potassium deficits can exist despite only a small decrease in the serum potassium concentration (a chronic decrease of 1 mEq/L can reflect a total body deficit of 600 to 800 mEq of potassium).

2. **Causes.** Hypokalemia is almost always due to drug-induced loss of potassium and less often as a result of shifts in potassium from extracellular to intracellular sites, inadequate intake, or abnormal losses through the kidneys (Table 21–5).

   a. **Drug-induced abnormal losses of potassium** are most often due to diuretic therapy. Diuretic-induced hypokalemia is often associated with metabolic alkalosis.

   b. **Drug-induced transcellular shifts of potassium** can occur acutely in response to β_2-adrenergic activity.

   c. **Non-drug-induced transcellular shifts of potassium** are most likely due to iatrogenic hyperventilation of the patient's lungs during surgery (0.5 mEq/L decrease in serum potassium concentration for every 10 mmHg decrease in $PaCO_2$). The sympathetic nervous system modulates the distribution of potassium between intracellular and extracellular sites (serum potassium concentrations measured immediately before induction of anesthesia are often lower than determinations 1 to 3 days preoperatively). The possible presence of stress-

Table 21–5 • Drug-Induced and Non-Drug-Induced Causes of Hypokalemia

Hypokalemia Due to Increased Renal Potassium Loss
Thiazide diuretics
Loop diuretics
Mineralocorticoids
High-dose glucocorticoids
High-dose antibiotics (penicillin, nafcillin, ampicillin)
Drugs associated with magnesium depletion (aminoglycosides)
Surgical trauma
Hyperglycemia
Aldosteronism

Hypokalemia Due to Transcellular Potassium Shift
β-Adrenergic agonists
   Epinephrine
   Decongestants (pseudoephedrine)
   Bronchodilators (albuterol, terbutaline, ephedrine, isoproterenol)
   Tocolytic drugs (ritodrine)
Verapamil overdose
Insulin overdose
Respiratory or metabolic alkalosis
Familial periodic paralysis
Hypercalcemia
Hypomagnesemia

Hypokalemia Due to Excess Gastrointestinal Loss of Potassium
Vomiting and diarrhea
Zollinger-Ellison syndrome
Jejunoileal bypass
Malabsorption
Chemotherapy
Nasogastric suction

Adapted from: Gennari JF. Hypokalemia. N Engl J Med 1998;339:451–8.

induced hypokalemia should be considered when interpreting serum potassium concentrations, as measured during the immediate preoperative period.

   d. **Nondrug causes of abnormal losses of potassium** often reflect surgical trauma (50 mEq daily lost in the urine for the first 2 days postoperatively).

3. **Signs and symptoms.** See Table 21–6 and Figure 21–2. Patients with serum potassium concentrations between 3.0 and 3.5 mEq/L often have no symptoms. The likelihood of symptoms appears to correlate with the rapidity of the decrease in serum potassium concentrations. In patients

≡ Table 21–6 • Signs and Symptoms of Hypokalemia

Skeletal muscle weakness (most prominent in legs)
Ileus
Polyuria (decreased concentrating ability)
Metabolic alkalosis
Orthostatic hypotension (autonomic nervous system dysfunction)
Poor myocardial contractility (most likely to be associated with chronic hypokalemia)
Cardiac conduction disturbances (most likely to be associated with abrupt additional decreases in serum potassium concentrations in the presence of chronic hypokalemia; increased automaticity due to more rapid rates of spontaneous depolarization; ventricular fibrillation is a common terminal dysrhythmia)

without underlying heart disease, abnormalities in cardiac conduction are unusual, even when the serum potassium concentration is < 3.0 mEq/L.

4. **Treatment** of hypokalemia is based on potassium replacement, recognizing that supplemental potassium administration is also the most important cause of severe hyperkalemia in hospitalized patients.

   a. When potassium is administered intravenously, the rate should be < 20 mEq/hr, with the patient's cardiac rhythm monitored continuously on the electrocardiogram (ECG). Total body potassium deficits (often 500 to 1000 mEq) cannot be replaced during the 12 to 24 hours preoperatively, but intravenous infusions of 0.2 mEq/kg/hr during the few hours preceding surgery may be beneficial (presumably even small amounts of potassium are helpful for normalizing the electrophysiology of cells). Repeat serum potassium concentration measurements every 12 to 24 hours are useful for guiding continued replacement and rates of intravenous infusion.

   b. Regardless of the cause of hypokalemia, the ability to correct potassium deficiency is impaired when magnesium deficiency is present.

5. **Management of anesthesia.** The advisability of proceeding with elective surgery in the presence of chronic serum potassium concentrations < 3.5 mEq/L is controversial (concern that an increased risk for intraoperative cardiac dysrhythmias exists but it is not possible to validate arbi-

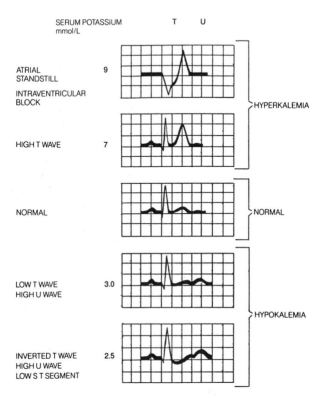

Fig. 21–2 • Manifestations on the electrocardiogram of changes in serum potassium concentrations. (From Goudsouzian NG, Karamanian A. The electrocardiogram. In: Physiology for the Anesthesiologist. Norwalk, CT: Appleton-Century-Crofts, 1977;37, with permission.)

trary serum potassium concentrations acceptable for elective surgery).

  a. Routine preoperative potassium repletion in otherwise asymptomatic patients (with or without cardiovascular disease) solely on the basis of preoperative serum potassium measurements is not recommended.
  b. Adverse effects of hypokalemia are most likely when acute decreases in serum potassium concentrations are

superimposed on co-existing chronic hypokalemia (hyperventilation of the patient's lungs, intravenous fluids contributing to hyperglycemia).

   c. The potential for prolonged responses to nondepolarizing muscle relaxants is a consideration (decrease initial doses and guide subsequent doses based on responses evoked by the peripheral nerve stimulator).

   d. No specific anesthetic drug or technique appears to be superior for use in hypokalemic patients. The association of chronic hypokalemia with decreased myocardial contractility and orthostatic hypotension could manifest as increased sensitivity to volatile anesthetics or responses to positive-pressure ventilation. Likewise, the association of chronic hypokalemia with polyuria may be considered when choosing volatile anesthetics metabolized to fluoride.

   e. Inclusion of epinephrine in local anesthetic solutions might act to accentuate co-existing hypokalemia.

   f. It is important to monitor the ECG for perioperative evidence of hypokalemia. Any new evidence of hypokalemia on the ECG requires prompt treatment with intravenous administration of potassium chloride, including considering injection of 0.5 to 1.0 mEq IV boluses until the ECG reverts to normal.

E. **Hyperkalemia** is defined as an increase in the serum potassium concentration to > 5.5 mEq/L.

   1. **Causes.** See Table 21–7.

   2. **Signs and symptoms.** Adverse effects of hyperkalemia are likely to accompany acute increases in the serum potassium concentration. In contrast, chronic hyperkalemia is more likely to be associated with normalization of gradients between intracellular and extracellular sites for potassium and subsequent return of resting membrane potentials to near normal.

   a. The most detrimental effect of hyperkalemia is on the cardiac conduction system (Fig. 21–2). The most likely cardiac event in the presence of hyperkalemia is cardiac standstill during diastole.

   b. Cardiac conduction abnormalities are frequently present when serum potassium concentrations are > 7.0 mEq/L. Peaking of T waves on the ECG, although diagnostic, occurs in fewer than 25% of patients in the presence of hyperkalemia.

▆ **Table 21–7 •** Causes of Hyperkalemia

Increased Total Body Potassium Content
Acute oliguric renal failure (classic cause)
Chronic renal failure (glomerular filtration rate < 15 ml/min)
Hypoaldosteronism
Drugs that impair potassium excretion
   Triamterene
   Spironolactone
   Nonsteroidal antiinflammatory drugs
Drugs that inhibit the renin-angiotensin-aldosterone system
   β-Antagonists
   Angiotensin-converting enzyme inhibitors
Altered Transcellular Potassium Shifts
Succinylcholine
Respiratory or metabolic acidosis (0.1 unit decrease in pH as
   produced by a 10 mmHg increase in $PaCO_2$ can increase serum
   potassium concentrations by about 0.5 mEq/L)
Hemolysis
Lysis of cells due to chemotherapy
Iatrogenic bolus
Pseudohyperkalemia

3. **Treatment.** Immediate treatment of hyperkalemia is indicated in the presence of abnormalities on the ECG or if the serum potassium concentration is > 6.5 mEq/L (Table 21–8). Initial treatment of hyperkalemia is directed at antagonizing the adverse effects of potassium on the heart (intravenous calcium) and facilitating movement of potassium from plasma into cells (intravenous glucose and insulin, sodium bicarbonate, hyperventilation).

4. **Management of anesthesia.** If it is not possible to decrease the serum potassium concentration to < 6.5 mEq/L before elective surgery, it is useful to adjust the anesthetic technique to facilitate recognition of adverse effects of hyperkalemia intraoperatively (ECG for evidence of hyperkalemia) and to minimize the likelihood of any additional increases in the serum potassium concentration (normocapnia or hypocapnia).

   a. Succinylcholine-induced potassium release may be undesirable.

   b. Perioperative intravenous fluids must be selected with the realization that most solutions contain potassium

Table 21–8 • Treatment of Hyperkalemia

Treatment	Dose	Mechanism	Onset	Duration
Calcium gluconate	10–20 ml of 10% solution IV	Direct antagonism	Rapid	15–30 minutes
Sodium bicarbonate	50–100 mEq IV	Intracellular shift	15–30 minutes	3–6 hours
Glucose and insulin	25–50 g with 10–20 units of insulin IV	Intracellular shift	15–30 minutes	
Hyperventilation	$PaCO_2$ 25–30 mmHg	Intracellular shift	Rapid	
Kayexelate		Remove	1–3 hours	
Peritoneal dialysis		Remove	1–3 hours	
Hemodialysis		Remove	Rapid	

(lactated Ringer's solution contains 4 mEq of potassium per liter).

F. Pseudohyperkalemia ("benign" or "spurious" hyperkalemia) is characterized by increased serum potassium concentrations (as high as 7 mEq/L) due to in vitro release of intracellular stores of this ion from leukocytes and platelets during the clotting or separation process (hemolysis or possibly an inherited trait). Clinically, pseudohyperkalemia is distinguished from hyperkalemia by measuring both the serum and plasma concentrations of potassium.

G. Hypocalcemia is defined as a decrease in the serum calcium concentration to < 4.5 mEq/L.

   1. Causes. The most common cause of hypocalcemia is decreased plasma albumin concentrations (critically ill patients with low plasma albumin concentrations characteristically have low plasma calcium concentrations, but ionized calcium levels may be normal). Hyperventilation of the lungs may result in a decreased plasma ionized calcium concentration due to alkalosis-induced increases in calcium binding to proteins.

   2. Signs and symptoms of hypocalcemia reflect actions of calcium on the central nervous system, heart, and neuromuscular junctions (Table 21–9).

   3. Treatment is intravenous infusion of calcium and correction of any co-existing alkalosis.

   4. Management of anesthesia. Alkalosis due to hyperventilation of the lungs is avoided. Intraoperative hypotension may reflect exaggerated drug-induced cardiac depression in the presence of decreased serum ionized calcium concentrations. Postoperatively, a sudden decrease in the serum calcium concentration can produce skeletal muscle spasm, including laryngospasm.

≡ Table 21–9 • Signs and Symptoms of Acute Hypocalcemia or Hypomagnesemia

Numbness and circumoral paresthesias
Skeletal muscle spasm (laryngospasm)
Hypotension (decreased myocardial contractility)
Confusion
Seizures
Prolonged QT interval (not a consistent observation)

H. **Hypercalcemia** is defined as an increase in the serum calcium concentration to > 5.5 mEq/L.
   1. **Causes.** The most common causes of hypercalcemia are hyperparathyroidism and neoplastic disorders with bone metastases.
   2. **Signs and symptoms** of hypercalcemia reflect actions of calcium on the central nervous system, heart, gastrointestinal tract, and neuromuscular junction (Table 21–10).
   3. **Treatment** of hypercalcemia is hydration with normal saline, 150 ml/hr (lowers serum calcium concentrations by dilution, and sodium acts to inhibit renal absorption of calcium). Diuresis produced with furosemide 40 to 80 mg IV every 2 to 4 hours (thiazide diuretics may enhance renal tubular reabsorption of calcium) minimizes the risk of overhydration and facilitates renal elimination of calcium. Ambulation is an important aspect of treatment, as it decreases calcium release from bone associated with immobilization.
      a. Bisphosphanates such as disodium etidronate are the drugs of choice for treating life-threatening hypercalcemia (they bind to hydroxyapatite in bone and inhibit osteoclastic bone resorption).
      b. Calcitonin is effective for prompt lowering of serum calcium concentrations, but the effects of this hormone are transient.
   4. **Management of anesthesia** in the presence of hypercalcemia includes intravenous hydration with sodium-containing crystalloid solutions to stimulate urine output. The preoperative presence of skeletal muscle weakness suggests the possibility of decreased dose requirements for muscle relaxants.
I. **Hypomagnesemia** is defined as a decrease in the serum magnesium concentration to < 1.5 mEq/L.

═ Table 21–10 • Signs and Symptoms of Hypercalcemia

Sedation
Vomiting
Polyuria
Cardiac conduction disturbances (prolonged PR interval, wide QRS, shortened QT interval)
Renal calculi

≡ Table 21–11 • Signs and Symptoms of Hypermagnesemia

Central nervous system depression (hyporeflexia, sedation)
Cardiac depression
Skeletal muscle weakness (apnea)

---

1. **Causes.** Hypomagnesemia is associated with chronic alcoholism, hyperalimentation therapy without added magnesium, and protracted vomiting or diarrhea. Hypokalemia resistant to treatment with potassium supplements may be caused by hypomagnesemia.
2. **Signs and symptoms.** See Table 21–9. Cardiac dysrhythmias attributed to diuretic-induced hypokalemia may in fact be due to hypomagnesemia.
3. **Treatment** of hypomagnesemia is with magnesium sulfate, 1 g IV, administered over 15 to 20 minutes. Depression or disappearance of patellar reflexes is an indication to stop magnesium replacement therapy.
4. **Management of anesthesia** includes consideration of disturbances likely to be associated with hypomagnesemia (alcoholism, malnutrition, hypovolemia).

J. **Hypermagnesemia** is defined as an increase in the serum magnesium concentration to > 2.5 mEq/L.
   1. **Causes.** The most important cause of hypermagnesemia is iatrogenic (treatment of pregnancy-induced hypertension, excessive use of antacids or laxatives).
   2. **Signs and symptoms.** See Table 21–11.
   3. **Treatment** of the acute manifestations of hypermagnesemia is the intravenous administration of calcium. The definitive therapy for persistent and life-threatening hypermagnesemia requires peritoneal dialysis or hemodialysis.
   4. **Management of anesthesia** includes avoidance of acidosis and dehydration (events that can lead to increased serum magnesium concentrations), maintenance of urine output, and recognition that responses to muscle relaxants may be prolonged.

II. ACID-BASE DISTURBANCES

Acid-base homeostasis exerts a major influence on enzyme function with subsequent effects on tissue and organ function. It is the condition that causes the change in pH more than the actual

Table 21–12 • Direction of Changes During Acute and Chronic Acid-Base Disturbances

Parameter	pHa	PaCO$_2$	HCO$_3$
Respiratory acidosis			
Acute	Moderate decrease	Marked increase	Slight increase
Chronic	Slight decrease	Marked increase	Moderate increase
Respiratory alkalosis			
Acute	Moderate increase	Marked decrease	Slight decrease
Chronic	Slight increase to no change	Marked decrease	Moderate decrease
Metabolic acidosis			
Acute	Moderate to marked decrease	Slight decrease	Marked decrease
Chronic	Slight decrease	Moderate decrease	Marked decrease
Metabolic alkalosis			
Acute	Marked increase	Moderate increase	Marked increase
Chronic	Marked increase	Moderate increase	Marked increase

pH value that determines the patient's status and prognosis. Management of serious acid-base disturbances always requires diagnosis and treatment of the underlying disease.

A. Classification. Acid-base disturbances are classified as respiratory or metabolic based on measurement of arterial hydrogen ion concentrations (pHa) and $PaCO_2$ and estimation of serum bicarbonate (HCO_3) concentrations from a nomogram (Table 21–12; Figs. 21–3, 21–4, 21–5).

   1. Henderson-Hasselbalch equation. The normal pHa is regulated over a narrow range of 7.35 to 7.45. In this regard, a normal pHa depends on maintaining an optimal $20:1$ HCO_3/CO_2 ratio (Henderson-Hasselbalch equation).

   2. Serum bicarbonate concentrations. Interpretation of nomogram-derived estimates of serum HCO_3 concentrations as a reflection of acid-base disturbances requires an adjustment for the impact of alveolar ventilation. For example, an increase in $PaCO_2$ leads to hydration of carbon dioxide to form carbonic acid with a subsequent increase in the serum HCO_3 concentration.

B. Signs and symptoms. Major adverse consequences of severe systemic acidosis (pHa < 7.2) can occur independently of whether the acidosis is of respiratory, metabolic, or mixed origin (Table 21–13). Major adverse consequences of severe

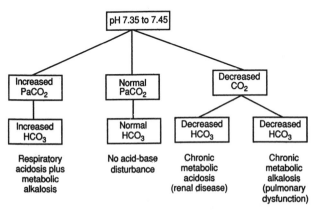

Fig. 21–3 • Diagnostic approach to the interpretation of a normal arterial pH based on the $PaCO_2$ and HCO_3 (bicarbonate) concentrations.

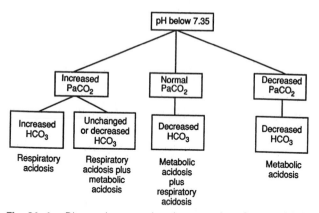

Fig. 21–4 • Diagnostic approach to interpretation of an arterial pH < 7.35 based on the $PaCO_2$ and HCO_3 (bicarbonate) concentrations.

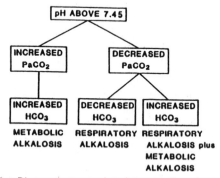

Fig. 21–5 • Diagnostic approach to interpretation of an arterial pH > 7.45 based on the $PaCO_2$ and HCO_3 (bicarbonate) concentrations.

≡ Table 21–13 • Adverse Consequences of Severe Acidosis

Nervous System
Obtundation
Coma
Cardiovascular System
Impaired myocardial contractility
Decreased cardiac output
Decreased arterial blood pressure
Sensitization to reentrant cardiac dysrhythmias
Decreased threshold for ventricular fibrillation
Decreased responsiveness to catecholamines
Ventilation
Hyperventilation
Dyspnea
Fatigue of muscles of breathing
Metabolic
Hyperkalemia
Insulin resistance
Inhibition of anaerobic glycolysis

Adapted from: Adrogue HJ, Madias NE. Management of life-threatening acid-base disorders. N Engl J Med 1998; 338:26–34.

systemic alkalosis (pHa > 7.60) reflect impairment of cerebral and coronary blood flow due to arteriolar vasoconstriction, an effect that is more pronounced with respiratory than metabolic alkalosis (Table 21–14).

C. **Respiratory acidosis** is present when decreases in alveolar ventilation result in increases in the $PaCO_2$ sufficient to decrease the pHa to < 7.35 (Table 21–15).

   1. **Treatment** of respiratory acidosis is correction of the disorder responsible for hypoventilation.

   2. Rapid lowering of a chronically elevated $PaCO_2$ decreases body stores of carbon dioxide more rapidly than the kidneys can excrete HCO_3, resulting in metabolic alkalosis (neuromuscular irritability, seizures).

D. **Respiratory alkalosis** is present when increases in alveolar ventilation result in decreases in the $PaCO_2$ sufficient to increase the pHa to > 7.45 (Table 21–16).

   1. **Treatment** of respiratory alkalosis is directed at correcting the underlying disorder responsible for alveolar hyperventilation.

   2. Hypokalemia and hypochloremia that characterize respiratory alkalosis may also require treatment.

≡ **Table 21–14 • Adverse Consequences of Alkalosis**

Nervous System
Decreased cerebral blood flow
Seizures
Lethargy
Delirium
Tetany
Cardiovascular System
Arteriolar vasoconstriction
Decreased coronary blood flow
Decreased threshold for angina pectoris
Predisposition to refractory supraventricular and ventricular cardiac
  dysrhythmias
Ventilation
Hypoventilation
Hypercarbia
Arterial hypoxemia
Metabolic
Hypokalemia
Decreased serum ionized calcium concentrations
Hypomagnesemia
Hypophosphatemia
Stimulation of anaerobic glycolysis and production of organic acids

Adapted from: Adrogue JH, Madias NE. Management of life-threatening acid-base disorders. N Engl J Med 1998;338:107–11.

    E. **Metabolic acidosis** is characterized by decreased pHa owing to accumulation of nonvolatile acids, as is likely to accompany major organ dysfunction, especially renal failure (Table 21–17).

        1. **Lactic acidosis** is most often caused by tissue hypoxia due to circulatory failure. In the presence of severe lactic acidosis, intravenous administration of sodium HCO_3 may

≡ **Table 21–15 • Causes of Respiratory Acidosis**

Drug-induced depression of ventilation (opioids, volatile anesthetics)
Permissive hypercapnia
Upper airway obstruction
Status asthmaticus
Restriction of ventilation (rib fractures with flail chest)
Disorders of neuromuscular function
Malignant hyperthermia
Hyperalimentation solutions

≡ **Table 21–16** • Causes of
Respiratory Alkalosis

Iatrogenic (mechanical hyperventilation)
Decreased barometric pressure
Arterial hypoxemia
Central nervous system injury
Hepatic disease
Pregnancy
Salicylate overdose

be indicated. The prognosis of patients with lactic acidosis is poor if the underlying cause cannot be effectively managed.

2. **Dilutional acidosis** may occur when serum HCO_3 concentrations are diluted by expanding the extracellular fluid volume due to administration of solutions (normal saline) that do not contain bicarbonate.

3. **Treatment** of metabolic acidosis is removal of nonvolatile acids in the circulation and administration of sodium HCO_3, especially if myocardial depression or cardiac dysrhythmias are present.

   a. A useful approach is to administer about one-half the calculated dose of sodium HCO_3 [body weight × deviation of serum HCO_3 concentration from normal × extracellular fluid volume as a fraction of the body mass (0.2)], followed in about 30 minutes by a repeat mea-

≡ **Table 21–17** • Causes of Metabolic
Acidosis

Lactic acidosis (inadequate tissue oxygenation)
Dilutional acidosis
Diabetic ketoacidosis
Renal failure
Hepatic failure
Methanol and ethylene glycol intoxication
Aspirin intoxication
Increased skeletal muscle activity
Cyanide poisoning
Carbon monoxide poisoning

☰ Table 21–18 • Causes of Metabolic Alkalosis

Hypovolemia
Vomiting
Nasogastric suction
Diuretic therapy
Iatrogenic
Hyperaldosteronism
Chloride-wasting diarrhea

---

surement of the pHa to evaluate the impact of treatment.

    b. Sodium HCO_3 administration results in endogenous carbon dioxide production, necessitating an increase in alveolar ventilation to prevent hypercarbia and worsening of the already existing acidosis.

F. Metabolic alkalosis is characterized by the loss of nonvolatile acids from the extracellular fluid (Table 21–18).

    1. Depletion of intravascular fluid volume is the most important factor in maintaining metabolic alkalosis. Skeletal muscle weakness and hypokalemia are often present when hypovolemia complicates metabolic alkalosis.

    2. Treatment of metabolic alkalosis is directed at resolution of the events responsible for the acid-base derangement and appropriate replacement of electrolytes. On occasion, intravenous infusion of hydrogen in the form of ammonium chloride or 0.1 N hydrochloric acid is used to facilitate return of pHa to near-normal levels.

22

Endocrine Diseases

Endocrine disease is characterized by the overproduction or underproduction of single or multiple hormones (Stoelting RK, Dierdorf SF. Endocrine diseases. In: Anesthesia and Co-Existing Disease, 4th ed. New York, Churchill Livingstone, 2002;395–440). The presence of unsuspected endocrine disease may be determined by seeking the answer to specific questions during the patient's preoperative evaluation (Table 22–1).

I. DIABETES MELLITUS

Diabetes mellitus is characterized by metabolic dysregulation, most notably that of glucose metabolism, accompanied by predictable long-term vascular and neurologic complications.

A. Classification of diabetes mellitus. See Table 22–2.

B. Pathogenesis of diabetes mellitus includes insulin deficiency, genetic factors, and insulin resistance.

1. **Absolute insulin deficiency** is characteristic of insulin-dependent diabetes mellitus (IDDM), making these patients dependent on exogenous insulin for survival. Clinical diabetes mellitus manifests when more than 90% of the islet beta cells have been destroyed.

2. **Genetics and IDDM.** It seems likely that environmental influences are superimposed on the inheritable component of IDDM.

3. **Insulin resistance.** Most patients with non-insulin-dependent diabetes mellitus (NIDDM) do not manifest any abnormality in the structure of insulin receptors. The principal sequela of insulin resistance is decreased skeletal muscle uptake of glucose. A common feature of NIDDM is that both insulin resistance and insulin secretion are improved if fasting blood glucose concentrations are normalized by diet or drugs. Abdominal obesity is associated with the development of NIDDM.

≡ Table 22–1 • Preoperative Evaluation of Endocrine Function

Does the urinalysis reveal glycosuria?
Are the systemic blood pressure and heart rate normal?
Is body weight unchanged?
Is sexual function normal?
Is there a history of treatment with hormone replacement drugs?

---

    4. Genetics and NIDDM. Insulin resistance, characteristic of NIDDM, appears to be inherited, manifesting as postprandial hyperglycemia.

  C. Metabolic abnormalities. See Table 22–3. Metabolic lability tends to be less severe in patients with NIDDM than in those with IDDM.

  D. Clinical presentation. The clinical presentation of IDDM is usually unmistakable (special diagnostic tests other than measurement of blood glucose concentrations and possibly serum ketones and electrolytes are not required). Compared with IDDM patients, patients with NIDDM are more likely to have no or fewer clinical symptoms (as many as 50% of patients are undiagnosed), and the diagnosis may require measurement of fasting blood glucose concentrations or an oral glucose tolerance test.

  E. Management of IDDM requires delivery of exogenous insulin, self-monitoring by the patient, and lifestyle adaptations including diet and exercise. Intensive exogenous insulin therapy intended to maintain normal blood glucose concentrations [glycosylated hemoglobin A_{1c} (HbA_{1c}) levels < 7.5%] decreases the development and progression of long-term diabetic complications (retinopathy, nephropathy, neuropathy). The disadvantage of more intensive control of hyperglycemia is an increased incidence of symptomatic hypoglycemia.

    1. Self-monitoring. Development of insulin delivery systems and attempts to provide more precise control of blood glucose concentrations require accurate self-monitoring of the metabolic status (urine glucose tests not sufficient).

    2. Glycosylated hemoglobin. HbA_{1c} concentrations reflect the mean blood glucose concentrations over approxi-

Table 22-2 • Classification of Diabetes Mellitus

Class	Prevalence	Clinical Characteristics	Diagnostic Criteria
Insulin-dependent diabetes mellitus (IDDM, type I)	0.4%	Absolute insulin deficiency Usual onset in youth Ketosis prone Anti-islet cell antibodies	Hyperglycemia Polyuria Polydipsia Weight loss
Non-insulin-dependent diabetes mellitus (NIDDM, type II)	6.6%	Insulin resistance often in the presence of adequate insulin secretion Usual onset after 40 years of age Ketosis-resistant Obese	Same as IDDM Fasting serum glucose > 140 mg/dl Abnormal oral glucose tolerance test
Gestational diabetes mellitus	2–3% of pregnancies	Glucose intolerance with usual onset at 24–30 weeks' gestation Increased perinatal complications Glucose intolerance corrects after delivery NIDDM develops in 30–50% within 10 years	Abnormal oral glucose tolerance test
Secondary diabetes		Pancreatic disease Drugs (glucocorticoids) Acromegaly Cushing's disease	Same as IDDM

☰ Table 22–3 • Metabolic Abnormalities Associated with Insulin Deficiency

Hyperglycemia (unrestrained hepatic glucose production due to glycogenolysis and gluconeogenesis and decreased skeletal muscle uptake)

Increased serum fatty acid concentrations (lipolysis)

Increased serum ketone concentrations (unrestrained hepatic ketogenesis from free fatty acids)

Increased serum triglyceride concentrations (decreased lipoprotein lipase activity resulting in increased synthesis of very low density lipoproteins)

Decreased protein synthesis

Dehydration (glucose acts as an osmotic diuretic)

mately 60 days. The HbA_{1c} assay provides the most accurate and objective assessment of long-term blood glucose control and the efficacy of therapeutic interventions (goal of intensive therapy in patients with IDDM is to maintain the HbA_{1c} at $< 7.5\%$).

   3. **Insulin** formulations may be classified as rapid-acting, intermediate-acting, or long-acting (Table 22–4). Insulin delivery devices (implantable pumps, mechanical syringes) may be used to facilitate frequent administration of regular insulin that is part of intensive treatment regimens. However, similar metabolic results can be achieved with three or more daily subcutaneous injections of regular insulin.

F. **Management of NIDDM.** Typically, normoglycemia in NIDDM patients can be achieved with less complex drug regimens and with lower risks of diabetic ketoacidosis and hypoglycemia than in IDDM patients. Diet is the most important initial treatment of NIDDM. Laboratory measurements of fasting blood glucose concentrations or HbA_{1c} every 3 to 6 months usually provides an accurate index of blood glucose concentrations in stable NIDDM patients.

   1. **Hypoglycemic medications.** See Table 22–5.

      a. **Sulfonylureas** are oral medications that act primarily by stimulating insulin secretion (Table 22–6).

      b. **Biguanides** are useful in the management of NIDDM by virtue of their ability to decrease hyperglycemia

Table 22–4 • Insulin Formulations*

Insulin Type	Onset (hours)	Duration (hours)	Peak (hours)	Other Characteristics
Regular-acting (regular, crystalline zinc insulin; CZI)	0.5–1.0	6–8	2–3	Subcutaneous injection does not produce a sharp peak CZI must be administered 30–60 minutes before meals
Very rapid-acting (lispro)	0.25–0.50	4–6	1–2	As a recombinant human insulin is more readily absorbed Administer 10–15 minutes before meals
Intermediate-acting (Lente, NPH)	2–4	10–14	4–8	
Long-acting (Ultralente)	8–14	18–24	10–14	Because of long half-life, a new steady state is not achieved for 3–4 days after a change in dose

* All available in animal and human formulations except for lispro and Ultralente, which are available only as human (recombinant) preparations.
Adapted from: Nathan DM. Diabetes mellitus. Sci Am Med 1997;1–24.

Table 22–5 • Comparison of Insulin with Oral Hypoglycemic Drugs for Treatment of NIDDM

Parameter	Insulin	Sulfonylurea	Metformin	Acarbose
Lowers HbA$_{1c}$	> 2%	1.5%–2.0%	1.5%–2.0%	0.5%–1.0%
Maximum daily dose	None	20–40 mg	25–50 mg	300 mg
Primary failure rate	None	10%–20%	10%–20%	10%–20%
Effect on lipids				
Triglycerides	Decreases	Decreases	Decreases	Decreases
Total cholesterol	Decreases	Minimal	Decreases	Minimal
HDL cholesterol	Increases	Minimal	Minimal	Minimal
Hypoglycemia	Rare but severe	Rare	No	No
Weight gain	Yes	No	No	No
May be combined with other antidiabetic medications	All	All	All	All

HbA$_{1c}$, hemoglobin A$_{1c}$; NIDDM, non-insulin-dependent diabetes mellitus; HDL, high density liproprotein.
Adapted from: Nathan DM. Diabetes mellitus. Sci Am Med 1997;1–24.

Table 22-6 • Classification of Sulfonylureas

Drug	Dose Range (mg)	Duration (hours)	Other Considerations
First Generation			
Chlorpropamide	100–750	> 36	Disulfiram-like effects
			Prolonged hypoglycemia
			Hyponatremia
Tolbutamide	500–3000	6–12	Metabolized in liver
			Use in patients with renal insufficiency
Acetohexamide	250–1500	12–18	Metabolized in liver to active metabolites
Tolazamide	100–1000	12–24	
Second Generation			
Glyburide	2.5–20.0	18–24	Fewer side effects than first-generation drugs
Glipizide	5–40	12–18	
Glimepiride	1–8	24	Administer once a day

Adapted from: Nathan DM. Diabetes mellitus. Sci Am Med 1997;1–24.

(inhibit gluconeogenesis in the liver and kidneys, increase glucose uptake into skeletal muscles) with low risks of hypoglycemia.

   i. **Metformin,** a biguanide, has a lower risk of causing lactic acidosis than the previously available biguanide, phenformin.

   ii. Lactic acidosis has been described following minor surgery in a patient treated with metformin. The risk of lactic acidosis is increased in elderly patients or those with a decreased glomerular filtration rate, congestive heart failure, or shock.

c. **Glycoside inhibitors.** Acarbose, an α-glycoside inhibitor, decreases the absorption of carbohydrate from the gastrointestinal tract, resulting in blunted glycemic responses during the postprandial period in all individuals, including those with IDDM.

d. **Insulin** is the most effective hypoglycemic drug, and its combination with sulfonylureas may result in acceptable blood glucose concentrations with lower insulin doses.

G. **Complications** of diabetes mellitus. See Table 22–7.

1. **Ketoacidosis.** Hyperglycemia in the presence of metabolic acidosis and a history of IDDM are sufficient to establish the diagnosis of ketoacidosis (Table 22–8).

   a. **Treatment.** See Table 22–9.

≡ **Table 22–7 • Complications of Diabetes Mellitus**

Metabolic
Ketoacidosis
Hypoglycemia
Macrovascular
Coronary artery disease
Cerebral vascular disease
Peripheral vascular disease
Microvascular
Retinopathy
Nephropathy
Nervous System
Autonomic nervous system neuropathy
Peripheral neuropathy

Table 22–8 • Signs and Symptoms of Diabetic Ketoacidosis

Clinical
Nausea and vomiting
Dehydration
  Hypotension
  Tachycardia
Kussmaul's respirations
Abdominal pain
Ileus
Somnolence or coma
Laboratory
Hyperglycemia
Metabolic acidosis
  Arterial pH < 7.3
  Bicarbonate < 15 mEq/L
Ketones present in urine and blood
Hyperosmolarity
Hypokalemia
Increased blood urea nitrogen and/or creatinine concentrations

Adapted from: Nathan DM. Diabetes mellitus. Sci Am Med 1997;1–24.

b. It is estimated that adult IDDM patients in diabetic ketoacidosis present with an intravascular fluid volume deficit of 5 to 8 L, a potassium deficit of 200 to 400 mEq, and a sodium chloride deficit of 350 to 600 mEq.

Table 22–9 • Treatment of Diabetic Ketoacidosis

Tracheal intubation if central nervous system depression is present
Administer intravenous regular insulin (10 units followed by 5–10 units/hr)
Restore intravascular fluid volume (normal saline 5–10 ml/kg/hr IV; add 5% glucose when blood glucose concentrations decrease to < 250 mg/dl)
Restore total body potassium (0.3–0.5 mEq/kg/hr IV)
Monitor blood glucose, serum potassium, arterial pH, and urine ketones concentration
Identify causes (sepsis, myocardial infarction, poor compliance)

≡ Table 22–10 • Signs and Symptoms of Hypoglycemia

Evidence of Autonomic Nervous System Activation
Diaphoresis
Tremulousness
Tachycardia
Evidence of Neuroglycopenia
Impaired cognition
Confusion
Headache
Irritability
Retrograde amnesia
Seizures
Unconsciousness

---

2. **Hypoglycemia.** The central nervous system, erythrocytes, and cells of the renal medulla are dependent on glucose as their primary and, in most circumstances, sole energy source.

   a. **Signs and symptoms.** See Table 22–10.

   b. **Treatment.** See Table 22–11.

3. **Retinopathy** is directly related to the degree and duration of hyperglycemia. Photocoagulation of leaking vessels in the retina with the argon laser may be an effective treatment.

4. **Nephropathy** ultimately manifests as end-stage renal disease requiring dialysis and perhaps renal transplantation.

5. **Cardiovascular disease** is not specific for diabetes, but the risk is significantly increased in NIDDM patients, especially obese and hypertensive women. The combination of peripheral vascular disease and peripheral neu-

---

≡ Table 22–11 • Treatment of Hypoglycemia

Orange juice 180 ml PO
Glucose 25 ml of 50% solution IV if unable to swallow
Glucagon 1 mg IV; alternative to intravenous glucose

ropathy involving the lower extremities may result in the need for amputation.

6. **Peripheral neuropathy** usually manifests as a symmetrical sensorimotor neuropathy that presents as numbness or tingling in the toes and feet, often at night. Nerve conduction abnormalities may precede the diagnosis of NIDDM, and the incidence of clinically detectable polyneuropathy increases progressively with the duration of NIDDM.

   a. Mononeuropathies are generally asymmetrical and affect cranial or peripheral nerves at sites of external pressure (radial nerve, peroneal nerve).

   b. Entrapment neuropathies (ulnar nerve at the cubital tunnel, median nerve at the carpal tunnel) occur more frequently in diabetics than nondiabetics. Diabetes is often present in patients who develop postoperative peripheral nerve injuries involving the arms or legs (unavoidable pressure during surgical positioning may exacerbate a previously asymptomatic neuropathy).

7. **Autonomic nervous system neuropathy** reflects dysfunction of the autonomic nervous system. It is estimated to be present in 20% to 40% of patients with long-standing diabetes mellitus (Table 22–12). The likelihood of autonomic nervous system neuropathy is even greater in the

---

Table 22–12 • Manifestations of Diabetic Autonomic Neuropathy

Resting tachycardia
Orthostatic hypotension
Absent beat-to-beat variation in heart rate with deep breathing
Cardiac dysrhythmias (QT abnormalities)
Sudden death syndrome (may occur coincidentally during the perioperative period)
Gastroparesis
    Vomiting
    Diarrhea
    Abdominal distension
Bladder atony
Impotence
Asymptomatic hypoglycemia (blood glucose concentrations < 50 mg/dl)

presence of systemic hypertension, renal failure, or peripheral sensory neuropathies.

8. **Stiff joint syndrome** reflects limited joint mobility (glycosylation of tissue proteins from chronic hyperglycemia) especially in the small joints of the digits and hands and the atlanto-occipital joint (difficult tracheal intubation is not predictably increased).

   a. **Diabetic scleredema** manifests as thickening and hardening of the skin characteristically over the back of the neck, shoulders, and upper back, although it can involve the hands, arms, and legs.

   b. In children with diabetes, associated findings may include carpal tunnel syndrome and limited mobility of the finger joints.

H. **Management of anesthesia.** The principal goal in the management of diabetic patients undergoing elective surgery is to mimic normal metabolism as closely as possible by avoiding hypoglycemia, excessive hyperglycemia, ketoacidosis, and electrolyte disturbances. Improved glycemic control has been shown to decrease perioperative morbidity and mortality in diabetic patients undergoing major surgery.

   1. **Preoperative evaluation.** See Table 22–13. The well controlled, diet-treated NIDDM patient does not require hospitalization or any special treatment (including insulin) before or during surgery. Likewise, patients with well controlled IDDM undergoing brief outpatient surgical

---

■ Table 22–13 • Preoperative Evaluation of Patients with Diabetes Mellitus

Measurement of HbA_{1c} concentrations ($<$ 7.5% suggests adequate control for approximately the last 60 days)

Seek evidence of ischemic heart disease (most common cause of perioperative morbidity in diabetic patients), cerebrovascular disease, and renal dysfunction (proteinuria)

Evaluate for joint mobility

Note presence of peripheral neuropathy (influences selection of regional anesthesia) and autonomic nervous system neuropathy

Consider impact of obesity (commonly present) on ease of tracheal intubation or performance of regional anesthesia

procedures may not require any adjustment in the usual subcutaneous insulin regimen. If oral hypoglycemic drugs are being administered, they may be continued until the evening before surgery, remembering that these drugs can produce hypoglycemia several hours after their administration in the absence of caloric intake. Pre-admission to the hospital is probably indicated only for patients with poorly controlled IDDM.

2. **Exogenous insulin.** There is a consensus that IDDM patients undergoing major surgery should be treated with insulin, but the accepted route of administration (subcutaneous, intravenous) remains unsettled. The most important factor in controlling the diabetic patient's blood glucose concentration during the perioperative period is not the method utilized for delivery of insulin but, rather, frequent measurements of blood glucose concentrations (as often as every 1 to 2 hours during major surgery and the early postoperative period).

   a. A traditional, effective approach to insulin delivery for diabetic patients undergoing elective surgery is subcutaneous administration of one-fourth to one-half the usual daily intermediate-acting dose of insulin on the morning of surgery. If regular insulin is part of the morning schedule, the intermediate-acting insulin dose may be increased by 0.5 unit for each unit of regular insulin. It is common practice to initiate intravenous infusions of glucose (5 to 10 g/hr) during the preoperative fasting period, along with the subcutaneous insulin, to minimize the likelihood of hypoglycemia.

   b. An alternative to subcutaneous delivery of insulin is the continuous intravenous infusion of low doses of regular insulin (circumvents the unpredictable absorption of subcutaneous insulin) typically beginning with 0.5 to 1.0 unit/hr (Table 22–14).

3. **Induction and maintenance.** The choice of drugs for induction and maintenance of anesthesia is less important than monitoring the blood glucose concentration and treating the potential physiologic derangements associated with diabetes. The increased incidence of peripheral neuropathies is a consideration when choosing regional anesthetic techniques in diabetic pa-

▭ Table 22–14 • Continuous Intravenous Infusion of Regular Insulin During the Perioperative Period

Mix 50 units of regular insulin in 500 ml of normal saline (1 unit/hr = 10 ml/hr)
Initiate intravenous infusion at 0.5–1.0 unit/hr
Measure blood glucose concentrations as necessary (every 1–2 hours) and adjust glucose infusion rates accordingly

< 80 mg/dl	Turn intravenous infusion off for 30 minutes; administer 25 ml of 50% glucose; remeasure the blood glucose concentration in 30 minutes
80–120 mg/dl	Decrease insulin infusion rate by 0.3 unit/hr
120–180 mg/dl	No change in insulin infusion rate
180–220 mg/dl	Increase insulin infusion rate by 0.3 unit/hr
> 220 mg/dl	Increase insulin infusion rate by 0.5 unit/hr

Provide sufficient glucose (5–10 g/hr) and potassium (2–4 mEq/L)

Adapted from: Hirsh IB, Magill JOB, Cryer EG, et al. Perioperative management of surgical patients with diabetes mellitus. Anesthesiology 1991;74:346–59.

tients. Prompt intervention with epinephrine is important for treating bradycardia that develops intraoperatively in patients with autonomic nervous system neuropathy.

I. **Emergency surgery.** It is useful to evaluate the patient's metabolic status (blood glucose concentrations, HbA$_{1c}$, electrolytes, pH, urine ketones) when preparing for anesthetic management. If diabetic ketoacidosis is present, surgery can be delayed for a short time to institute treatment (Table 22–9).

J. **Hyperosmolar, hyperglycemic nonketotic coma** is associated with severe hyperglycemia, but by definition it is not associated with ketoacidosis (Table 22–15).

K. **Anesthetic considerations in pancreas transplant patients** includes the possible loss of bicarbonate in the urine (grafts are drained into the bladder) leading to dehydration and metabolic acidosis.

▬ **Table 22–15** • Hyperosmolar Hyperglycemic Nonketotic Coma

Hyperglycemia (> 600 mg/dl)
Hyperosmolarity (> 350 mOsm/L)
Normal pHa
Osmotic diuresis (hypokalemia)
Hypovolemia (hemoconcentration)
Central nervous system depression
Elderly

II. HYPOGLYCEMIC DISORDERS

Hypoglycemic disorders may be categorized as drug-induced (relative excess of insulin in diabetic patients treated with exogenous insulin; sulfonylureas), fasting (parturients), and reactive.

A. Insulinoma is suggested by hypoglycemia that follows an overnight fast in association with increased circulating concentrations of insulin.

B. Management of anesthesia. The principal challenge during anesthesia for surgical excision of an insulinoma is the avoidance of hypoglycemia, as may occur during manipulation of the tumor. Because evidence of hypoglycemia (systemic hypertension, tachycardia, diaphoresis) may be masked during anesthesia, it is probably prudent to include glucose in the intravenous fluids administered intraoperatively.

III. THYROID GLAND DYSFUNCTION

Thyroid gland dysfunction reflects the overproduction or underproduction of triiodothyronine (T_3) and/or thyroxine (T_4). These two hormones act on cells through the adenylate cyclase system, producing changes in the speed of biochemical reactions, total body oxygen consumption, and energy (heat production).

A. Hyperthyroidism is estimated to affect approximately 2.0% of women and 0.2% of men. The presence of normal serum thyrotropin concentrations nearly always excludes the diagnosis of hyperthyroidism.

1. **Causes.** Among the many possible causes of hyperthyroidism, Graves' disease (diffuse goiter and ophthalmopathy) is the most common explanation, occurring most often in women 20 to 40 years of age.
2. **Signs and symptoms.** See Table 22–16.
3. **Treatment** of hyperthyroidism includes administration of drugs, radiation therapy, and surgical removal of a portion of the gland (subtotal thyroidectomy) (Table 22–17).
   a. **Subtotal thyroidectomy** is appropriate treatment of Graves' disease only when radioiodine therapy is refused and for rare patients with large goiters causing tracheal compression or cosmetic concerns. Patients with hyperthyroidism scheduled for elective thyroidectomy should first be rendered euthyroid with drugs (Table 22–18). In an emergency, patients can be prepared for surgery in less than 1 hour by intravenous administration of esmolol or propranolol.
   b. **Side effects.** See Table 22–19.
4. **Thyrotoxic crisis (thyroid storm)** is a medical emergency characterized by the abrupt appearance of clinical signs of hyperthyroidism (tachycardia, hyperthermia, agitation, skeletal muscle weakness, congestive heart failure, dehydration, shock) due to abrupt release of T_4 and T_3.
   a. Thyrotoxic crisis associated with surgery can occur intraoperatively (mimic malignant hyperthermia) but is more likely to occur 6 to 18 hours postoperatively.

≡ Table 22–16 • Signs and Symptoms of Hyperthyroidism

Goiter
Tachycardia
Anxiety
Tremor
Heat intolerance
Fatigue
Weight loss
Eye signs
Skeletal muscle weakness
Atrial fibrillation

Table 22–17 • Medical Treatment of Hyperthyroidism

Drug	Mechanism of Action	Indications	Side Effects
Antithyroid drugs Propylthiouracil Methimazole Carbimazole	Inhibit thyroid hormone synthesis	Initial therapy for Graves' disease	Agranulocytosis; increased aminotransferases; intraoperative bleeding; hypothyroidism
β-Adrenergic antagonists Propranolol Metoprolol Atenolol Nadalol	Ameliorate actions of T_3 and T_4 in tissues	Adjunctive therapy and may be only treatment needed for thyroiditis	Asthma; congestive heart failure
Iodine-containing compounds Potassium iodide Lugol's solution	Inhibit T_3 and T_4 release for a limited time (days to weeks)	Preparation for surgery; thyrotoxic crisis	
Radioiodine therapy	Destroys thyroid tissue	Graves' disease; recurrent hyperthyroidism	Permanent hypothyroidism
Lithium	Inhibits T_3 and T_4 release	Severe subacute thyroiditis; thyrotoxic crisis; Graves' disease	
Glucocorticoids	Ameliorates actions of T_3 and T_4 in tissues Immunosuppressive actions		

T_3, triiodothyronine; T_4, thyroxine.
Adapted from: Franklyn JA. The management of hyperthyroidism. N Engl J Med 1994;330:1731–9.

Table 22–18 • Treatments to Render Hyperthyroid Patients Euthyroid Prior to Surgery

Emergency Surgery
Esmolol 100–300 μg/kg/min IV until heart rate < 100 beats/min
Elective Surgery
Oral administration of β-adrenergic antagonists (propranolol, nadolol, atenolol) until heart rate is < 100 beats/min
Antithyroid drugs
Antithyroid drugs plus potassium iodide
Potassium iodide plus β-adrenergic receptor antagonists

---

       b. Treatment of thyrotoxic crisis is with intravenous infusion of cooled crystalloid solutions and continuous infusion of esmolol to maintain the heart rate at an acceptable level (usually < 100 beats/min). When hypotension is persistent, administration of cortisol (100 to 200 mg IV) may be considered.

    5. Management of anesthesia. See Table 22–20.

  B. Hypothyroidism is estimated to be present in 0.5% to 0.8% of the adult population. Subclinical hypothyroidism manifesting only as increased plasma thyrotropin concentrations

---

Table 22–19 • Side Effects of Subtotal Thyroidectomy

Nerve damage (abductor fibers of the recurrent laryngeal nerves; characterized by hoarseness and a paralyzed vocal cord if unilateral and aphonia and paralyzed vocal cords, which can collapse together producing airway obstruction if bilateral)
Postoperative bleeding into the neck (tracheal compression in the postanesthesia care unit requiring prompt opening of the surgical incision)
Hypoparathyroidism (hypocalcemia develops 24–72 hours postoperatively but may manifest as early as 1–3 hours after surgery)
Relapse of hyperthyroidism
Permanent hypothyroidism

≡ Table 22–20 • Management of Anesthesia in Patients with Hyperthyroidism

Render euthyroid before elective surgery (when emergency can control hyperdynamic cardiovascular system with esmolol)

Avoid anticholinergic drugs in preoperative medication

Evaluate upper airway for obstruction from goiter (computed tomography)

Induction of anesthesia (thiopental plus succinylcholine or nondepolarizing drugs that lack cardiovascular effects)

Maintenance of anesthesia (isoflurane, desflurane, or sevoflurane plus nitrous oxide; anesthetic requirements not greatly altered)

Monitor for signs of thyroid storm (body temperature, heart rate)

Treatment of hypotension (possible exaggerated responses to indirect-acting vasopressors)

Regional anesthesia (associated blockade of sympathetic nervous system is potentially useful)

is present in about 5% of the population, with a prevalence of 13.2% in otherwise healthy elderly patients, especially women.

1. **Causes** of hypothyroidism are categorized as primary [destruction of the thyroid gland most often due to chronic thyroiditis (Hashimoto's thyroiditis)] or secondary [central nervous system dysfunction (hypothalamic or anterior pituitary)].

2. **Signs and symptoms.** The onset of hypothyroidism in adult patients is insidious and may go unrecognized (Table 22–21). Cardiovascular impairment is minimal to absent in the presence of subclinical hypothyroidism.

3. **Treatment** is with oral administration of T_4. It is not unusual to encounter patients previously started on thyroid hormone replacement without convincing laboratory confirmation of hypothyroidism.

4. **Myxedema coma** is a rare complication of hypothyroidism, manifesting as loss of deep tendon reflexes, spontaneous hypothermia, hypoventilation, cardiovascular collapse, coma, and death. Treatment is with intravenous administration of T_3 and cortisol if adrenal insufficiency is suspected.

5. **Management of anesthesia** should consider possible adverse responses associated with hypothyroidism (Table

≡ **Table 22–21 • Signs and Symptoms of Hypothyroidism**

Lethargy
Intolerance to cold
Bradycardia
Peripheral vasoconstriction (conserve heat)
Atrophy of the adrenal cortex
Hyponatremia

22–22). Controlled clinical studies do not confirm an increased risk to patients with mild to moderate hypothyroidism who are undergoing elective surgery.

  a. **Preoperative preparation.** Most patients with hypothyroidism are receiving thyroid hormone replacement and are euthyroid at the time of surgery.
  b. **Preoperative medication** may include supplemental cortisol.

≡ **Table 22–22 • Possible Adverse Responses of Hypothyroid Patients During the Perioperative Period**

Increased sensitivity to depressant drugs
Hypodynamic cardiovascular system
Decreased heart rate
Decreased cardiac output
Slowed metabolism of drugs
Unresponsive baroreceptor reflexes
Impaired ventilatory responses to arterial hypoxemia or hypercarbia
Hypovolemia
Delayed gastric emptying time
Hyponatremia
Hypothermia
Anemia
Hypoglycemia
Adrenal insufficiency

    c. **Induction of anesthesia** is often with intravenous administration of ketamine.

    d. **Maintenance of anesthesia** is often achieved by inhalation of nitrous oxide plus supplementation, if necessary, with short-acting opioids, benzodiazepines, or ketamine. Decreased skeletal muscle activity associated with hypothyroidism suggests the possibility of prolonged responses when traditional doses of muscle relaxants are administered to hypothyroid patients. Monitoring hypothyroid patients during anesthesia is intended to facilitate prompt recognition of exaggerated cardiovascular depression and detection of the onset of hypothermia (raise ambient temperatures of the operating rooms, use warming devices placed over patients, warm the inhaled gases, and pass intravenous fluids through a warmer).

    e. **Postoperative management.** Recovery from the sedative effects of anesthetic drugs may be delayed in hypothyroid patients. Tracheal extubation is deferred until hypothyroid patients are responding appropriately and body temperature is near 37°C.

    f. **Regional anesthesia** is an appropriate selection, provided intravascular fluid volume is well maintained.

IV. PARATHYROID GLAND DYSFUNCTION

  A. **Hyperparathyroidism** is present when the secretion of parathormone is increased (serum calcium concentrations may be increased, decreased, or unchanged).

    1. **Primary hyperparathyroidism** results from excessive secretion of parathormone owing to benign parathyroid adenomas (responsible for 90% of affected patients), carcinoma of a parathyroid gland, or hyperplasia of the parathyroid glands.

      a. **Diagnosis.** Primary hyperparathyroidism is the most common cause of hypercalcemia in the general population (serum calcium concentrations > 5.5 mEq/L and ionized calcium concentrations > 2.5 mEq/L).

      b. **Signs and symptoms.** See Table 22–23.

      c. **Treatment.** See Table 22–24.

      d. **Management of anesthesia.** There is no evidence that specific anesthetic drugs or techniques are indicated. Maintenance of hydration and urine output is important during perioperative management of hypercalce-

Table 22–3 • Signs and Symptoms of Hypercalcemia Due to Hyperparathyroidism

Organ System	Signs and Symptoms
Neuromuscular	Skeletal muscle weakness
Renal	Polyuria and polydipsia
	Decreased glomerular filtration rate
	Kidney stones
Hematopoietic	Anemia
Cardiac	Prolonged PR interval
	Short QT interval
	Systemic hypertension
Gastrointestinal	Vomiting
	Abdominal pain
	Peptic ulcers
	Pancreatitis
Skeletal	Skeletal demineralization
	Collapse of vertebral bodies
	Pathologic fractures
Nervous	Somnolence
	Decreased pain sensation
	Psychosis
Ocular	Calcifications (band keratopathy)
	Conjunctivitis

Table 22–24 • Treatment of Primary Hyperparathyroidism and Associated Hypercalcemia

Medical Management
Saline infusion (150 ml/hr) to produce a daily urine output of 3–5 L
Furosemide (40–80 mg IV every 2 hours) after intravascular fluid volume is reestablished as reflected by central venous pressure
Bisphosphonate (disodium etidronate) administered intravenously for life-threatening hypercalcemia
Surgical Management
Removal of diseased or abnormal portions of the parathyroid glands (serum calcium concentrations normalize within 3–4 days)

mia. Somnolence and skeletal muscle weakness suggest possible decreased requirements for anesthetic drugs and muscle relaxants.

2. **Secondary hyperparathyroidism** reflects appropriate compensatory responses of the parathyroid glands to secrete more parathormone to counteract a disease process (chronic renal disease) that produces hypocalcemia.

3. **Ectopic hyperparathyroidism** is due to secretion of parathormone (lung, breast, pancreas, or kidney cancer; lymphoproliferative disease).

B. **Hypoparathyroidism** is present when secretion of parathormone is deficient or absent (most often due to inadvertent removal of the parathyroid glands during thyroidectomy) or peripheral tissues are resistant to the effects of the hormone.

1. **Diagnosis.** Serum calcium concentrations < 4.5 mEq/L and ionized calcium concentrations < 2.0 mEq/L are indicative of hypoparathyroidism.

2. **Signs and symptoms** depend on the rapidity of onset of hypocalcemia (Table 22–25).

3. **Treatment** of acute hypocalcemia consists of an infusion of calcium (10 ml of 10% calcium gluconate IV) until signs of neuromuscular irritability disappear. Thiazide diuretics may be useful, as these drugs cause sodium depletion without proportional potassium excretion, thus tending to increase serum calcium concentrations.

☰ Table 22–25 • Signs and Symptoms of Hypocalcemia Due to Hypoparathyroidism

---

Acute Hypocalcemia (accidental surgical removal)
Perioral paresthesias
Restlessness
Neuromuscular irritability (positive Chvostek or Trousseau sign, inspiratory stridor)
Chronic Hypocalcemia (renal failure)
Fatigue
Skeletal muscle weakness
Prolonged QT interval
Cataracts

---

      4. Management of anesthesia in the presence of hypocalcemia is designed to prevent any further decreases in serum calcium concentrations (avoid hyperventilation) and to treat adverse effects of hypocalcemia, particularly on the heart.

  C. DiGeorge syndrome is characterized by hypoplasia or aplasia of the parathyroid glands and thymus gland resulting in secondary hypocalcemia and a propensity to develop infections.

      1. Management of anesthesia. Micrognathia may interfere with adequate exposure of the glottic opening during direct laryngoscopy. Iatrogenic hyperventilation is avoided, and responses to neuromuscular blocking drugs may be altered in the presence of hypocalcemia.

      2. Ability to measure serum calcium concentrations, particularly the ionized fraction, is helpful for perioperative management of these patients.

V. ADRENAL GLAND DYSFUNCTION

  A. Hypercortisolism (Cushing syndrome) is categorized as corticotropin-dependent Cushing syndrome (pituitary adenomas) or corticotropin-independent Cushing syndrome (adrenocortical tumors).

      1. Diagnosis. There are no pathognomonic signs or symptoms (sudden weight gain, moon facies, systemic hypertension, glucose intolerance, skeletal muscle weakness) that confirm the diagnosis of Cushing syndrome. The diagnosis is confirmed by demonstrating cortisol hypersecretion based on 24-hour urinary secretion of cortisol.

      2. Treatment. The treatment of choice for patients with Cushing's disease is transsphenoidal microadenomectomy.

      3. Management of anesthesia is influenced by the physiologic effects of excess cortisol secretion (systemic blood pressure, electrolyte balance, blood glucose concentrations). Osteoporosis is a consideration when positioning the patient for the operative procedure. The choice of drugs for preoperative medication, induction of anesthesia, and maintenance of anesthesia is not influenced by the presence of hypercortisolism. Muscle relaxant doses should probably be decreased initially in view of skeletal muscle weakness, which frequently accompanies hypercortisolism. Continuous infusions of cortisol (100 mg daily IV) may be initiated intraoperatively as plasma cortisol concentrations decrease promptly after microadenomectomy or bilateral adrenalectomy.

B. Hypocortisolism (Addison's disease) reflects the absence of cortisol and aldosterone owing to destruction of the adrenal cortex.

1. **Signs and symptoms.** See Table 22–26.

2. **Treatment** of life-threatening hypocortisolism is administration of cortisol, 100 mg IV, followed by continuous infusions of 10 mg/hr IV.

   a. **Surgery and suppression of the pituitary adrenal axis.** Corticosteroid supplementation should be provided for patients being treated for chronic hypocortisolism who undergo surgical procedures. More controversial is the management of patients who display suppression of the pituitary-adrenal axis owing to current or previous treatment with corticosteroids (dose or duration of therapy to produce suppression or the time necessary for recovery is not known) for treatment of diseases (asthma, rheumatoid arthritis) unrelated to pathology in the anterior pituitary or adrenal cortex.

   b. Original recommendations for supplemental corticosteroid dosages were excessive and based on anecdotal information.

      i. **Steroid coverage based on physiologic responses to stress.** A recommended regimen for corticosteroid supplementation during the perioperative period for patients being treated with corticoste-

---

≡ Table 22–26 • Signs and Symptoms of Hypocortisolism

Weight loss
Skeletal muscle weakness
Systemic hypotension (indistinguishable from shock due to loss of intravascular fluid volume)
Hyperkalemia
Hypoglycemia
Hyperpigmentation over palmar surfaces and pressure points

roids or who have been treated more than 1 month during the immediately preceding 6 to 12 months is administration of cortisol, 25 mg IV, at induction of anesthesia followed by continuous infusions of cortisol, 100 mg IV, during the next 24 hours.

ii. An alternative to this physiologic replacement regimen is administration of cortisol 25 mg IV, every 4 hours.

iii. In addition to cortisol supplementation, patients receiving daily maintenance doses of corticosteroids should also receive this dose with the preoperative mediation on the day of surgery.

iv. Continuation of corticosteroid supplementation into the postoperative period is based on the magnitude of the surgical stress and the known corticosteroid production rates associated with this stress [endogenous cortisol production produced by intense physiologic stress (burns) is 75 to 150 mg daily].

3. **Management of anesthesia** for patients with known hypocortisolism introduces no unique considerations other than provision of exogenous corticosteroid supplementation and a high index of suspicion for primary adrenal failure if unexplained intraoperative hypotension occurs.

C. **Primary hyperaldosteronism (Conn syndrome)** is present when there is excess secretion of aldosterone from functional tumors (aldosteronoma) independent of a physiologic stimulus.

1. **Signs and symptoms** of primary aldosteronism may reflect systemic hypertension (sodium retention, increased extracellular fluid volume) and hypokalemia (skeletal muscle weakness, nephropathy, metabolic alkalosis).

2. **Diagnosis.** Spontaneous hypokalemia in patients with systemic hypertension is highly suggestive of aldosteronism.

3. **Treatment** of hyperaldosteronism consists of supplemental potassium and administration of competitive aldosterone antagonists, such as spironolactone. Definitive treatment for an aldosterone-secreting tumor is surgical excision.

4. **Management of anesthesia** for the treatment of hyperaldosteronism is facilitated by preoperative correction of hypokalemia and treatment of systemic hypertension.

D. **Hypoaldosteronism** is suggested by the presence of hyperkalemia in the absence of renal insufficiency.

E. **Pheochromocytomas** are catecholamine-secreting tumors that may occur independently or as part of an autosomal dominant multiglandular neoplastic syndrome (Table 22–27). Pheochromocytomas and associated systemic hypertension and hypermetabolism may mimic other diseases, including malignant hyperthermia.

1. **Diagnosis.** Computed tomography and magnetic resonance imaging provides accurate identification and localization of most pheochromocytomas, especially when the tumors are suprarenal. Diagnosis of pheochromocytoma requires chemical confirmation of excessive catecholamine release into the systemic circulation (free norepinephrine in a 24-hour urine collection). Clonidine, 0.3 mg PO, suppresses plasma concentrations of catecholamines in hypertensive patients but not in those with pheochromocytomas (blocks neurogenic release but not diffusion into systemic circulation).

2. **Signs and symptoms.** The triad of diaphoresis, tachycardia, and headache in hypertensive patients is highly suggestive of pheochromocytoma. Hyperglycemia reflects a predominance of α-adrenergic activity (inhibition of insulin release) over β-adrenergic effects (insulin release). Orthostatic hypotension is a common finding and reflects

Table 22–27 • Manifestations of Multiple Endocrine Neoplasia

Syndrome	Manifestations
MEN type 2a (Sipple syndrome)	Medullary thyroid cancer
	Parathyroid adenoma
	Pheochromocytoma
MEN type 2b	Medullary thyroid cancer
	Mucosal adenomas
	Marfan appearance
	Pheochromocytoma
Von Hippel-Lindau syndrome	Hemangioblastoma involving the central nervous system
	Pheochromocytoma

decreased in intravascular fluid volume associated with sustained systemic hypertension. Sustained increases in plasma catecholamine concentrations can result in focal necrosis of cardiac muscle and the development of dilated cardiomyopathy and congestive heart failure. Death resulting from pheochromocytomas is often due to congestive heart failure, myocardial infarction, or intracerebral hemorrhage.

3. **Treatment** of pheochromocytomas is surgical excision of the catecholamine-secreting tumor (or tumors) but only after medical control is optimized by instituting α-adrenergic blockade (phenoxybenzamine) to stabilize the systemic blood pressure, expand intravascular fluid volume, and normalize myocardial performance. Persistence of tachycardia or cardiac dysrhythmias despite α-blockade is an indication for preoperative administration of drugs such as propranolol. Echocardiography may be

---

Table 22–28 • Management of Anesthesia for Excising a Pheochromocytoma

Continue α- and β-antagonist therapy

Consider the need for supplemental cortisol

Place an intra-arterial catheter

Intravenous induction of anesthesia, followed by establishment of a surgical level of anesthesia with volatile anesthetics (isoflurane, desflurane, sevoflurane)

Skeletal muscle paralysis with nondepolarizing muscle relaxants devoid of circulatory effects

Minimize circulatory responses to direct laryngoscopy and tracheal intubation (nitroprusside or phentolamine readily available)

Maintenance of anesthesia with volatile anesthetics (isoflurane, desflurane, sevoflurane) plus nitrous oxide (opioids, nitroprusside, esmolol, lidocaine as needed)

Pulmonary artery catheter for monitoring status of intravascular fluid volume (transesophageal echocardiography provides much of the same information and is less invasive)

Monitor arterial blood gases, electrolytes, blood glucose concentrations

Postoperatively continue invasive monitoring and provide pain relief (neuraxial opioids)

useful for recognizing patients with suspected cardiomyopathy.

4. **Management of anesthesia** for patients requiring excision of pheochromocytomas is based on the administration of drugs that do not stimulate the sympathetic nervous system plus the use of invasive monitoring techniques to facilitate early, appropriate interventions if catecholamine-induced changes in cardiovascular function occur (Table 22–28). Regional anesthesia is not protective, as postsynaptic α-receptors can still respond to sudden increases in the circulating concentrations of catecholamines.

VI. DYSFUNCTION OF THE TESTES OR OVARIES

See Table 22–29.

VII. PITUITARY GLAND DYSFUNCTION

See Table 22–30.

A. **Acromegaly** is due to excess secretion of growth hormone in adults, most often from an adenoma in the anterior pituitary gland.

1. **Signs and symptoms.** See Table 22–31.
2. **Treatment** is transsphenoidal surgical excision of the pituitary adenoma.

≡ **Table 22–29** • Dysfunction of the Testes and Ovaries

Klinefelter syndrome (XXY chromosomal defect, most common expression of testicular dysfunction)

Physiologic menopause (absence of estrogen levels leads to osteoporosis)

Premenstrual syndrome (prostaglandins)

Ovarian hyperstimulation syndrome (ascites, hypovolemia)

Turner syndrome (primary amenorrhea, difficult airway management)

Noonan syndrome (resembles Turner syndrome but mental retardation and congenital heart disease likely)

Stein-Leventhal syndrome (primary amenorrhea, hirsutism, and increased skeletal muscle development)

Table 22–30 • Hypothalamic and Related Pituitary Hormones

Hypothalamic Hormone	Action	Pituitary Hormone or Organ Affected	Action
Corticotropin-releasing hormone	Stimulatory	Corticotropin	Stimulates secretion of cortisol
Thyrotropin-releasing hormone	Stimulatory	Thyrotropin	Stimulates secretion of androgens Stimulates secretion of thyroxine Stimulates secretion of triiodothyronine
Gonadotropin-releasing hormone	Stimulatory	Follicle-stimulating hormone Luteinizing hormone	Stimulates estradiol secretion* Stimulates progesterone secretion* Stimulates ovulation* Stimulates testosterone secretion† Stimulates spermatogenesis†
Growth hormone-releasing hormone	Stimulatory	Growth hormone	Stimulates production of insulin-like growth factor
Dopamine	Inhibitory	Prolactin	Stimulates lactation*
Somatostatin	Inhibitory	Growth hormone	
Vasopressin (antidiuretic hormone)	Stimulatory	Kidneys	Stimulates free-water reabsorption
Oxytocin	Stimulatory	Uterus Breasts	Stimulates uterine contractions* Stimulates milk ejection*

* Actions in females.
† Actions in males.
Adapted from Vance ML. Hypopituitarism. N Engl J Med 1994;330:1651–62.

☰ Table 22–31 • Manifestations of Acromegaly

Parasellar
Enlarged sella turcica
Headache
Visual field defects
Rhinorrhea
Excess Growth Hormone
Skeletal overgrowth (prognathism)
Soft tissue overgrowth (lips, tongue, epiglottis, vocal cords)
Connective tissue overgrowth (recurrent laryngeal nerve paralysis)
Peripheral neuropathy (carpal tunnel syndrome)
Visceromegaly
Glucose intolerance
Osteoarthritis
Osteoporosis
Hyperhydrosis
Skeletal muscle weakness

3. **Management of anesthesia** considers the potential for difficult upper airway management and anticipation of the possible need to insert a small-diameter tracheal tube. When placing a catheter in the radial artery, it is important to consider the possibility of inadequate collateral circulation at the wrist. Monitoring blood glucose concentrations is useful if diabetes mellitus accompanies acromegaly.

B. **Diabetes insipidus** reflects the absence of antidiuretic hormone due to destruction of the posterior pituitary (neurogenic diabetes insipidus) or failure of the renal tubules to respond to the hormone (nephrogenic diabetes mellitus accompanies acromegaly).

1. **Treatment** is intravenous infusion of electrolyte solutions if oral intake cannot offset polyuria. Chlorpropamide is useful for treating nephrogenic diabetes insipidus, and intramuscular or intranasal vasopressin is useful for managing neurogenic diabetes insipidus.

2. **Management of anesthesia** for patients with diabetes insipidus includes monitoring the urine output and serum electrolyte concentrations during the perioperative period.

C. **Inappropriate secretion of antidiuretic hormone** accompanies diverse pathologic processes (intracranial tumors, hypothyroidism, carcinoma of the lung) and is common after surgery. Inappropriately increased urinary sodium concentrations and osmolarity in the presence of hyponatremia and decreased plasma osmolarity are diagnostic. Initial treatment is restriction of fluid intake.

23

Nutritional Diseases and Inborn Errors of Metabolism

The presence of nutritional diseases and inborn errors of metabolism may influence the management of anesthesia (Table 23–1) (Stoelting RK, Dierdorf SF. Nutritional diseases and inborn errors of metabolism. In: Anesthesia and Co-Existing Disease, 4th ed. New York, Churchill Livingstone, 2002;441–470).

I. OBESITY

Obesity (body weight 20% or more above ideal weight) is a disorder of energy balance. It represents the most common and costly nutritional disorder in the United States, affecting an estimated one-third of the adult population. Obesity is associated with increased morbidity and mortality and a wide spectrum of medical and surgical diseases (Table 23–2). A measure of obesity is the body-mass index (BMI) in which a value of 28 for males and 27 for females corresponds to 20% above ideal body weight (Table 23–3).

A. **Pathogenesis.** Obesity is a complex, multifactorial disease (mechanisms are fat storage, genetic, psychological), but in simple terms it occurs when net energy intake exceeds net energy expenditure over a prolonged period of time.

1. **Fat storage.** Surplus calories are converted to triglyceride and stored in adipocytes. Central or android distribution of fat (abdominal obesity) is more common in men. Abdominal fat deposits are metabolically more active than peripheral or gynecoid fat deposits (hips, buttocks, thighs) and thus are associated with a higher incidence of metabolic complications (dyslipidemia, glucose intolerance, diabetes mellitus, ischemic heart disease, congestive heart failure, stroke).

2. **Metabolic effects of weight changes.** Small decreases in body weight result in decreased energy expenditures such that persistent decreases in caloric intake may be associated with weight gain.

⬛ Table 23–1 • Nutritional Disorders and Inborn Errors of Metabolism

Nutritional
Obesity
Malnutrition
Anorexia nervosa
Bulimia nervosa
Binge-eating disorders
Vitamin imbalance disorders
Inborn Errors of Metabolism
Porphyria
Gout
Pseudogout
Hyperlipidemia
Carbohydrate metabolism disorders
Amino acid disorders
Mucopolysaccharidoses
Gangliosidoses

B. **Treatment** of obesity is intended to result in weight reduction that decreases morbidity. A weight loss of 5 to 20 kg may decrease the systemic blood pressure and plasma lipid concentrations and enhance the control of diabetes mellitus. Gastroplasty is the most commonly performed surgical procedure for treatment of obesity (usually reserved for those with a BMI > 40).

C. **Physiologic disturbances associated with obesity.** See Table 23–2. Many obese individuals choose to sleep sitting in a chair to avoid symptoms of orthopnea and paroxysmal nocturnal dyspnea.

   1. **Obstructive sleep apnea** is present in 2% to 4% of middle-age adults, especially men (Table 23–4). An estimated 5% of obese subjects develop obstructive sleep apnea.

      a. **Pathogenesis.** Apnea occurs when the pharyngeal airway collapses.

      b. **Risk Factors.** See Table 23–4.

      c. **Treatment.** Positive airway pressure delivered through a nasal mask is the initial treatment of choice in the presence of clinically significant obstructive

▬ Table 23–2 • Medical and Surgical Conditions Associated with Obesity

Organ System	Side Effects
Respiratory system	Obstructive sleep apnea
	Obesity hypoventilation syndrome
	Restrictive lung disease
Cardiovascular system	Systemic hypertension
	Cardiomegaly
	Congestive heart failure
	Ischemic heart disease
	Cerebrovascular disease
	Peripheral vascular disease
	Pulmonary hypertension
	Deep vein thrombosis
	Pulmonary embolism
	Hypercholesterolemia
	Hypertriglyceridemia
	Sudden death
Endocrine system	Diabetes mellitus
	Cushing syndrome
	Hypothyroidism
Gastrointestinal system	Hiatus hernia
	Inguinal hernia
	Gallstones
	Fatty liver infiltration
Musculoskeletal system	Osteoarthritis of weight-bearing joints
	Back pain
Malignancy	Breast
	Prostate
	Cervical
	Uterine
	Colorectal

Adapted from: Adams JP, Murphy PG. Obesity in anaesthesia and intensive care. Br J Anaesth 2000;85:91–108.

▬ Table 23–3 • Calculation of Body Mass Index

$$\text{Body mass index (BMI)} = \frac{\text{weight (kg)}}{\text{height}^2\text{ (m)}}$$

Example: A 150 kg, 1.8 meter tall man has a BMI of 47 (more than 100% above ideal body weight). A similar patient weighing 80 kg has a BMI of 25.

▤ Table 23–4 • Manifestations and Risk Factors of Obstructive Sleep Apnea

Manifestations

Frequent episodes of obstructive sleep apnea (10 seconds or longer occurring five times per hour or more during sleep) or hypopnea (50% decrease in airflow or a decrease sufficient to decrease arterial oxygen saturation by 4%)

Snoring

Daytime somnolence most likely reflecting sleep fragmentation (memory and concentration deficits, motor vehicle accidents)

Physiologic changes
    Arterial hypoxemia
    Polycythemia
    Arterial hypercarbia
    Systemic hypertension (ischemic heart disease, cerebrovascular disease)

Pulmonary hypertension

Risk Factors

Male gender

Middle age

Obesity (body mass index > 30)

Alcohol (evening ingestion; decreases pharyngeal muscle tone)

Drug-induced sleep

---

sleep apnea. Nocturnal oxygen therapy is a consideration for patients who experience severe arterial oxygen desaturation. Surgical treatment of obstructive sleep apnea includes tracheostomy, palatal surgery (laser-assisted uvulopalatopharyngoplasty), and maxillofacial surgical procedures to enhance upper airway patency during sleep (genioglossal advancement).

    d. **Management of anesthesia.** See Table 23–5.

        i. **Specialized surgical procedures** to treat obstructive sleep apnea are often prolonged (general anesthesia with muscle relaxants). A tracheostomy is mandatory before surgery that involves the base of the tongue.

        ii. **Uvulopalatopharyngoplasty** is performed with patients supine and the head slightly elevated to enhance venous drainage. Worsening of upper air-

---

≡ Table 23–5 • Management of Anesthesia in Patients with Obstructive Sleep Apnea

Exquisitely sensitive to central nervous system depressant drugs (upper airway obstruction or apnea possible with even minimal doses of these drugs)

Possible difficult exposure of glottic opening (decreased anatomic space to accommodate anterior displacement of the tongue)

Use short-acting inhaled and injected anesthetics

Use short-acting neuromuscular blocking drugs

Regional anesthesia is useful

Tracheal extubation when fully awake

Increased risk of arterial hypoxemia during the postoperative period (may occur early as well as up to 5 days postoperatively)

Management of postoperative pain must consider exquisite sensitivity to ventilatory depressant effects of opioids including neuraxial opioids (regional analgesia is useful; nonsteroidal antiinflammatory drugs)

---

way obstruction is possible during the early postoperative period due to residual effects of anesthetic drugs and/or surgically induced upper airway edema. Acute upper airway obstruction may occur immediately following tracheal extubation. Postoperative analgesia with nonsteroidal antiinflammatory drugs is often recommended.

2. **Obesity hypoventilation syndrome** is the long-term consequence of obstructive sleep apnea (nocturnal alterations in the control of breathing manifesting as central apneic events). It culminates in *pickwickian syndrome.*

3. **Lung volumes.** Obesity imposes a restrictive ventilation defect because of the weight added to the thoracic cage and the abdominal weight impeding the motion of the diaphragm, especially with assumption of the supine position. Anesthesia accentuates decreases in functional residual capacity (FRC) in obese anesthetized patients compared to that in nonobese individuals (Fig. 23–1). The decrease in FRC impairs the ability of obese patients to tolerate even brief periods of apnea, as during direct laryngoscopy for tracheal intubation.

4. **Gas exchange.** Arterial oxygenation may deteriorate markedly on induction of anesthesia, and increased con-

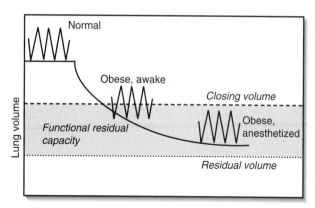

Fig. 23–1 • Effects of severe obesity on functional residual capacity (FRC). Anesthesia and obesity are associated with decreases in FRC resulting in small airway closure, ventilation-to-perfusion mismatching, and impaired arterial oxygenation. (From Adams JP, Murphy PG. Obesity in anaesthesia and intensive care. Br J Anaesth 2000;85:91–108. © The Board of Management and Trustees of the British Journal of Anaesthesia. Reproduced by permission of Oxford University Press/British Journal of Anaesthesia.

centrations of delivered oxygen are needed to maintain an acceptable PaO_2.

5. **Lung compliance and resistance.** Changes in lung compliance and resistance result in rapid shallow breathing patterns and increased work of breathing, which is most marked when obese individuals assume the supine position.

6. **Work of breathing.** Obese patients typically breathe rapidly and shallowly, as this pattern results in the least oxygen cost of breathing.

7. **Systemic hypertension.** Mild to moderate systemic hypertension is present in most obese patients (increased extracellular fluid volume, increased cardiac output, hyperinsulinemia). Pulmonary hypertension is common in obese patients and most likely reflects the impact of chronic arterial hypoxemia and/or increased pulmonary blood volume.

8. **Ischemic heart disease.** Obesity seems to be an independent risk factor for the development of ischemic heart

disease and is more common in obese individuals with central distributions of fat.

9. **Congestive heart failure.** Systemic hypertension leads to concentric left ventricular hypertrophy and a progressively noncompliant left ventricle, which when combined with hypervolemia increases the risk of congestive heart failure. Obesity-induced cardiomyopathy is associated with hypervolemia and increased cardiac output; it reflects interactions with systemic hypertension and ischemic heart disease (Fig. 23–2).

10. **Gastric emptying.** The notion that obese patients are at increased risk for aspiration based on delayed gastric emptying, is questionable.

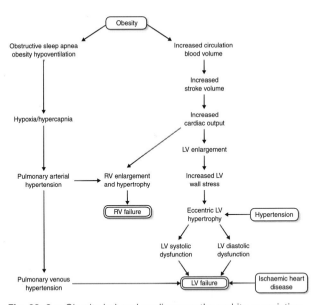

Fig. 23–2 • Obesity-induced cardiomyopathy and its association with congestive heart failure [right ventricular (RV), left ventricular (LV)], systemic hypertension, and ischemic heart disease. (From Adams JP, Murphy PG. Obesity in anaesthesia and intensive care. Br J Anaesth 2000;85:91–108. © The Board of Management and Trustees of the British Journal of Anaesthesia. Reproduced by permission of Oxford University Press/British Journal of Anaesthesia.)

11. **Diabetes mellitus.** Glucose tolerance curves are often abnormal, and the incidence of diabetes mellitus is increased severalfold in obese patients (resistance of peripheral tissues to the effects of insulin in the presence of increased adipose tissue).

12. **Hepatobiliary disease.** Abnormal liver function tests and fatty liver infiltration are frequent findings in obese patients. The risk of developing gallbladder and biliary tract disease is increased in obese patients.

13. **Thromboembolic disease.** The risk of deep vein thrombosis in obese patients undergoing surgery is increased (polycythemia, increased abdominal pressure, immobilization).

14. **Pharmacokinetics of drugs.** See Table 23–6.

D. **Management of anesthesia** is influenced by obesity-induced alterations in physiologic function (Table 23–2).

1. **Induction of anesthesia.** Difficulties with mask ventilation and tracheal intubation may be considerable based on the presence of unique anatomic features (fat face and cheeks, short neck, large tongue, excessive palatal and pharyngeal soft tissue, large breasts). Obese patients are traditionally presumed to be at increased risk for pulmonary aspiration during the induction of anesthesia, but the greater risk of pulmonary aspiration is more related to difficult tracheal intubation. The low FRC associated with obesity means that rapid decreases in arterial

---

Table 23–6 • Pharmacokinetics of Drugs and Physiologic Changes Associated with Obesity

Volume of distribution increased (increased blood volume and cardiac output)

Decreased total body water (fat contains less water)

Congestive heart failure and decreased hepatic blood flow

Calculate initial dose for injected drugs for administration to obese patients based on ideal body weight (80 kg for women, 100 kg for men)

Recovery times from general anesthesia are not influenced by obesity

---

oxygenation may accompany direct laryngoscopy for tracheal intubation (Fig. 23–3).

2. **Maintenance of anesthesia.** The best choice of drugs or techniques for maintenance of anesthesia in obese patients is not known. Storage of anesthetic drugs in fat has not been documented to delay awakening of obese versus nonobese patients.

   a. **Spinal and epidural anesthesia** may be technically difficult to perform in obese patients, as landmarks may be obscured (local anesthetic requirements may be decreased, presumably reflecting fatty infiltration and vascular engorgement of the epidural space).

   b. **Management of ventilation** may include positive end-expiratory pressure to improve oxygenation (effects on cardiac output may offset beneficial effects). Assumption of the supine position by spontaneously breathing obese patients can decrease the PaO_2 (cardiac arrest is a remote risk).

   c. **Tracheal extubation** is considered when obese patients are fully recovered from the depressant effects of anesthetics. Ideally, obese patients are allowed to recover in a head-up to sitting position. A history of

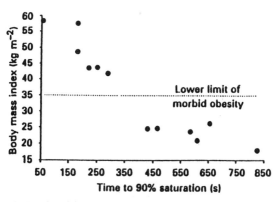

Fig. 23–3 • Arterial oxygen saturation decreases to 90% more rapidly in morbidly obese patients, as quantitated by the body mass index. (From Berthoud MC, Peacock JE, Reilly CS. Effectiveness of preoxygenation in morbidly obese patients. Br J Anaesth 1991;67:464–6, with permission.)

▬ Table 23-7 • Postoperative Complications in Obese Patients

Hypoventilation (especially following abdominal operations)
Arterial hypoxemia (use semisitting position when possible)
Obstructive sleep apnea
Obesity hypoventilation syndrome
Wound infection
Deep vein thrombosis
Pulmonary embolism

---

obstructive sleep apnea or obesity hypoventilation syndrome mandates intense postoperative monitoring.

3. **Postoperative analgesia.** Opioid-induced depression of ventilation in obese patients is a concern, and the intramuscular route of administration may be unreliable owing to unpredictable absorption of drugs. Patient-controlled analgesia and neuraxial opioids are commonly selected.

4. **Postoperative complications.** See Table 23-7.

II. EATING DISORDERS

Eating disorders typically occur in adolescent girls or young women (Table 23-8).

A. **Anorexia nervosa** is a relatively rare disorder, with an incidence of 5 to 10 cases per 100,000 persons and a mortality of 5% to 10% (medical complications are associated with malnutrition, suicide).

1. **Signs and symptoms.** See Table 23-9.

2. **Management of anesthesia** is based on the known pathophysiologic effects evoked by starvation (cardiac dysfunction, hypokalemia, hypovolemia, delayed gastric emptying, intraoperative cardiac dysrhythmias).

B. **Bulimia nervosa** is often triggered by emotional experiences (depression, anxiety disorders, and substance abuse commonly accompany this disorder). Metabolic alkalosis secondary to purging is frequently present with increased serum bicarbonate concentrations, hypochloremia, and occasionally hypokalemia. Dental complications, including periodontal disease, are likely.

Table 23–8 • Diagnostic Criteria for Eating Disorders

Anorexia Nervosa
Body mass index < 17.5
Fear of weight gain
Inaccurate perception of body shape and weight
Amenorrhea
Bulimia Nervosa
Recurrent binge eating (2 days a week for 3 months)
Recurrent purging, excessive exercise, or fasting
Excessive concern about body weight or shape
Binge-Eating Disorders
Recurrent binge eating (2 days per week for 6 months)
Eating rapidly
Eating until uncomfortably full
Eating when not hungry
Eating alone
Feeling guilty after a binge
No purging or excessive exercise

Adapted from: Becker AE, Grinspoon SK, Klibanski A, et al. Eating disorders. N Engl J Med 1999;340:1092–8.

Table 23–9 • Signs and Symptoms of Anorexia Nervosa

Unexplained weight loss in an adolescent girl
Decreased cardiac mass and contractility
Cardiomyopathy (starvation)
Sudden death (ventricular cardiac dysrhythmias)
Amenorrhea
Decreased body temperature
Orthostatic hypotension (altered autonomic nervous system activity)
Bradycardia
Osteoporosis
Slowed gastric emptying
Impaired cognitive functioning
Hypokalemia (self-induced vomiting, abuse of laxatives)
Fatty liver infiltration

C. **Binge-eating disorders** resemble bulimia nervosa; but in contrast to patients with bulimia nervosa, these patients do not purge and the periods of dietary restriction are less striking. The diagnosis of binge-eating disorders should be suspected in morbidly obese patients, particularly those with continued weight gain or marked weight cycling.

III. MALNUTRITION AND VITAMIN DEFICIENCIES

A. **Malnutrition** is a medically distinct syndrome that is responsive to caloric support provided by enteral or total parenteral nutrition (hyperalimentation). Malnourished patients are identified by the presence of serum albumin concentrations < 3 g/dl and transferrin levels < 200 mg/dl. Critically ill patients often experience negative caloric intake complicated by hypermetabolic states due to increased caloric needs produced by trauma (fractures, burns), fever (1°C elevation increases the daily caloric requirements by about 15%), sepsis, and wound healing.

1. **Treatment.** It is often recommended that patients who have lost more than 20% of their body weight be treated nutritionally before undergoing elective surgery.

   a. **Enteral nutrition.** When the gastrointestinal tract is functioning, enteral nutrition can be provided by

---

≡ **Table 23–10 •** Complications Associated with Total Parenteral Nutrition

Hyperglycemia (may require exogenous insulin)
Nonketotic hyperosmolar hyperglycemic coma
Hypoglycemia (a risk if infusion abruptly discontinued)
Hyperchloremic metabolic acidosis (reflects liberation of hydrochloric acid from metabolism of amino acids present in solutions)
Fluid overload (congestive heart failure in patients with compromised cardiac function)
Increased carbon dioxide production (reflects metabolism of large amounts of glucose; may interfere with weaning from mechanical ventilation)
Catheter-related sepsis
Electrolyte abnormalities
Renal dysfunction
Hepatic dysfunction
Thrombosis of central veins

≡ Table 23–11 • Disorders Related to Vitamin Deficiencies

Thiamine deficiency (high-output congestive heart failure with mental confusion and polyneuropathy; most likely to occur in chronic alcoholic patients with poor dietary intake)

Ascorbic acid deficiency (scurvy)

Nicotinic acid deficiency (pellagra characterized by mental confusion and peripheral neuropathy; may occur in chronic alcohol abuse patients or in the presence of carcinoid tumors)

Vitamin A deficiency (conjunctival drying and anemia)

Vitamin D deficiency (thoracic kyphosis)

Vitamin K deficiency (prolonged antibiotic therapy or absence of bile salts; prolonged prothrombin times)

---

means of nasogastric or gastrostomy tube feedings. Complications of enteral feedings are infrequent but may include hyperglycemia leading to osmotic diuresis and hypovolemia (exogenous insulin administration is a consideration).

    b. Total parenteral nutrition is indicated when the gastrointestinal tract is not functioning. When daily caloric requirements exceed 2000 calories or prolonged support is anticipated (> 14 days), a catheter is placed in the subclavian vein to permit infusion of hypertonic parenteral solutions.

  2. Potential complications of total parenteral nutrition are numerous (Table 23–10).

 B. Vitamin deficiencies. See Table 23–11.

IV. INBORN ERRORS OF METABOLISM

See Table 23–12.

 A. Porphyrias are a group of inborn errors of metabolism characterized by the overproduction of porphyrins (essential for many vital physiologic functions including oxygen transport and storage) and their precursors. The synthetic pathway involved in the production of porphyrins is determined by a sequence of enzymes, and a defect in any of these enzymes results in accumulation of the preceding intermediaries and produces a form of porphyria (Fig. 23–4). Heme is the most important porphyrin (hemoglobin, cytochrome P_{450}), and its production is controlled by aminolevulinic acid (ALA) synthetase (an inducible enzyme).

Table 23–13; Fig. 23–4

≡ **Table 23–12 •** Inborn Errors of Metabolism
Porphyria
Gout
Pseudogout
Hyperlipidemia
Carbohydrate metabolism disorders
Amino acid disorders
Mucopolysaccharidoses
Gangliosidoses

1. **Classification** (Table 23–13; Fig. 23–4). Only acute forms of porphyria are relevant to the management of anesthesia, as they are the only forms of porphyria that may result in life-threatening reactions in response to certain drugs.
2. **Acute porphyrias** are most commonly precipitated by events that decrease the heme concentration, thus increasing the activity of ALA synthetase and stimulating production of porphyrinogens (Fig. 23–4). Enzyme-inducing drugs are the most important triggering factors for the development of acute porphyrias.
   a. **Signs and symptoms.** See Table 23–14. Complete and prolonged remissions are likely between attacks, and many patients with the genetic defect never develop symptoms (first symptoms may be in response to inadvertent administration of triggering drugs during the perioperative period). ALA synthetase concentrations are increased during all acute attacks of porphyria.
   b. **Triggering drugs.** See Table 23–15.
   c. **Acute intermittent porphyria** affecting the central nervous system and peripheral nervous system produces the most serious symptoms (systemic hypertension, renal dysfunction) and is the form of porphyria that is most likely to be life-threatening.
   d. **Variegate porphyria and hereditary coproporphyria** are characterized by neurotoxicity and cutaneous photosensitivity.
   e. **Porphyria cutanea tarda** appears most often as photosensitivity, and drugs do not trigger attacks (anesthe-

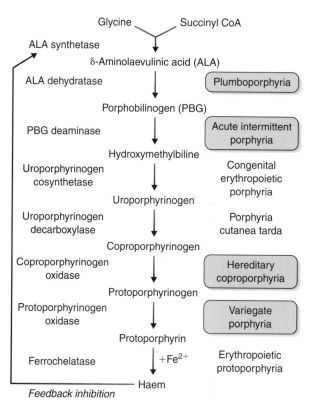

Fig. 23–4 • Metabolic pathways for heme synthesis. Enzymes are noted on the feedback inhibition loop of the sequence, and the type of porphyria associated with the enzyme deficiency is designated on the right. Examples of acute porphyrias are indicated in the boxes. (From James MFM, Hift RJ. Porphyrias. Br J Anaesth 2000;85:143–53. © The Board of Management and Trustees of the British Journal of Anaesthesia. Reproduced by permission of Oxford University Press/British Journal of Anaesthesia.)

sia is not a hazard, although the presence of liver disease is a consideration).

    f. Erythropoietic uroporphyria. In contrast to porphyrin synthesis in the liver, porphyrin synthesis in the erythropoietic system is responsive to changes in hematocrit and tissue oxygenation. Hemolytic anemia,

---

≡ Table 23–13 • Classification of Porphyrias

> *Acute*
> Acute intermittent porphyria
> Variegate porphyria
> Hereditary coproporphyria
> Plumboporphyria
> *Nonacute*
> Porphyria cutanea tarda
> Erythropoietic porphyrias
> > Erythropoietic uroporphyria
> > Erythropoietic protoporphyria

Adapted from: James MFM, Hift RJ. Porphyrias. Br J Anaesth 2000;85:143–53.

bone marrow hyperplasia, and splenomegaly are often present. Repeated infections are common, and photosensitivity is severe. Neurotoxicity and abdominal pain do not occur.

  g. **Erythropoietic protoporphyria,** a less debilitating form of porphyria, is characterized by photosensitivity. Administration of barbiturates does not adversely affect the course of this disease, and survival to adulthood is common.

3. **Management of anesthesia.** Most patients with porphyria can be anesthetized with safety assuming that appropriate precautions are taken (exposure to multiple potential enzyme-inducing drugs may be more dangerous than exposure to any one drug).

≡ Table 23–14 • Signs and Symptoms of Acute Porphyria

Severe abdominal pain (may mimic appendicitis, acute cholecystitis, renal colic)
Autonomic nervous system instability
Electrolyte disturbances
Dehydration
Neuropsychiatric manifestations
Skeletal muscle weakness (quadriparesis and respiratory failure)
Tachycardia
Systemic hypertension (less often hypotension)
Seizures

☰ Table 23–15 • Recommendations Regarding Use of Anesthetic Drugs in the Presence of Acute Porphyrias

Drug Class	Drug	Recommendation
Inhaled anesthetics	Nitrous oxide	Safe
	Isoflurane	Probably safe*
	Sevoflurane	Probably safe*
	Desflurane	Probably safe*
Intravenous anesthetics	Propofol	Safe
	Ketamine	Probably safe*
	Thiopental	Avoid
	Etomidate	Avoid
Analgesics	Acetaminophen	Safe
	Fentanyl	Safe
	Sufentanil	Safe
	Ketorolac	Probably avoid†
	Pentazocine	Avoid
Opioid antagonists	Naloxone	Safe
Neuromuscular blocking drugs	Succinylcholine	Safe
	Pancuronium	Safe
	Atracurium	Probably safe*
	Cisatracurium	Probably safe*
	Vecuronium	Probably safe*
	Rocuronium	Probably safe*
	Mivacurium	Probably safe*
Anticholinergics	Atropine	Safe
Anticholinesterases	Neostigmine	Safe
Local anesthetics	Lidocaine	Safe
	Bupivacaine	Safe
	Mepivacaine	Safe
	Ropivacaine	No data
Sedatives and antiemetics	Droperidol	Safe
	Midazolam	Probably safe*
	Cimetidine	Probably safe*
	Metoclopramide	Probably safe*
	Ondansetron	Probably safe*
Cardiovascular drugs	Epinephrine	Safe
	α-Agonists	Safe
	β-Agonists	Safe
	Diltiazem	Probably safe*
	Nitroprusside	Probably safe*
	Nifedipine	Probably avoid†

* Although safety is not conclusively established, the drug is unlikely to provoke acute porphyria.
† Use only if expected benefits outweigh the risks.
Adapted from: James MFM, Hift RJ. Porphyrias. Br J Anaesth 2000;85:143–53.

a. **Preoperative evaluation.** In addition to a careful family history and thorough physical examination (often no clinical evidence or subtle skin lesions), the presence of peripheral neuropathy and autonomic nervous system instability is noted. Preoperative preparation in patients experiencing an acute porphyric crisis should include careful assessment of fluid balance and electrolyte status. Preoperative starvation should be minimized, but if prolonged fasts are unavoidable, intravenous administration of glucose-saline infusions may be considered, as caloric restriction has been linked to the precipitation of acute porphyria attacks.

b. **Preoperative medication** is commonly with benzodiazepines. Aspiration prophylaxis including antacids and/or H_2-receptor antagonists are acceptable.

c. **Prophylactic therapy.** No specific prophylactic therapy is of proven benefit. Carbohydrate administration can suppress porphyrin synthesis, so oral carbohydrate supplements (20 g/hr) preoperatively may be recommended.

d. **Regional anesthesia.** If a regional anesthetic is considered, it is essential to perform a neurologic examination before initiating the block to minimize the likelihood that worsening of any neuropathy would be erroneously attributed to the regional anesthetic. The use of regional anesthesia for patients experiencing acute intermittent porphyria is not a likely selection based on concerns related to hemodynamic instability, mental confusion, and associated neuropathy.

e. **General anesthesia.** The total dose of the drugs administered and the length of exposure may influence the risk of triggering a porphyric crisis in vulnerable patients (use short-acting drugs) (Table 23–15). Perioperative monitoring should consider the frequent presence of autonomic nervous system dysfunction and the possibility of labile systemic blood pressure.

   i. **Induction of anesthesia** has been safely performed with propofol, although the use of prolonged continuous infusions of this drug are of unproven safety in these patients.

   ii. **Maintenance of anesthesia** includes nitrous oxide and volatile anesthetics with or without opi-

☰ Table 23–16 • Treatment of a Porphyric Crisis

Removal of any known triggering factors
Adequate hydration
Carbohydrate administration
Antiemetics
β-Blockers (tachycardia and systemic hypertension)
Benzodiazepines (treat seizures)
Treat electrolyte abnormalities
Hematin 3–4 mg/kg IV over 20 minutes (only specific form of
  therapy)

oids. Neuromuscular blocking drugs are acceptable.
  iii. **Cardiopulmonary bypass** is a potential risk for
       development of acute porphyria in susceptible
       patients (stress introduced by hypothermia, he-
       molysis, large number of drugs administered).
  4. **Treatment of a porphyric crisis.** See Table 23–16.
B. **Gout** is a disorder of purine metabolism characterized by
   hyperuricemia and recurrent acute arthritis. The incidence of
   systemic hypertension, ischemic heart disease, and diabetes
   mellitus is increased in patients with gout.
   1. **Treatment.** See Table 23–17.
   2. **Management of anesthesia.** See Table 23–18.
C. **Lesch-Nyhan syndrome** is a genetically determined disorder
   of purine metabolism manifesting exclusively in males as
   mental retardation, spasticity, seizures, and self-mutilation
   (oral scarring and associated difficulties during tracheal intubation).
D. **Hyperlipoproteinemia.** See Table 23–19.

☰ Table 23–17 • Treatment of Gout

Decreased plasma concentrations of uric acid
  Probenecid (uricosuric)
  Allopurinol (inhibits xanthine oxidase and conversion of purines
    to uric acid)
Relieve joint pain
  Colchicine (side effects include nausea, vomiting, hepatorenal
    dysfunction, agranulocytosis)

≣ **Table 23–18** • Management of Anesthesia in the Presence of Gout

Prehydration
Evaluate renal function
Consider co-existing diseases
   Systemic hypertension
   Ischemic heart disease
   Diabetes mellitus
Possibility of temporomandibular arthritis
Adverse effects of drug therapy

1. **Treatment** of hyperlipoproteinemia includes diet, smoking cessation, and drug therapy ("statin drugs"). It is possible that beneficial effects of the statin drugs extend beyond their lipid-lowering effects, perhaps reflecting antiinflammatory effects that reduce the likelihood of an atherosclerotic plaque rupturing.

2. **Management of anesthesia** in the presence of hyperlipoproteinemia is influenced by the possible presence of ischemic heart disease in these patients (not in familial lipoprotein lipase deficiency).

E. **Carnitine deficiency** may manifest as recurrent attacks of nausea and vomiting (systemic form) or skeletal muscle weakness and cardiomyopathy (myopathic form). Intravenous glucose infusions are included in the perioperative management of these patients.

F. **Tangier disease** is characterized by the absence or marked deficiency of normal high density lipoproteins and accumulation of cholesterol esters in multiple tissues: tonsils (may affect the airway), spleen, lymph nodes, thymus, intestinal mucosa, nerves (peripheral neuropathy), cornea.

G. **Propionic acidemia** is an inborn error of metabolism characterized by relapsing metabolic ketoacidosis usually precipitated by excessive protein intake or concurrent infections. Avoidance of events during the perioperative period that precipitate metabolic acidosis (fasting, arterial hypoxemia, dehydration, hypotension) are important.

H. **Disorders of carbohydrate metabolism** usually reflect genetically determined enzymatic defects (Table 23–20).

I. **Mucopolysaccharidoses** are progressive familial diseases of connective tissue metabolism caused by an absence or insuf-

Table 23–19 • Characteristics of Hyperlipoproteinemia

Lipid Abnormality	Cholesterol	Triglycerides	Xanthomas	Risk of Ischemic Heart Disease
Familial lipoprotein lipase deficiency (hyperchylomicronemia)	Normal	Increased	Eruptive	Very low
Familial dysbetalipoproteinemia	Increased	Increased	Palmar Plantar Tendon	Very high
Familial hypercholesterolemia	Increased	Normal to increased	Tendon	Very high
Familial hypertriglyceridemia	Normal	Increased	Eruptive	Low
Familial combined hyperlipidemia	Markedly increased	Markedly increased	Palmar Plantar Tendon	High
Polygenic hypercholesterolemia	Increased	Normal	Tendon	Moderate

▬ Table 23–20 • Disorders of Carbohydrate Metabolism

Glycogen storage disease type 1a (von Gierke's disease) (cannot convert glycogen to glucose and hypoglycemia may occur; provide glucose intraoperatively and minimize preoperative fasting)

Glycogen storage disease type 1b (hypoglycemia and lactic acidosis; provide glucose intraoperatively and minimize preoperative fasting)

Pompe's disease (glycogen deposition in heart and upper airway; upper airway obstruction may occur with onset of unconsciousness)

McArdle's disease (glycogen is not broken down to glucose; myoglobinuria may lead to renal failure; intraoperatively may develop hypoglycemia, and rhabdomyolysis may occur)

Galactosemia (cataracts, cirrhosis of the liver, and mental retardation reflect tissue accumulation of galactose)

Fructose 1,6-diphosphate deficiency (hypoglycemia, metabolic acidosis, and skeletal muscle hypotonia are common; use of lactated Ringer's solution is questionable)

Pyruvate dehydrogenase deficiency (chronic metabolic acidosis; use of lactated Ringer's solution questionable)

---

ficiency of key enzymes catalyzing the metabolism of three main components of connective tissue: dermatan sulfate, heparan sulfate, heratan sulfate (Table 23–21).

1. **Management of anesthesia.** Extensive preoperative evaluation of the upper airway, lungs, cervical spine, heart, and lungs and a thorough neurologic evaluation are recommended in patients with mucopolysaccharidoses scheduled for elective surgery. Perioperative morbidity and mortality are common in these patients and are most often related to difficult airway management (cervical spine instability) and tracheal intubation (awake fiberoptic intubation).

2. General anesthesia is most likely to be selected considering the young age of most of these patients and the predictable presence of mental retardation.

J. **Gangliosidoses.** The gangliosidoses (Gaucher's disease, Fabry's disease, Tay-Sachs disease, Niemann-Pick disease) are characterized by abnormalities of sphingolecithin metabolism resulting in damage to nerve membranes.

K. **Disorders of amino acid metabolism.** See Table 23–22.

Table 23–21 • Classification and Characteristics of Mucopolysaccharidoses

Eponym	Prevalence	Progressive Craniofacial Deformities	Progressive Joint and Skeletal Deformities	Progressive Cardiac Involvement
Hurler	1 : 100,000	Macrocephaly	Stiff joints	Coronary intimal and valvular thickening
		Coarse facies	Thoracolumbar kyphosis	
		Macroglossia	Odontoid hypoplasia	Mitral regurgitation
		Hydrocephalus	Short neck	Cardiomegaly
			Short stature	
Scheie	1 : 500,000	Coarse facies	Short neck	Aortic regurgitation
		Macroglossia	Normal stature	
		Prognathia		
Hurler-Scheie	1 : 100,000	Macrocephaly	Diffuse joint limitation	Mitral and aortic valvular thickening and regurgitation
		Coarse facies	Short neck	
		Macroglossia	Short stature	
		Micrognathia		
Hunter	1 : 150,000	Macrocephaly	Diffuse joint limitation	Coronary intimal thickening
		Coarse facies	Short neck	
		Hydrocephalus	Short stature	
San Filippo	1 : 24,000	Coarse facies	Stiff joints	Ischemic cardiomyopathy
			Lumbar vertebral dysplasia	Minimal to none
			Short stature	

Table continued on following page

Table 23–21 • Classification and Characteristics of Mucopolysaccharidoses *Continued*

Eponym	Prevalence	Progressive Craniofacial Deformities	Progressive Joint and Skeletal Deformities	Progressive Cardiac Involvement
Morquio	1 : 100,000	Coarse facies	Joint laxity Kyphoscoliosis Odontoid hypoplasia Short neck C1-2 and C2-3 subluxation Short stature	Aortic regurgitation
Maroteaux-Lamy	1 : 100,000	Macrocephaly Coarse facies Macroglossia	Joint stiffness Kyphoscoliosis Odontoid hypoplasia Short stature	Mitral and aortic valvular thickening and regurgitation
Sly	Rare	Macrocephaly Coarse facies	Joint flexion contractures Thoracolumbar gibbus Hip dysplasia	Mitral and aortic valvular thickening Aortic dissection

Adapted from: Diaz JH, Belani KG. Perioperative management of children with mucopolysaccharidoses. Anesth Analg 1993;77:1261–70.

Table 23–22 • Disorders of Amino Acid Metabolism

Disorder	Mental Retardation	Seizures	Metabolic Acidosis	Hyper-ammonemia	Hepatic Failure	Thrombo-embolism	Other
Phenylketonuria	Yes	Yes	No	No	No	No	Friable skin
Homocystinuria	Yes/no	Yes	No	No	No	Yes	
Hypervalinemia	Yes	Yes	Yes	No	No	No	Hypoglycemia
Citrullinemia	Yes	Yes	No	Yes	Yes	No	Hypoglycemia
Branched-chain aciduria (maple syrup urine disease)	Yes	Yes	Yes	No		Yes	Neurologic deterioration during the perioperative period Acidosis intraoperatively
Methylmalonyl coenzyme A mutase deficiency			Yes	Yes			Avoid nitrous oxide? Hypovolemia
Isoleucinemia	Yes	Yes	Yes	Yes	Yes	No	
Methioninemia	Yes	No	No	No	No	No	Thermal instability
Histidinuria	Yes	Yes/no	No	No	No	No	Erythrocyte fragility
Neutral aminoaciduria (Hartnup's disease)	Yes/no		Yes	No	No	No	Dermatitis
Argininemia	Yes		No	Yes	Yes	No	

1. **Management of anesthesia** in patients with disorders of amino acid metabolism is directed toward maintenance of intravascular fluid volume and acid-base homeostasis.
2. Use of anesthetics that could evoke seizures may be questionable in view of the likely presence of seizure disorders in these patients.

24

Diseases Due to Altered Hemoglobin Concentrations or Structures

Disease states may be related to abnormal concentrations (anemia, polycythemia) or structures (sickle cell disease) of hemoglobin (Stoelting RK, Dierdorf SF. Diseases due to altered hemoglobin concentrations or structures. In: Anesthesia and Co-Existing Disease, 4th ed. New York, Churchill Livingstone, 2002;471–488). Oxygen-carrying capacity and adequacy of tissue oxygen delivery are often the most important clinical manifestations of these derangements.

I. ANEMIA

Anemia is a disease manifesting clinically as a numerical deficiency of erythrocytes (Table 24–1). There is no single laboratory value that defines anemia, but it is usually considered present when the hemoglobin concentration is < 11.5 g/dl (hematocrit 36%) in females and < 12.5 g/dl (hematocrit 40%) in males. The most important adverse effect of anemia is decreased tissue oxygen delivery owing to an associated decrease in arterial content of oxygen (CaO_2). Compensation for decreased CaO_2 is accomplished by a rightward shift of the oxyhemoglobin dissociation curve and increased cardiac output as a reflection of decreased blood viscosity (Fig. 24–1).

A. Iron deficiency anemia.
Nutritional deficiency of iron is a cause of anemia only in infants and small children. In adults, iron deficiency anemia can only reflect depletion of iron stores due to chronic blood loss, most likely from the gastrointestinal tract or from the female genital tract (menstruation). Parturients are susceptible to the development of iron deficiency anemia because of increased erythrocyte (RBC) mass during gestation and the needs of the fetus for iron.

1. **Diagnosis.** The presence of RBCs with too little hemoglobin (insufficient iron) results in microcytic hypochromic anemia. Demonstration of a decreased serum ferritin concentration serves as a cost-effective alternative test to bone

≡ Table 24–1 • Causes of Anemia

Iron Deficiency Anemia
Anemia of Chronic Disease
Thalassemia
β-Thalassemia major
β-Thalassemia minor
α-Thalassemia
Acute Blood Loss
Aplastic Anemia
Fanconi syndrome
Diamond-Blackfan syndrome
Megaloblastic Anemia
Vitamin B_{12} deficiency
Folic acid deficiency
Hemolytic Anemia
Sickle cell disease
Hereditary spherocytosis
Paroxysmal nocturnal hemoglobinuria
Glucose-6-phosphate dehydrogenase deficiency
Pyruvate kinase deficiency
Immune hemolytic anemia
Altered Ability of Hemoglobin to Bind Oxygen
Methemoglobinemia
Sulfhemoglobinemia

marrow examination for diagnosing iron deficiency anemia.

2. **Treatment** of iron deficiency anemia is with iron salts administered orally for at least 1 year. A favorable response to iron therapy is characterized by an increase in the hemoglobin concentration of about 2 g/dl in 3 weeks or return of hemoglobin concentrations to normal levels in 6 weeks. Recombinant human erythropoietin may be used to treat drug-induced anemia or to improve the hemoglobin concentration before elective surgery.

   a. **Perioperative treatment.** Minimum acceptable hemoglobin concentrations that should be present before proceeding with elective surgery in patients with chronic anemia cannot be recommended (there is no evidence that a hemoglobin concentration < 10 g/dl mandates the need for preoperative RBC transfusion). Ultimately, the decision to administer RBCs during the perioperative period is influenced by the risk of anemia

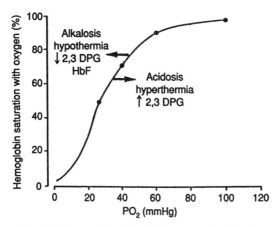

Fig. 24–1 • Oxyhemoglobin dissociation curve describes the relation between the SaO_2 and the PaO_2. The PaO_2 at which SaO_2 is 50% is designated the P_{50} (normally 26 mmHg). Increases in the P_{50} reflect shifts of the oxyhemoglobin dissociation curve to the right [increased levels of 2,3-diphosphoglycerate in erythrocytes (RBCs), acidosis, increased body temperature]; thus binding of oxygen to hemoglobin is less avid, facilitating its release to peripheral tissues. Decreases in the P_{50} reflect shifts in the oxyhemoglobin dissociation curve to the left (decreased levels of 2,3-diphosphoglycerate in the RBCs, alkalosis, decreased body temperature); thus binding of oxygen to hemoglobin is more avid, impairing its release to peripheral tissues. Mixed venous blood has an SvO_2 of about 75% and a corresponding PvO_2 close to 40 mmHg. When the SaO_2 is about 90%, the corresponding PaO_2 is close to 60 mmHg.

(decreased oxygen-carrying capacity) and the risks associated with transfusions (transmissible diseases, hemolytic and nonhemolytic transfusion reactions, immunosuppression) (Table 24–2).

b. The ability of the cardiovascular system to compensate for decreases in CaO_2 by increasing the cardiac output is an important compensatory mechanism for maintaining tissue oxygen delivery, especially in acutely anemic patients.

c. Preoperative transfusions of packed RBCs can be administered to increase hemoglobin concentrations, recognizing that about 24 hours are needed to restore

---

≡ **Table 24–2 • Guidelines for Blood Transfusions and Management of Blood Loss During the Perioperative Period**

Hemoglobin concentration > 10 g/dl—transfusions rarely indicated

Hemoglobin concentration < 6 g/dl—transfusions almost always indicated especially when the anemia is acute

Hemoglobin concentration of 6–10 g/dl—decision to transfuse is determined by individual patient's risks for complications of decreased tissue oxygenation (patients with ischemic heart disease)

Transfusion trigger—not recommended for application to all patients, as it ignores physiologic and surgical factors unique to individual patients

Preoperative autologous donation in selected patients

Intraoperative blood salvage when appropriate

Acute normovolemic hemodilution when appropriate

---

intravascular fluid volume (compared with similar volumes of whole blood, packed RBCs produce about twice the increase in hemoglobin concentration) (Table 24–3).

3. **Management of anesthesia.** If elective surgery is performed in the presence of chronic anemia, it seems prudent to minimize the likelihood of significant changes that

---

≡ **Table 24–3 • Basis for Administering Transfusions Preoperatively**

Cause of anemia
Degree of anemia
Duration of anemia
Intravascular fluid volume
Urgency of surgery
Likelihood of intraoperative blood loss
Age of patient
Co-existing diseases
  Ischemic heart disease
  Cerebrovascular disease
  Peripheral vascular disease
  Lung disease

could further interfere with oxygen delivery to tissues (drug-induced decreases in cardiac output, leftward shifts of the oxyhemoglobin dissociation curve) (Fig. 24–1). Monitoring cardiac function with transesophageal echocardiography may be useful for evaluating the effects of anemia during the intraoperative course.

  a. Although supporting evidence is not available, it is likely that intraoperative blood loss will be replaced with whole blood or packed RBCs when the hemoglobin concentration decreases acutely to 7 g/dl.

  b. During the postoperative period, it is important to minimize the occurrence of shivering or increases in body temperature, as these changes could increase total body oxygen requirements.

B. **Anemia of chronic disease.** See Table 24–4.

  1. **Treatment** with iron replacement is not effective.

  2. This form of anemia is usually mild; identifying and treating the underlying disease is the most effective therapy.

C. **Thalassemia** is an inherited disorder of hemoglobin synthesis (β-thalassemia major, β-thalassemia minor, α-thalassemia) resulting in anemia that may require treatment with blood transfusions.

D. **Acute blood loss.** See Table 24–5. The hematocrit may not reflect anemia due to acute blood loss, as physiologic mechanisms for restoring the plasma volume operate slowly. The obvious treatment of anemia due to acute blood loss is correction of the cause and prompt restoration of intravascular fluid volume with RBCs plus colloid or crystalloid solutions (crystalloid is administered at about 3 ml for every 1 ml of colloid).

≡ Table 24–4 • Chronic Diseases Associated with Anemia

Infections
Cancer
Connective tissue disorders
Acquired immunodeficiency syndrome
Alcoholic liver disease
Renal failure
Diabetes mellitus

Table 24–5 • Clinical Signs Associated with Anemia Owing to Acute Blood Loss

Blood Volume Lost (%)	Signs
10	None
20–30	Orthostatic hypotension
	Tachycardia
	Low central venous pressure
40	Hypotension
	Tachycardia
	Tachypnea
	Diaphoresis

1. **Hemorrhagic shock** (systolic blood pressure < 90 mmHg, tachycardia, oliguria, metabolic acidosis, restlessness) is a potential complication of acute blood loss.
    a. **Treatment** of hemorrhagic shock is with infusion of whole blood and crystalloid solutions (interstitial fluid shifts accompany acute hemorrhage). Invasive monitoring is often necessary to guide the adequacy of intravascular fluid volume replacement and to evaluate the response to inotropes (vasopressors are used sparingly, although it may be necessary to maintain cerebral and cardiac perfusion pressures with a vasopressor until intravascular fluid volume can be replaced). Persistent metabolic acidosis probably reflects the continued presence of hypovolemia and inadequate oxygen delivery to tissues.
    b. **Management of anesthesia.** Induction and maintenance of anesthesia in the presence of hemorrhagic shock requires invasive monitoring of systemic blood pressure and often includes ketamine administration.
E. **Aplastic anemia** is most often due to destruction of bone marrow stem cells by cancer chemotherapeutic drugs resulting in pancytopenia.
    1. **Fanconi syndrome** is congenital aplastic anemia plus numerous associated anomalies (microcephaly, short stature, cleft palate, cardiac defects).
    2. **Diamond-Blackfan syndrome** is a form of pure RBC aplasia treated with RBC transfusions and corticosteroids. Splenectomy may be necessary for patients who are unresponsive to corticosteroids.

3. **Management of anesthesia** in the presence of aplastic anemia includes consideration of drugs used during treatment, susceptibility to infection, and occurrence of hemorrhage with minor trauma (tracheal intubation must be atraumatic).

F. **Megaloblastic anemia** is most often due to deficiencies of vitamin B_{12} and/or folic acid. Both vitamins must be supplied by diet, as neither is produced in adequate amounts by intrinsic synthesis.

1. **Vitamin B_{12} deficiency** is associated with bilateral peripheral neuropathy due to degeneration of the lateral and posterior columns of the spinal cord (symmetrical paresthesias with loss of proprioceptive and vibratory sensations, especially in the lower extremities). Gait is unsteady, and memory impairment may be prominent.

   a. Nonmedical use of nitrous oxide may be associated with neurologic findings similar to those that accompany vitamin B_{12} deficiency.

   b. **Management of anesthesia** may be influenced by the presence of neurologic changes and the use of nitrous oxide.

2. **Folic acid deficiency** is the most common of the vitamin deficiencies (smooth tongue, hyperpigmentation, mental depression, peripheral edema). Peripheral neuropathy may or may not be present. Liver dysfunction occurs frequently. Oral folic acid is effective in reversing megaloblastic anemia due to deficiencies of this vitamin.

G. **Hemolytic anemias.** Anemia due to intravascular hemolysis is characterized by rapid decreases in the patient's hematocrit and increased plasma concentrations of bilirubin. Causes of hemolysis include abnormalities in the structure of hemoglobin, abnormalities of RBC membranes, and RBC enzyme defects. These changes make RBCs so fragile they rupture easily as they pass through capillaries, especially in the spleen.

1. **Sickle cell disease** represents an inherited disorder that ranges in severity from the usually benign sickle cell trait to the debilitating, often fatal sickle cell anemia (chronic hemolysis and acute episodic vaso-occlusive crises that may cause organ failure).

   a. **Pathogenesis.** Sickle cell disease is due to the presence of a mutant hemoglobin S, which has the property of forming insoluble globulin polymers when deoxygenated (fundamental molecular event leading to clinical

---

≡ Table 24–6 • Possible Initiating Events of Sickle Cell Crises

---

$PaO_2 < 40$ mmHg
Acidosis
Hypothermia
Increased blood viscosity (dehydration)

---

manifestations of sickle cell disease) (Table 24–6). Among hemolytic anemias, the vaso-occlusive features of sickle cell disease are unique.

  b. **Signs and symptoms** of sickle cell disease are due to chronic hemolysis and occlusion of blood vessels with sickle cells.

   i. **Vaso-occlusion** is the single most important pathophysiologic process that results in most of the acute complications of sickle cell disease (Table 24–7).

≡ Table 24–7 • Signs and Symptoms of Sickle Cell Disease

Vaso-occlusive Complications
Painful episodes
Stroke (cerebral infarction in children and intracranial hemorrhage in adults)
Acute chest syndrome
Renal insufficiency
Liver disease
Splenic sequestration
Proliferative retinopathy
Priapism
Spontaneous abortion
Leg ulcers
Osteonecrosis
Complications Related to Hemolysis
Anemia (hematocrit 15–30%)
Cholelithiasis (chronic bilirubin overload)
Acute aplastic episodes
Infectious Complications
Streptococcus pneumoniae sepsis
Escherichia coli sepsis
Osteomyelitis

Adapted from: Steinberg MH. Management of sickle cell disease. N Engl J Med 1999;340:1021–30.

Multiple organ system dysfunction produced by infarctive events (pulmonary emboli, cerebral emboli, renal emboli) is the major reason that prolonged survival is unlikely.

ii. **Acute chest syndrome** is a medical emergency (mortality approaches 10%) characterized by an acute pain crisis, often affecting the lower chest wall. Fever, cough, pleuritic chest pain, arterial hypoxemia, pulmonary hypertension, and radiologic evidence of lung infiltrates are likely. Recurrent episodes of the acute chest syndrome are accompanied by progressive pulmonary fibrosis and chronic respiratory insufficiency. Treatment may include mechanical support of ventilation and exchange transfusions to achieve hemoglobin S concentrations < 30%. Inhaled nitric oxide is beneficial in some patients.

c. **Treatment.** See Table 24–8.

d. **Management of anesthesia.** See Table 24–9.

2. **Hereditary spherocytosis** is characterized by abnormalities of RBC membranes manifesting as anemia, reticulocytosis, and mild jaundice. Splenectomy may be necessary if anemia is severe (pneumococcal vaccine may be indicated subsequently as the incidence of bacterial infections is increased).

≡ Table 24–8 • Treatment of Sickle Cell Disease

General Measures
Pneumococcal vaccine
Antibiotics
Folic acid
Acute Pain Episodes
Fluid replacement (3–4 L daily in adults)
Initiate analgesics (morphine, nonsteroidal antiinflammatory drugs, consider patient-controlled analgesia)
Chronic Pain Episodes
Acetaminophen with codeine
Fentanyl patches
Nonsteroidal antiinflammatory drugs
Transfusions
Decrease hemoglobin S concentrations to < 30%
Hydroxyurea (stimulates production of hemoglobin F)
Bone Marrow Transplantation

Table 24–9 • Management of Anesthesia in Patients with Sickle Cell Disease

Preoperative Period
Admit to hospital 12–24 hours before surgery to permit optimal hydration with intravenous fluids
Treat obstructive lung disease with bronchodilators
Transfuse to increase the hematocrit to 30% (not necessary before minor operations)
Intraoperative Period
Maintain arterial oxygenation
Maintain hydration
Maintain body temperature
Replace blood loss when necessary
Postoperative Period
Maintain arterial oxygenation
Continue intravenous fluids for hydration
Consider incentive spirometry
Consider overnight observation in the hospital

Adapted from: Steinberg MH. Management of sickle cell disease. N Engl J Med 1999;340:1021–30.

3. **Paroxysmal nocturnal hemoglobinuria** is characterized by acute episodes of thrombosis and complement-mediated hemolysis superimposed on a background of chronic hemolysis. Anesthesia may be a risk factor for hemoglobinuria in these patients should acidosis develop.

4. **Glucose-6-phosphate dehydrogenase deficiency** is the most common inherited RBC enzyme disorder (affects 10% of African-American males in the United States).
   a. **Signs and symptoms.** Chronic hemolytic anemia is the most common clinical manifestation of glucose-6-phosphate dehydrogenase deficiency. Drugs that form peroxides by interaction with oxyhemoglobin can trigger hemolysis in these patients (Table 24–10). Disseminated intravascular coagulation may accompany drug-induced hemolysis.
   b. Although drugs used during anesthesia have not been incriminated as triggering agents, the onset of hemolysis and jaundice during the early postoperative period, especially in African-American males, suggests consideration of this diagnosis.

5. **Pyruvate kinase deficiency** is characterized by RBC membranes that are highly permeable to potassium and vulnerable to rupture as evidenced by the development of hemolytic anemia.

Table 24–10 • Drugs that May Induce Hemolysis in Patients with Glucose-6-Phosphate Dehydrogenase Deficiency

Nonopioid Analgesics
Phenacetin
Acetaminophen
Antibiotics
Nitrofurans
Penicillin
Streptomycin
Chloramphenicol
Isoniazid
Sulfonamides
Antimalarial Drugs
Miscellaneous
Probenecid
Quinidine
Vitamin K analogues
Methylene blue
Nitroprusside (?)

6. **Immune hemolytic anemia** is characterized by immunologic alterations in RBC membranes (diagnosed by the presence of Coombs' antibody) due to drugs, diseases, or sensitization of RBCs.
   a. **Drug-induced hemolysis** may occur in patients treated with α-methyldopa (stimulates production of immunoglobulin G antibodies directed against Rh antigens on the surface of RBCs), high doses of penicillin, and levodopa.
   b. **Disease-induced hemolysis** may accompany hypersplenism necessitating splenectomy (platelets may be needed intraoperatively if thrombocytopenia is present).
   c. **Sensitization of RBCs** manifests most often as hemolytic disease of the newborn. Administration of Rh-immune globulin (RhoGAM) within 72 hours of delivery destroys fetal RBCs in the maternal circulation, preventing the subsequent development of sensitization.
7. **Hemoglobin Hammersmith** is a rare, unstable hemoglobin with low oxygen affinity (hemolytic anemia is severe,

requiring frequent transfusions). Monitoring during anesthesia may be complicated by interference of hemoglobin Hammersmith with accurate functioning of conventional pulse oximetry (falsely low SpO_2 values).

H. **Anemia due to temporary formation of abnormal hemoglobins.** Acute exposure to certain drugs may predispose genetically susceptible patients to the formation of hemoglobins that cannot optimally bind hemoglobin. Altered absorption spectra result in erroneously low SpO_2 readings (methemoglobinemia, sulfhemoglobinemia) or are interpreted erroneously as oxyhemoglobin (carboxyhemoglobin).

   1. **Methemoglobinemia** cannot bind oxygen, and the oxygen-carrying capacity of blood is decreased. Congenital absence of methemoglobin reductase enzyme may predispose to the development of methemoglobinemia in patients receiving nitrate-containing compounds (nitroglycerin, benzocaine).

      a. **Diagnosis** of methemoglobinemia is suggested by cyanosis (methemoglobin concentrations about 15%) in the presence of normal PaO_2 levels but low measured SaO_2 concentrations (calculation of SaO_2 based on the measured PaO_2 using a nomogram does not detect methemoglobinemia). The presence of desaturation based on pulse oximetry readings (SpO_2 reads 85%) that is associated with normal PaO_2 values may alert the anesthesiologist to the possible presence of methemoglobinemia.

      b. Treatment of cyanosis owing to methemoglobinemia is with methylene blue, 1 mg/kg IV.

   2. **Sulfhemoglobinemia** is a rare cause of cyanosis that is usually drug-induced (often the same drugs that cause methemoglobinemia). There is no pharmacologic treatment for sulfhemoglobinemia.

I. **Myelodysplastic syndrome** is a hematologic disorder characterized by cytopenia in the peripheral blood and normal cellularity to hypercellularity in the bone marrow. Hemorrhage due to thrombocytopenia (uncontrolled bleeding may accompany surgery) and infection secondary to leukopenia are the principal causes of morbidity in affected individuals.

II. POLYCYTHEMIA

Polycythemia (erythrocytosis) is defined as an increase in the number of circulating RBCs as reflected by an increase in the hematocrit and hemoglobin concentrations.

A. **Relative polycythemia** occurs most often in middle-age, obese, hypertensive men who have a chronic history of smoking (hematocrit usually > 55%).

    1. **Smoker's polycythemia** is confirmed by measurements of plasma carboxyhemoglobin concentrations (5% to 7% in those who smoke 30 cigarettes daily) at the end of the day.

    2. Cessation of smoking for about 5 days usually corrects the decreased plasma volume, and the hematocrit decreases.

B. **Secondary polycythemia** may occur when erythropoietin production is increased as a result of appropriate compensatory responses to chronic tissue hypoxia, as associated with existence at high altitude, cardiopulmonary disease, obesity-hypoventilation syndrome, obstructive sleep apnea, and increased serum concentrations of carboxyhemoglobin.

C. **Primary polycythemia (polycythemia vera)** is a neoplastic (myeloproliferative) disorder that originates from a single neoplastic hematopoietic stem cell.

    1. **Signs and symptoms** are related to hyperviscosity (headache, cognitive dysfunction, weakness) and hypermetabolic changes (fever, weight loss, excessive diaphoresis).

    2. **Laboratory diagnosis.** Hematocrit values of > 60% in males and > 57% in females are virtually diagnostic of primary or secondary polycythemia. Leukocytosis and thrombocytosis are common.

Table 24–11 • Complications of Polycythemia Vera

Bleeding and thrombosis during surgery [optimize patient's hematocrit (< 46%) prior to elective surgery; platelets may not function properly]
Myocardial infarction
Ischemic stroke
Transient ischemic attacks
Peripheral arterial thrombosis
Deep vein thrombosis
Hepatic vein thrombosis (Budd-Chiari syndrome)
Acute myeloid leukemia
Gout and nephrolithiasis
Postpolycythemic myeloid metaplasia (hepatosplenomegaly may be massive)

Table 24–12 • Leukocytes and Clinical Importance

Leukocytes	Range (cells/mm³)	Total (%)	Physiologic Significance
All leukocytes	4300–10,000	100	
Neutrophils	1800–7200	55	Defense against bacterial infections; neutropenia common in patients with infectious mononucleosis and AIDS
Lymphocytes	1500–4000	36	Production of immunoglobulins; lymphocytosis is associated with viral infections; lymphocytopenia is a common finding in patients with AIDS
Eosinophils	0–700	2	Response to allergic reactions and fungal infections; Loeffler syndrome is eosinophilia in the presence of pulmonary infiltrates; hypereosinophilic syndrome is associated with cardiomyopathy, ataxia, peripheral neuropathy, and recurrent thromboembolism
Basophils	0–150	1	Release chemical mediators including tryptase; tissue counterparts are mast cells
Monocytes	200–900	6	Modify immune response; phagocytosis; tissue counterparts are macrophages

AIDS, acquired immunodeficiency syndrome.

3. **Treatment** includes phlebotomy until a target hematocrit value (< 46%) is reached plus administration of a myelo-suppressive drug (hydroxyurea, busulfan).
4. **Complications.** See Table 24–11.

III. DISORDERS OF LEUKOCYTES

See Table 24–12.

25

Coagulopathies

Coagulopathies may be hereditary or acquired (Table 25–1) (Stoelting RK, Dierdorf SF. Coagulopathies. In: Anesthesia and Co-Existing Disease, 4th ed. New York, Churchill Livingstone, 2002;489–504). One of the most important questions to ask preoperatively deals with hemostatic responses to prior operations (tonsillectomy, dental extractions). There is no evidence that preoperative coagulation tests in asymptomatic patients are of any value (Table 25–2). Thromboelastography (TEG) may be considered in selected patients, especially if rapid preoperative evaluation of coagulation is desired (Fig. 25–1).

I. HEREDITARY COAGULATION DISORDERS

Hereditary coagulation disorders are usually due to the congenital absence or decreased presence of a single procoagulant.

A. **Hemophilia A** is an X-linked recessive genetic disorder (recent genetic mutations in approximately one-third of patients so there is no family history of a bleeding disorder). It affects approximately 2 per 10,000 males, making it the most common hereditary coagulation disorder. The genetic defect results in the absence, severe deficiency, or defective functioning of plasma coagulation factor VIII (antihemophiliac factor).

1. **Signs and symptoms.** The clinical manifestations of hemophilia A are joint (hemarthroses) and skeletal muscle hemorrhages, easy bruising, and prolonged and potentially fatal hemorrhage after trauma or surgery, but no excessive bleeding after minor cuts or abrasions. Bleeding into closed spaces can result in compression of peripheral nerves or vascular or airway obstruction. Intracranial bleeding may be a cause of death.

2. **Diagnosis** of hemophilia A is suspected when unusual bleeding is encountered in male patients [normal platelet counts, prothrombin time (PT), prolonged activated par-

☰ Table 25–1 • Categorization of Coagulation Disorders

Hereditary Disorders
Hemophilia A
Hemophilia B
Von Willebrand's disease
Afibrinogenemia
Factor V deficiency
Factor VIII deficiency
Hereditary hemorrhagic telangiectasia
Protein C deficiency
Antithrombin III deficiency
Acquired Disorders
Disseminated intravascular coagulation
Perioperative anticoagulation
Intraoperative coagulopathies
   Dilutional thrombocytopenia
   Dilution of procoagulants
   Massive blood transfusions
   Type of surgery (cardiopulmonary bypass, brain trauma,
     orthopedic surgery, urologic surgery, obstetric delivery)
Drug-induced hemorrhage
Drug-induced platelet dysfunction
Idiopathic thrombocytopenic purpura
Thrombotic thrombocytopenic purpura
Catheter-induced thrombocytopenia
Vitamin K deficiency

tial thromboplastin time (PTT)]. Specific assays for factor VIII are necessary to distinguish hemophilia A from hemophilia B (factor IX).

3. **Treatment** of hemophilia A is with factor VIII concentrates (recombinant derived factor VIII is comparable to plasma derived factor VIII and does not introduce the risk of transmitting viral diseases). In cases of major surgery or life-threatening bleeding, normal circulating factor VIII levels must be maintained [short elimination half-time (8 hours) means that repeated doses are needed]. Desmopressin increases plasma levels of factor VIII and von Willebrand factor and can be administered to treat patients with mild to moderate hemophilia and von Willebrand's disease.

4. **Management of anesthesia.** Preoperative medication of patients with hemophilia A is ideally achieved with drugs

Table 25–2 • Tests of Coagulation

Test	Normal Values	Measures
Bleeding time (Ivy)	3–10 minutes	Platelet function Vascular integrity
Platelet count	150,000–400,000 cells/mm³	
Prothrombin time	10–12 seconds	Factors I, II, V, VII, X
Partial thromboplastin time	25–35 seconds	Factors I, II, V, VII, IX, X, XI, XII
Activated clotting time	90–120 seconds	Factors I, II, V, VII, IX, X, XI, XII
Thrombin time	9–11 seconds	Factors I, II
Fibrinogen	160–350 mg/dl	
Fibrin degradation products	< 4 µg/ml	
Thromboelastography	See Fig. 25–1	Procoagulants Platelets

administered orally. Maintenance of anesthesia is most often with general anesthesia, as the risk of uncontrolled bleeding detracts from the selection of regional anesthetic techniques. Tracheal intubation is acceptable, although hemorrhage into the tongue and neck could impair upper airway patency. The high incidence of liver disease due

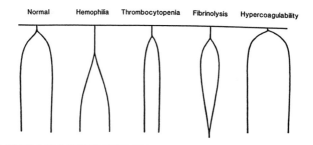

Fig. 25–1 • Coagulopathy as reflected by thromboelastography.

to hepatitis from prior blood or factor VIII transfusions and the possible presence of acquired immunodeficiency syndrome (AIDS) are considerations in these patients.

B. Hemophilia B is an X-linked genetic disorder caused by a defective or deficient factor IX molecule.

    1. Diagnosis of hemophilia B depends on demonstration of low or absent plasma IX concentrations in the presence of normal factor VIII activity.

    2. Treatment of hemophilia B is with factor IX concentrates, and the dosing interval is based on an elimination half-time of 24 hours.

C. Von Willebrand's disease affects both genders and is due to deficient or defective amounts of von Willebrand factor (vWF), which is necessary for adherence of platelets to exposed endothelium.

    1. Diagnosis of von Willebrand's disease is suggested by the patient's history [lifelong history of bruising and mild bleeding usually from mucosal surfaces (epistaxis)]. Excessive bleeding due to surgery or trauma is localized to the site of surgery.

    2. Treatment of von Willebrand's disease consists of replacing vWF with cryoprecipitate. Alternatively, desmopressin may stimulate the release of vWF, serving as an effective treatment in some patients.

D. Afibrinogenemia. Bleeding times, PT, and PTT are prolonged; and determination of serum fibrinogen concentrations reveals only trace amounts or the total absence of this procoagulant. Treatment is with fibrinogen or cryoprecipitate.

E. Factor V deficiency is inherited as an autosomal recessive trait affecting both genders. Bleeding is most often from mucosal surfaces, and treatment is with fresh frozen plasma.

F. Factor XII deficiency (Hageman factor) is not associated with excessive bleeding after trauma or surgery, and no substitution therapy is needed for these patients even during surgery. Standard tests to monitor heparin activity depend on in vitro activation of factor XII, making it impossible to monitor heparin activity intraoperatively in these patients.

G. Factor XIII deficiency can result in delayed hemorrhage after accidental trauma or surgery. Central nervous system hemorrhage is common. Treatment is with fresh frozen plasma or cryoprecipitate.

H. Heredity hemorrhagic telangiectasia (Osler-Weber-Rendu syndrome) is characterized by the development of arteriovenous fistulas, especially in the lungs (air embolism, arterial hypoxemia) and systemic circulation (high-output congestive heart failure). Epistaxis is common.

1. **Management of anesthesia** must consider the possibility of hemorrhage from telangiectatic lesions that may be present in the oropharynx, trachea, and esophagus.
2. Epidural anesthesia has been utilized in these patients, but the risk of neurologic sequelae should be kept in mind in the event that the bleeding tendency leads to formation of an epidural hematoma.

I. **Hereditary thrombocytopenia**
   1. **May-Hegglin anomaly** is a rare inherited disorder characterized by thrombocytopenia and a bleeding diathesis manifesting as purpura and epistaxis.
   2. **Fechtner syndrome** is characterized by hematologic abnormalities similar to those of May-Hegglin anomaly. Easy bruising, renal impairment, and hearing loss may be present.

J. **Grey platelet syndrome** is a rare inherited qualitative disorder of platelet dysfunction manifesting as bruising, ecchymosis, recurrent epistaxis, and menorrhagia, but severe hemorrhage has most commonly been reported following surgical procedures and vaginal delivery.

K. **α_2-Antiplasmin deficiency** is a rare congenital disease that results in activation of fibrinolysis. It requires specific treatment with antifibrinolytic drugs.

L. **Prekallikrein deficiency** is not associated with clinically significant impairment of hemostasis or increased risk of central neuraxial bleeding should epidural or spinal anesthesia be utilized.

M. **Hypercoagulable states** (congenital or acquired) occur when there is an imbalance between the anticoagulant and procoagulant activities of plasma in which the procoagulant activities predominate, often resulting in an increased incidence of deep vein thrombosis (Table 25–3).
   1. **Antithrombin III deficiency** is associated with an increased incidence of thromboembolic disease and resistance to the anticoagulant effects of exogenously administered heparin (treat with specific concentrate preparations containing antithrombin III or cryoprecipitate or with fresh frozen plasma).
   2. **Protein C deficiency** most often presents as a tendency for recurrent thromboembolic disease, including myocardial infarction, cerebral infarction, and pulmonary embolism.

≡ Table 25–3 • Hypercoagulable States and Associated Vascular Bed-Specific Thrombosis Sites

Hypercoagulable State	Vascular Bed-Specific Thrombosis Site
Congenital	
Antithrombin III deficiency	
Heterozygous	Deep veins of legs
Homozygous	Deep veins and arteries
Protein C deficiency	Deep veins of legs
Protein S deficiency	Deep veins of legs
Factor V Leiden presence	Deep veins of legs and brain Coronary arteries (?)
Acquired	
Paroxysmal nocturnal hemoglobinuria	Portal and hepatic veins
Myeloproliferative diseases	Portal and hepatic veins
Anti-phospholipid antibody syndrome	Arteries and veins
Warfarin-induced skin necrosis	Subcutaneous microvessels
Thrombotic thrombocytopenic purpura	All microvessels except those of brain and lungs
Acute coronary artery syndrome	Coronary arteries presumed to reflect interplay of plaque rupture and alteration of a vascular bed-specific hemostatic circuit

Adapted from: Rosenberg RD, Aird WC. Vascular-bed-specific hemostasis and hypercoagulable states. N Engl J Med 1999;340:1555–64.

Thrombosis may be initiated by events associated with the perioperative period, including endothelial damage, immobility, and stasis of blood flow.

3. **Protein S deficiency** may be associated with an increased risk of thromboembolism.

4. **Antiphospholipid syndrome** is an autoimmune disorder (estimated to be present in 2% of the general population) characterized by venous and/or arterial thromboses, thrombocytopenia, and recurrent fetal losses reflecting the presence of autoantibodies directed against phospholipid–protein complexes.

   a. **Management of anesthesia.** Patients with a history of antiphospholipid syndrome and at least one thrombotic episode are likely to present during the preoperative period while being treated with anticoagulants (regional anesthesia is not a likely selection).

  b. Prophylactic measures are taken to prevent thromboses, including use of elastic stockings, avoidance of dehydration, and attempts to maintain normothermia.

II. ACQUIRED COAGULATION DISORDERS

See Table 25–1.

A. Disseminated intravascular coagulation (DIC) is characterized by widespread systemic activation of coagulation that results in the intravascular formation of fibrin (thrombotic occlusion of small and midsize vessels resulting in multiple organ system failure) and consumption of platelets and coagulation factors (severe bleeding) (Fig. 25–2).

  1. Causes. See Table 25–4.

  2. Diagnosis. There is no single laboratory test that can establish or rule out the diagnosis of DIC (Table 25–5).

  3. Treatment. The most important initial step in the treatment of DIC is management of the underlying clinical disorder responsible for triggering the coagulation process.

  a. Anticoagulation. Interruption of the coagulation process is with intravenous administration of low doses (300 to 500 units/hr) of unfractionated heparin (low-molecular-weight heparin an alternative selection).

  b. Platelets and plasma. Patients experiencing DIC characterized by low platelet counts and decreased circulat-

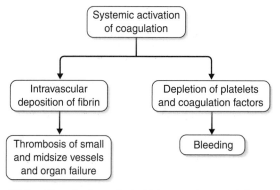

Fig. 25–2 • Steps in disseminated intravascular coagulation. (From Levi M, ten Cate H. Disseminated intravascular coagulation. N Engl J Med 1999;341;586–92. Copyright 1999 Massachusetts Medical Society, with permission.)

▬ **Table 25–4** • Clinical Conditions Associated with Disseminated Intravascular Coagulation

Sepsis
Gram-negative sepsis
Gram-positive sepsis
Trauma
Head injury
Fat embolism
Cancer
Myeloproliferative disorders
Solid tumors (pancreatic cancer, prostate cancer)
Obstetric Complications
Abruptio placentae
Amniotic fluid embolism
Pregnancy-induced hypertension
Vascular Disorders
Aortic aneurysms
Immunologic Disorders
Allergic reactions
Hemolytic transfusion reactions
Transplant rejection

Adapted from: Levi M, ten Cate H. Disseminated intravascular coagulation. N Engl J Med 1999;341:586–92. Copyright 1999 Massachusetts Medical Society, with permission.

▬ **Table 25–5** • Diagnosis of Disseminated Intravascular Coagulation

Presence of clinical conditions known to be associated with disseminated intravascular coagulation
Platelet counts < 100,000 cells/mm^3 and/or a rapid decrease in platelet count
Prolonged prothrombin time
Prolonged activated partial thromboplastin time
Presence of fibrin degradation products
Low plasma concentrations of coagulation inhibitors (antithrombin III)
Hypofibrinogenemia (severe cases)

ing concentrations of procoagulant factors benefit from treatment with platelet concentrates and fresh frozen plasma.

   c. **Antifibrinolytic drugs** are effective in patients with bleeding, but administration to patients with DIC is generally not recommended because the deposition of fibrin in patients with DIC appears to be due in part to insufficient fibrinolysis.

B. Perioperative anticoagulation. Long-term anticoagulation (thromboembolism, hypercoagulable states, cancer, mechanical heart valves, atrial fibrillation) may introduce the risk of increased intraoperative and postoperative bleeding, whereas events associated with surgery may predispose to thromboembolism, especially if oral anticoagulants are discontinued preoperatively resulting in rebound hypercoagulable states.

  1. Recommendations. Overall, there is no consensus on the appropriate perioperative management of anticoagulation for patients who have been receiving long-term warfarin therapy.

    a. **Warfarin.** Management of patients being treated with warfarin preoperatively may include discontinuing the oral anticoagulant prior to elective surgery and instituting intravenous or subcutaneous heparin in selected patients (Table 25–6). An INR of 1.5 is often considered acceptable for performing elective surgery.

    b. **History of venous thromboembolism.** Elective surgery should be avoided the first 30 days after an acute episode of venous thromboembolism. If this is not possible, intravenous heparin is administered before and after the surgical procedure while the INR is < 2.0. Mechanical methods of prophylaxis, such as graduated compression stockings or intermittent pneumatic compression stockings are combined with pharmacologic therapy.

    c. **History of arterial thromboembolism.** Elective surgery should be avoided during the first 30 days after an acute episode of arterial thromboembolism. If this is not possible, preoperative intravenous heparin therapy is recommended.

    d. **Regional anesthesia and neuraxial analgesia.** The prospect of administering spinal or epidural anesthetics or placing epidural catheters for postoperative neuraxial analgesia in patients who are to receive heparin

≡ Table 25–6 • Recommendations for Preoperative and Postoperative Anticoagulation in Patients Being Treated with Oral Anticoagulants

Indication	Before Surgery	After Surgery
Acute venous thromboembolism		
First 30 days	Heparin IV	Heparin IV
After 30 days	No change	Heparin IV
Recurrent venous thromboembolism	No change	Heparin SC
Acute arterial thromboembolism during first 30 days	Heparin IV	Heparin IV
Mechanical heart valve	No change	Heparin SC
Nonvalvular atrial fibrillation	No change	Heparin SC

IV, intravenous; SC, subcutaneous.
Adapted from: Kearon C, Hirsh J. Management of anticoagulation before and after elective surgery. N Engl J Med 1997;336:1506–11.

as prophylaxis against thromboembolic complications is a controversial clinical issue (benefits must outweigh the risk of epidural hematoma formation) (Table 25–7). Even more controversial is use of a spinal or epidural anesthetic in patients who are already anticoagulated (Table 25–7). The timing for removing the epidural catheter is also considered critical, as epidural bleeding could be initiated at this time (Table 25–7).

C. **Intraoperative coagulopathies**
   1. **Dilutional thrombocytopenia** is the most common cause of intraoperative coagulopathy, although as much as 80% of the patient's estimated blood volume may have to be replaced before clinically significant thrombocytopenia occurs. The presence of intraoperative thrombocytopenia is suggested by an abnormal thromboelastogram. There is no justification for prophylactic administration of platelets to massively transfused patients.
   2. **Dilution of procoagulants,** as with platelets, may occur with intraoperative fluid and blood administration (most procoagulant concentrations are needed in only 30% of their normal concentrations for coagulation to continue). There is no justification for prophylactic administration of fresh frozen plasma to massively transfused patients

≡ Table 25–7 • Recommendations for Performance of Neuraxial Analgesia and/or Anesthesia in the Presence of Anticoagulants Administered for Thromboembolism Prophylaxis or Intraoperative Coagulation

---

Unfractionated (Standard) Minidose Subcutaneous Heparin
No contraindication to neuraxial block
May consider delaying initiation of heparin therapy until after institution of the neuraxial block

Unfractionated (Standard) Intravenous Heparin for Intraoperative Coagulation
Delay initiating heparin administration for 1 hour after needle placement for the neuraxial block
Remove the epidural catheter 1 hour before any subsequent intravenous doses of heparin (assumes 12-hour dosing intervals) or 2–4 hours after the last dose of heparin
Consider the use of minimal concentrations of local anesthetics to permit early clinical detection of neurologic changes
Difficult neuraxial needle placement and/or appearance of blood in the needle or catheter does not mandate cancellation of the planned surgery; if the operation proceeds, it is important to perform frequent postoperative monitoring of neurologic status

Low-Molecular-Weight Heparin
Decision to perform neuraxial blocks is made on an individual basis
Difficult neuraxial needle placement and/or appearance of blood in the needle or catheter does not mandate cancellation of the planned surgery; if the operation proceeds it is important to delay initiation of low-molecular-weight heparin therapy for 24 hours
Delay epidural catheter removal for 10–12 hours after the last dose of low-molecular-weight heparin and do not administer any subsequent doses for 2 hours
Consider single-dose spinal anesthesia if regional anesthesia is required in patients being treated with low-molecular-weight heparin preoperatively
Perform frequent postoperative monitoring of neurologic status

Oral Anticoagulants
Stop anticoagulant and allow normalization of prothrombin time (INR) before performance of neuraxial blocks

Antiplatelet Drugs
Treatment with these drugs does not interfere with performance of neuraxial blocks

Fibrinolytic and Thrombolytic Drugs
Neuraxial blocks not recommended within 10 days of receiving these drugs

---

Adapted from: Neuraxial Anesthesia and Anticoagulation, Consensus Statements. American Society of Regional Anesthesia, 1998.

(each unit of platelets also contains 50 to 70 ml of plasma containing procoagulants).

3. **Metabolic changes.** Metabolic acidosis, as may accompany hypotension and poor tissue blood flow, can inhibit circulating procoagulants and platelet function. In patients with normal liver function, the citrate present in stored blood is readily metabolized to bicarbonate.

4. **Effects of surgery.** Surgery causes most patients to become hypercoagulable, whereas intraoperative hypothermia may prolong the PT and PTT and interfere with normal platelet function.

5. **Type of surgery.** See Table 25–8.

D. **Drug-induced hemorrhage.** Heparin overdose manifests as subcutaneous hemorrhage and deep tissue hematomas (prolonged effects of heparin accompany hepatorenal disease and hypothermia). Overdoses of warfarin manifest as ecchymosis formation, mucosal hemorrhage, and subserosal bleeding into the walls of the gastrointestinal tract.

E. **Drug-induced platelet dysfunction.** Aspirin and related nonsteroidal antiinflammatory drugs irreversibly inhibit cyclooxygenase, which is responsible for the platelet release of adenosine diphosphate (ADP), necessary for platelet aggregation (persists for the life of the platelets). Treatment of acute aspirin-induced hemorrhage consists of transfusion of platelets that can release ADP.

1. **Aspirin and elective surgery.** Despite the concern that operative blood loss could be increased, there is evidence that perioperative blood loss is not increased in patients receiving daily aspirin and undergoing hip replacement.

▬ Table 25–8 • Intraoperative Coagulopathies and Type of Surgery

---

Cardiopulmonary bypass (bleeding most often due to platelet dysfunction or heparin overdose; administration of hetastarch may increase bleeding)

Orthopedic surgery (trauma to long bones may cause extrusion of marrow fat resulting in DIC)

Brain surgery (release of lipids and tissue thromboplastins from cerebral trauma results in a high incidence of DIC)

Prostate surgery (release of urokinase)

Amniotic fluid embolism (triggers DIC)

DIC, disseminated intravascular coagulation.

2. There is no evidence that spinal or epidural anesthesia should be avoided in patients receiving antiplatelet drugs (neurologic monitoring is recommended for prompt detection of signs of spinal cord compression attributable to epidural hematoma formation).

F. **Idiopathic thrombocytopenic purpura** (ITP) is characterized by persistent thrombocytopenia caused by anti-platelet immunoglobulins that bind to platelet membranes, causing their premature rupture. Formation of petechiae, characteristically at sites of increased internal or external pressures (oral mucosa, constricting clothing) is likely, and intracranial hemorrhage is the principal cause of mortality in patients with ITP.

1. **Causes.** See Table 25–9.

2. **Heparin-induced thrombocytopenia** may manifest as modest nonprogressive decreases in platelet counts that require no intervention or as severe thrombocytopenia (due to heparin-dependent antibodies) often to $< 50,000$ cells/mm^3 (frequently associated with arterial thromboembolism).

3. **Treatment** of ITP is initially with corticosteroids. Splenectomy is indicated if the platelet response to corticosteroids is inadequate or not sustained.

4. **Management of anesthesia.** See Table 25–10.

G. **Thrombotic thrombocytopenic purpura** (TTP) is characterized by disseminated intravascular aggregation of platelets resulting in thrombocytopenia, severe hemolytic anemia, central nervous system disturbances (seizures), renal dys-

---

≡ **Table 25–9** • Factors Associated with Thrombocytopenia

Idiopathic
Heparin
Infectious mononucleosis
Acquired immunodeficiency syndrome
Hodgkin's disease
Systemic lupus erythematosus
Rheumatoid arthritis
Raynaud's phenomenon
Hyperthyroidism
Sepsis
Quinidine
Thiazide diuretics

≡ Table 25–10 • Management of Anesthesia for
Patients with Idiopathic Thrombocytopenic Purpura

Preoperative corticosteroids (platelet counts > 50,000 cells/mm^3
  at the induction of anesthesia)
Administer platelet concentrates at induction of anesthesia and
  with ligation of splenic pedicle if platelet counts < 50,000 cells/
  mm^3
Minimize trauma to upper airway during direct laryngoscopy
Regional anesthesia rarely selected
Continue corticosteroids postoperatively

---

function, and jaundice. Treatment of TPP is with antiplatelet
drugs (aspirin) and exchange plasmapheresis.

H. **Catheter-induced thrombocytopenia.** Thrombus formation
   on catheters placed in the systemic circulation is a predictable
   event (prevent with heparin-incorporated catheters). Thrombocytopenia may reflect increased platelet consumption
   owing to thrombus formation.

I. **Vitamin K deficiency** occurs in the presence of malnutrition,
   gastrointestinal malabsorption, antibiotic-induced elimination of intestinal flora necessary for the synthesis of vitamin K,
   and obstructive jaundice. Diagnosis of vitamin K deficiency is
   based on determination of a prolonged PT in the presence
   of a normal PTT. Treatment is determined by the urgency
   of the situation (parenteral vitamin K analogues require 6 to
   24 hours to exert beneficial effects versus prompt responses
   to fresh frozen plasma).

26

Skin and Musculoskeletal Diseases

Diseases of the skin and musculoskeletal system manifest with obvious clinical signs, as both systems are readily visible (Stoelting RK, Dierdorf SF. Skin and musculoskeletal diseases. In: Anesthesia and Co-Existing Disease, 4th ed. New York, Churchill Livingstone, 2002;505–549).

I. EPIDERMOLYSIS BULLOSA

Epidermolysis bullosa is a rare hereditary disorder of the skin that may also involve mucous membranes, particularly of the oropharynx and esophagus.

A. **Signs and symptoms.** Epidermolysis bullosa is characterized by bulla formation (blistering) due to separation within the epidermis followed by fluid accumulation. Bulla formation is typically initiated when lateral shearing forces are applied to the affected patient's skin (pressure applied perpendicular to the skin is not as great a hazard).

B. **Treatment** is symptomatic and often includes corticosteroids.

C. **Management of anesthesia.** See Table 26–1.

II. PEMPHIGUS

Pemphigus is a group of chronic autoimmune blistering (vesiculobullous) diseases that may involve extensive areas of the skin and mucous membranes. Cutaneous pemphigus closely resembles the oral manifestations of epidermolysis bullosa (eating is painful, and malnutrition may be present).

A. **Treatment** is with corticosteroids. Azathioprine, methotrexate, cyclophosphamide, and cyclosporine may be useful for early treatment.

B. **Management of anesthesia** is similar to that described for patients with epidermolysis bullosa (Table 26–1).

≡ **Table 26–1** • Management of Anesthesia in the Presence of Epidermolysis Bullosa

Consider preoperative drug therapy (corticosteroids, chemotherapeutic drugs)

Avoid trauma to skin and mucous membranes (suture catheters or hold in place with gauze wrap)

Consider cortisol ointment application to face mask

Minimize frictional trauma to oropharynx (lubricate laryngoscope blade)

Tracheal intubation is acceptable (ketamine an alternative drug when controlled ventilation of the lungs is not required)

Increased incidence of porphyria may influence selection of drugs

Succinylcholine is acceptable

Regional anesthesia is acceptable

Avoid suctioning of pharynx at time of tracheal extubation, as it may induce bulla formation

Risk of aspiration is increased in presence of esophageal strictures

III. PSORIASIS

Psoriasis is a common (affects 1% to 3% of the world's population) chronic dermatologic disorder. It is characterized by accelerated epidermal growth that results in inflammatory erythematous papules covered with loosely adherent scales (chronic plaque psoriasis). An inflammatory asymmetrical arthropathy occurs in about 20% of patients with psoriasis.

  A. **Treatment** of psoriasis is directed at slowing the rapid proliferation of epidermal cells (crude coal tar, salicylic acid, topical corticosteroids).

  B. **Management of anesthesia** must include consideration of drugs being used for treatment of psoriasis. Skin trauma (venipuncture) may accentuate psoriasis in some patients.

IV. MASTOCYTOSIS

Mastocytosis is a rare disorder of mast cell proliferation that occurs in both cutaneous (urticaria pigmentosa) and systemic forms.

A. **Signs and symptoms** reflect degranulation of mast cells and release of histamine, heparin, and prostaglandins into the systemic circulation (pruritus, urticaria, cutaneous flushing, hypotension, tachycardia). Bleeding is unusual in these patients, even though mast cells contain heparin.

B. **Management of anesthesia** is usually uneventful, although there are reports of life-threatening anaphylactoid reactions occurring with even minor surgical procedures (epinephrine must be readily available). Monitoring of serum tryptase concentrations during the perioperative period is useful for determining the occurrence of mast cell degranulation.

V. ATOPIC DERMATITIS

Atopic dermatitis is the cutaneous manifestation of the atopic state (dry, scaly eczematous, pruritic patches).

VI. URTICARIA

Urticaria is categorized as chronic urticaria (hives and associated angioedema) and physical urticaria (application of physical stimulation to the skin results in formation of local weals and itching) (Table 26–2).

A. **Chronic urticaria** is characterized by circumscribed wheals and localized areas of edema produced by extravasation of fluid through blood vessel walls (affects twice as many women as men).

1. **Angioedema** describes urticaria involving the mucous membranes, particularly those of the mouth, pharynx, and larynx.

2. **Treatment** is avoidance of identifiable causes and symptomatic management utilizing antihistamines (H_1-receptor antagonists) such as terfenadine. These patients should avoid angiotensin-converting enzyme inhibitors, aspirin, and nonsteroidal antiinflammatory drugs.

B. **Cold urticaria** is characterized by development of urticaria and angioedema following exposure to local or environmental cold. Life-threatening laryngeal edema, bronchospasm, and hypotension may occur.

1. **Treatment** is avoidance of known triggering mechanisms and administration of antihistamines.

Table 26–2 • Features of Common Types of Chronic Urticaria

Type of Urticaria	Age Range (years)	Clinical Features	Angioedema	Diagnostic Test
Chronic idiopathic	20–50	Pink or pale edematous papules or wheals Wheals often annular Pruritus	Yes	
Symptomatic dermatographism	20–50	Linear wheals with a surrounding bright-red flare at sites of stimulation Pruritus	No	Light stroking of skin causes wheal
Physical urticarias Cold	10–40	Pale or red swelling at sites of contact with cold surfaces or fluids Pruritus	Yes	Application of ice pack causes a wheal within 5 minutes of removing the ice (cold stimulation test)

Pressure	20–50	Swelling at sites of pressure (soles, palms, waist) lasting 24 hours or longer Painful Pruritus	No	Application of pressure perpendicular to skin produces persistent red swelling after a latent period of 1–4 hours
Solar	20–50	Pale or red swelling at site of exposure to ultraviolet or visible light Pruritus	Yes	Radiation by a solar simulator for 30–120 seconds causes wheals in 30 minutes
Cholinergic	10–50	Monomorphic pale or pink wheals on trunk, neck, and limbs Pruritus	Yes	Exercise or hot shower elicits wheals

Adapted from: Greaves MW. Chronic urticaria. N Engl J Med 1995;332:1767–72.

2. **Management of anesthesia** includes avoiding drugs likely to evoke the release of histamine, warming infused fluids, and increasing ambient temperatures in the operating rooms.

VII. ERYTHEMA MULTIFORME

Erythema multiforme is an acute recurrent disorder of the skin and mucous membranes characterized by lesions ranging from edematous macules to bullous lesions.

A. **Stevens-Johnson syndrome** is a severe manifestation of erythema multiforme associated with multisystem involvement (fever, tachycardia, tachypnea). Drugs associated with the onset of this syndrome include antibiotics and analgesics. Treatment is with corticosteroids.

B. **Management of anesthesia** for patients with Stevens-Johnson syndrome introduces risks similar to those in patients with epidermolysis bullosa (upper airway involvement, pulmonary blebs, and use of nitrous oxide and positive-pressure ventilation).

VIII. SCLERODERMA

Scleroderma is characterized by inflammation, vascular sclerosis, and fibrosis of the skin and viscera (may evolve into the CREST syndrome). Prognosis is poor and related to the extent of visceral involvement. Corticosteroids are not administered to patients with scleroderma.

A. **Signs and symptoms.** See Table 26–3.

B. **Management of anesthesia** is influenced by the multiple organ systems likely to be involved by the progressive changes associated with this disease (Table 26–3).

IX. PSEUDOXANTHOMA ELASTICUM

Pseudoxanthoma elasticum is a rare hereditary disorder of elastic tissues (degeneration and calcification) leading to loss of visual acuity, gastrointestinal hemorrhage, systemic hypertension, and ischemic heart disease.

A. **Management of anesthesia** in the presence of pseudoxanthoma elasticum is based on an appreciation of the abnormalities associated with this disease (cardiovascular derangements most important).

B. Use of a noninvasive blood pressure device is an acceptable alternative to placing an intra-arterial catheter.

≡ **Table 26–3 •** Signs and Symptoms
of Scleroderma

Skin and Musculoskeletal System
Flexion contractures (fingers, mouth)
Proximal skeletal muscle weakness
Nervous System
Nerve compression
Trigeminal neuralgia
Cardiovascular System
Dysrhythmias
Conduction abnormalities
Congestive heart failure
Lungs
Pulmonary fibrosis
Arterial hypoxemia
Kidneys
Accelerated systemic hypertension
Gastrointestinal Tract
Dysphagia
Hypomotility

X. EHLERS-DANLOS SYNDROME

Ehlers-Danlos syndrome consists of a group of inherited
connective tissue disorders due to abnormalities of metabolism in collagen. The only form of this syndrome associated
with an increased risk of death is designated type IV, which
may be complicated by sudden rupture of large blood vessels or disruption of the bowel.

A. **Signs and symptoms** include joint hypermobility, skin
fragility, bruising, musculoskeletal discomfort, and susceptibility to osteoarthritis. Dilation of the trachea is
often present. Ecchymosis may accompany even minor
trauma, but a specific coagulation defect has not
been identified.

B. **Management of anesthesia.** See Table 26–4.

XI. POLYMYOSITIS

Polymyositis (dermatomyositis) is a multisystem disease
of unknown etiology. It manifests as nonsuppurative inflammation of skeletal muscles (inflammatory myopathy).

Table 26–4 • Management of Anesthesia in Patients with Ehlers-Danlos Syndrome

---

Prophylactic antibiotics if cardiac murmur is present

Avoid intramuscular injections

Minimize trauma during direct laryngoscopy

Hematoma may accompany placement of arterial and/or venous catheters

Avoid esophageal instrumentation

Intravenous fluid extravasation may go unnoticed because of the extreme distensibility of the skin

Increased incidence of pneumothorax (avoid high airway pressures)

Increased incidence of ischemic heart disease

Regional anesthesia not recommended

Surgical bleeding may be excessive

A. **Signs and symptoms.** See Table 26–5.
B. **Diagnosis** of polymyositis is confirmed by proximal skeletal muscle weakness, increased serum creatine kinase concentrations, and the presence of characteristic skin rashes.
C. **Treatment** is with corticosteroids.

Table 26–5 • Signs and Symptoms of Polymyositis

Proximal skeletal muscle weakness [neck, shoulders, hips (difficulty climbing stairs)]

Dysphagia and pulmonary aspiration (paresis of pharyngeal and respiratory muscles)

Ventilatory insufficiency (weakness of intercostal muscles and diaphragm)

Increased serum creatine kinase concentrations

Heart block

Left ventricular dysfunction

Myocarditis

Associated with systemic lupus erythematosus, scleroderma, and rheumatoid arthritis

---

D. **Management of anesthesia** considers the vulnerability of these patients to pulmonary aspiration. Drugs capable of triggering malignant hyperthermia may be avoided. Responses to nondepolarizing muscle relaxants seem to be unchanged despite the presence of skeletal muscle weakness.

XII. SYSTEMIC LUPUS ERYTHEMATOSUS

Systemic lupus erythematosus (SLE) is a multisystem inflammatory disease characterized by antinuclear antibody production, most often manifesting in young women (may affect as many as 1 in 1000). The onset of SLE may be drug-induced (procainamide, hydralazine, isoniazid) and is related to the patient's acetylator phenotype (more likely to occur in slow acetylators). Pregnancy may exacerbate SLE.

A. **Diagnosis** of SLE is likely in the presence of antinuclear antibodies, characteristic skin rash, thrombocytopenia, and serositis or nephritis.

B. **Signs and symptoms.** See Table 26–6.

C. **Treatment** of SLE often includes corticosteroids.

D. **Management of anesthesia** is influenced by drugs used to treat SLE and by the magnitude of dysfunction of those organs damaged by the disease. Laryngeal involvement, including mucosal ulceration, cricoarytenoid arthritis, and recurrent laryngeal nerve palsy may be present.

XIII. URBACH-WIETHE DISEASE

Urbach-Wiethe disease is characterized by deposition of hyaline, leading to thickening of the skin or mucosa (laryngeal scarring manifests as hoarseness and may cause difficulties with tracheal intubation). A decrease in diastolic compliance, manifesting as impaired filling of the left ventricle during diastole, may be part of any type of left ventricular dysfunction.

XIV. CORNELIA de LANGE SYNDROME

Cornelia de Lange syndrome is a rare disorder due to hypoplasia of the mesenchyma (mental retardation, aspiration related to hiatal hernia, difficult tracheal intubation due to a short neck, small mouth, and high arched palate).

≡ **Table 26–6 •** Signs and Symptoms of Systemic Lupus Erythematosus

---

Articular Manifestations
Symmetrical arthritis (episodic and migratory)
Avascular necrosis
Systemic Manifestations
Central nervous system
  Cognitive dysfunction (mood disturbances)
  Atypical migraine headaches
  Aseptic meningitis
Heart
  Pericarditis
  Myocarditis
  Tachycardia
  Congestive heart failure
  Valvular abnormalities
Lungs
  Lupus pneumonia
  Recurrent atelectasis (phrenic nerve neuropathy)
  Lung hemorrhage
  Pulmonary hypertension
Kidneys
  Glomerulonephritis
  Hematuria
Liver
Neuromuscular
  Proximal skeletal muscle weakness
  Tendinitis
Hematologic
  Thromboembolism
  Leukopenia
  Thrombocytopenia
  Hemolytic anemia
Cutaneous
  Butterfly nasal malar erythema rash
  Alopecia

XV. TUMORAL CALCINOSIS

Tumoral calcinosis usually presents as multiple soft tissue masses adjacent to large joints (involvement of hyoid bone and cervical intervertebral joints may interfere with direct laryngoscopy for tracheal intubation).

XVI. MUSCULAR DYSTROPHY

Muscular dystrophy is a hereditary disease characterized by painless degeneration and atrophy of skeletal muscles.

A. **Pseudohypertrophic muscular dystrophy (Duchenne's muscular dystrophy)** is the most common (3 per 10,000 births) and most severe form of childhood progressive muscular dystrophy. The disease is caused by an X-linked recessive gene, becoming apparent in males aged 2 to 5 years (difficulty climbing stairs, kyphoscoliosis, increased serum creatine kinase concentrations).

   1. **Cardiopulmonary dysfunction.** Degeneration of cardiac muscle invariably accompanies muscular dystrophy. Chronic weakness of inspiratory muscles and decreased ability to cough can predispose to recurrent pneumonia.

   2. **Management of anesthesia.** See Table 26–7.

B. **Limb-girdle muscular dystrophy** is a slowly progressive and relatively benign disease.

C. **Facioscapulohumeral muscular dystrophy** is characterized by slowly progressive wasting of facial, pectoral, and shoulder girdle skeletal muscles that begins during adolescence. The heart is not involved, and serum creatine kinase concentrations are seldom increased.

D. **Nemaline rod muscular dystrophy** is characterized by slowly progressive to nonprogressive symmetrical dystrophy of skeletal and smooth muscles.

Table 26–7 • Management of Anesthesia in Patients with Pseudohypertrophic Muscular Dystrophy

Increased risk of aspiration (weak laryngeal reflexes and gastrointestinal hypomotility)
Succinylcholine contraindicated (risk of rhabdomyolysis, hyperkalemia, cardiac arrest)
Response to nondepolarizing muscle relaxants normal to prolonged
Volatile anesthetics may be associated with rhabdomyolysis
Increased incidence of malignant hyperthermia
Regional anesthesia acceptable
Monitors to detect malignant hyperthermia and cardiac depression
Anticipate postoperative pulmonary dysfunction

Table 26–8 • Management of Anesthesia in Patients with Nemaline Rod Muscular Dystrophy

---

Anticipated difficult tracheal intubation (awake fiberoptic)
Exaggerated respiratory depressant effects of drugs [intercostal muscle weakness and chest wall abnormalities (scoliosis, kyphoscoliosis)] or high sensory block produced by regional anesthesia
Risk of aspiration (bulbar palsy)
Unpredictable responses to muscle relaxants
Malignant hyperthermia (?)
Myocardial depression due to volatile anesthetics

---

1. **Signs and symptoms.** Micrognathia and dental malocclusion are common. Restrictive lung disease may result from myopathy and scoliosis.
2. **Management of anesthesia.** See Table 26–8.
    E. **Oculopharyngeal dystrophy** is characterized by progressive dysphagia and ptosis.
    F. **Emery-Dreifuss muscular dystrophy** is an X-linked recessive disorder characterized by the development of skeletal muscle contractures that precede the onset of skeletal muscle weakness in a humeroperoneal distribution. Cardiac involvement and associated cardiomyopathy (congestive heart failure, thromboembolism) may be life-threatening.

XVII. MYOTONIC DYSTROPHY

Myotonic dystrophy designates a group of hereditary degenerative diseases of skeletal muscles characterized by persistent contractures (myotonia) of skeletal muscles after voluntary contraction or following electrical stimulation (electromyographic findings are diagnostic). Peripheral nerves and the neuromuscular junctions are not affected.

A. **Myotonia dystrophica** is the most common and most serious form of myotonic dystrophy afflicting adults. Treatment is symptomatic and may include the use of quinine and phenytoin. Death due to pneumonia or congestive heart failure usually occurs by the sixth decade of life.

1. **Signs and symptoms.** See Table 26–9.
2. **Management of anesthesia.** See Table 26–10.

≡ Table 26-9 • Signs and Symptoms of Myotonic Dystrophy

Facial weakness ("expressionless facies")
Wasting of sternocleidomastoid muscles
Ptosis
Dysarthria
Dysphagia
Inability to relax handgrip
Mental retardation
Frontal baldness
Cataract formation
Endocrine gland dysfunction (gonadal atrophy, diabetes mellitus, decreased thyroid gland function, adrenal insufficiency)
Slowed gastric emptying
Central sleep apnea (hypersomnolence)
Cardiac dysrhythmias and conduction abnormalities (sudden death)
Mitral valve prolapse
Pulmonary aspiration

    B. Myotonia congenita does not involve other organ systems and does not result in decreased life expectancy.

    C. Paramyotonia congenita is characterized by generalized myotonia that may be exacerbated by exercise or cold.

    D. Hyperkalemic periodic paralysis is characterized by episodes of flaccid skeletal muscle paralysis associated with increased serum potassium concentrations. It is precipitated by cold, hunger, and emotional stress.

≡ Table 26-10 • Management of Anesthesia in Patients with Myotonia Dystrophica

Myocardial depression produced by volatile anesthetics may be exaggerated (presence of cardiomyopathy)
Succinylcholine produces prolonged skeletal muscle contractions
Responses to nondepolarizing neuromuscular blocking drugs are normal
Reversal of neuromuscular blockade with anticholinesterase drugs is acceptable
Exaggerated ventilatory depression produced by injected anesthetic drugs
Malignant hyperthermia susceptibility (?)
Postoperative shivering may induce myotonia

1. **Management of anesthesia** includes avoidance of potassium-containing fluids and drugs that evoke the release of potassium. Intravenous glucose infusions are administered during fasting to minimize carbohydrate depletion.
2. Calcium gluconate administered intravenously is suggested for emergency treatment of hyperkalemia-induced weakness.

E. **Acid-maltase deficiency** is a glycogen storage disease (Pompe's disease) presenting as pelvic girdle weakness and respiratory failure.

F. **Schwartz-Jampel syndrome** is a rare progressive disorder that manifests during childhood as skeletal muscle stiffness, myotonia, and skeletal abnormalities (micrognathia). These children may be susceptible to malignant hyperthermia.

XVIII. DYSKALEMIC FAMILIAL PERIODIC PARALYSIS

See Table 26–11.

A. **Management of anesthesia** is influenced by the nature of the potassium sensitivity (Table 26–11). Hypothermia is avoided regardless of the nature of the potassium sensitivity (warm intravenous fluids and increase the ambient temperatures of the operating rooms). Nondepolarizing muscle relaxants are acceptable.

1. **Hypokalemic periodic paralysis.** See Table 26–12.
2. **Hyperkalemic periodic paralysis.** See Table 26–13.

XIX. MYASTHENIA GRAVIS

Myasthenia gravis is an acquired chronic autoimmune disorder caused by decreases in functioning acetylcholine receptors at the neuromuscular junctions owing to their destruction or inactivation by circulating antibodies (Fig. 26–1). Loss of acetylcholine receptors manifests as weakness and rapid exhaustion of voluntary skeletal muscles with repetitive use. Skeletal muscles innervated by cranial nerves (ocular, pharyngeal, laryngeal muscles representing bulbar muscles) are especially vulnerable, as reflected by ptosis, diplopia, and dysphagia, which may be initial symptoms of the disease. Other conditions that cause weakness of the cranial and somatic musculature must be considered in the differential diagnosis of myasthenia gravis (Table 26–14).

Text continued on page 408

Table 26–11 • Clinical Features of Familial Periodic Paralysis

Type	Serum Potassium Concentrations During Symptoms	Precipitating Factors	Other Features
Hypokalemia	< 3 mEq/L	Large glucose meals Strenuous exercise Glucose-insulin infusions Stress Menstruation Pregnancy Anesthesia Hypothermia	Cardiac dysrhythmias Signs of hypokalemia on the ECG
Hyperkalemia	> 5.5 mEq/L	Exercise Potassium infusions Metabolic acidosis Hypothermia	Skeletal muscle weakness may be localized to tongue and eyelids

ECG, electrocardiogram.

☰ Table 26–12 • Management of Anesthesia in Patients with Hypokalemia Periodic Paralysis

Avoid events known to trigger hypokalemic attacks
    Psychological stress
    Cold
    Carbohydrate loads
    β-Adrenergic agonists
Monitor serum potassium concentrations (every 15–60 minutes)
Treat hypokalemia with potassium chloride (up to 40 mEq/hr)
Administer short-acting nondepolarizing muscle relaxants
Risk of malignant hyperthermia (?)

☰ Table 26–13 • Management of Anesthesia in Patients with Hyperkalemia Periodic Paralysis

Preoperative potassium depletion with furosemide-induced diuresis
Prevent carbohydrate depletion during fasting (administer glucose-containing solutions)
Avoid potassium-containing intravenous solutions
Avoid potassium-releasing drugs
Frequent monitoring of serum potassium concentrations
Ready availability calcium to treat signs of hyperkalemia

Normal

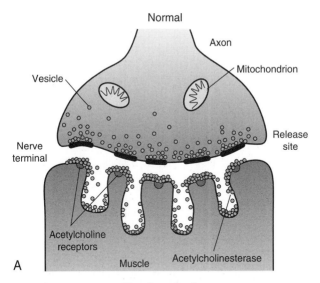

Axon

Mitochondrion

Vesicle

Release site

Nerve terminal

Acetylcholine receptors

Acetylcholinesterase

Muscle

A

Myasthena gravis

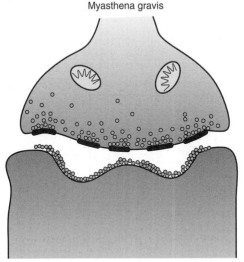

B

Fig. 26–1 • Normal (*A*) and myasthenic (*B*) neuromuscular junctions. Compared with normal neuromuscular junctions, myasthenic neuromuscular junctions have fewer acetylcholine receptors, simplified synaptic folds, and widened synaptic spaces. (From Drachman DB. Myasthenia gravis. N Engl J Med 1994;330:1797–1810. Copyright 1994 Massachusetts Medical Society, with permission.)

Table 26–14 • Differential Diagnosis of Myasthenia Gravis

Condition	Symptoms and Characteristics	Comments
Congenital myasthenic syndromes	Rare Early onset Not autoimmune	Electrophysiologic and immunocytochemical tests required for diagnosis
Drug-induced myasthenia gravis Penicillamine	Triggers autoimmune myasthenia gravis	Recovery within weeks of discontinuing the drug
Nondepolarizing muscle relaxants Aminoglycosides Procainamide	Increased sensitivity	Recovery after drug discontinuation
Lambert-Eaton syndrome	Oat cell cancer Fatigue	Incremental response on repetitive nerve stimulation Antibodies to calcium channels

Hyperthyroidism	Exacerbation of myasthenia gravis	Thyroid function normal
Graves' disease	Diplopia Exophthalmos	Thyroid-stimulating immunoglobulin present
Botulism	Generalized weakness Ophthalmoplegia	Incremental response on repetitive nerve stimulation
Progressive external ophthalmoplegia	Ptosis Diplopia Generalized weakness in some cases	Mitochondrial abnormalities
Intracranial mass compressing	Ophthalmoplegia Cranial nerve weakness	Abnormalities on CT or MRI

CT, computed tomography; MRI, magnetic resonance imaging.
Adapted from: Drachman DB. Myasthenia gravis. N Engl J Med 1994;330:1797–1810.

▬ **Table 26–15** • Classification of Myasthenia Gravis Based on Skeletal Muscles Involved and Severity of Symptoms

Type	Characteristics
I	Limited to extraocular muscles (ocular myasthenia gravis)
IIA	Slowly progressive and spares muscles of respiration
	Response to anticholinesterase drugs is good
IIB	More severe and rapidly progressive skeletal muscle weakness
	Muscles of respiration may be involved
	Response to anticholinesterase drugs may not be good
III	Acute onset and rapid deterioration
IV	Severe form of skeletal muscle weakness that results from progression of type I or II

  A. **Classification.** See Table 26–15.
  B. **Signs and symptoms.** See Table 26–16.
  C. **Treatment.** See Table 26–17.
  D. **Management of anesthesia** is most often required for elective surgical procedures (Table 26–18).

XX. **MYASTHENIC SYNDROME**

  Myasthenic syndrome (Eaton-Lambert syndrome) is a rare disorder of neuromuscular transmission resembling myasthenia gravis (Table 26–19).

▬ **Table 26–16** • Signs and Symptoms of Myasthenia Gravis

Ptosis and diplopia (most common initial complaints)
Dysphagia and dysarthria (weakness of pharyngeal and laryngeal muscles)
Asymmetrical skeletal muscle weakness with exercise
Myocarditis (cardiomyopathy, atrial fibrillation, heart block)
Hypothyroidism
Isolated respiratory failure

▤ Table 26–17 • Treatment of Myasthenia Gravis

Anticholinesterase Drugs
Pyridostigmine 60 mg PO (effect in 30 minutes and peak effect in about 120 minutes) equivalent to 2 mg IM or IV
Beneficial effects usually incomplete and wane after months or weeks of treatment

Thymectomy
Induces remissions or decreases dose of immunosuppressive medication needed
If vital capacity is < 2 L it may be helpful to perform plasmapheresis before surgery to improve the likelihood of adequate spontaneous ventilation during the postoperative period
Surgical approach is median sternotomy (optimizes removal of entire gland) or mediastinoscopy (less postoperative pain)

Immunosuppressive Therapy (when weakness not controlled by anticholinesterase drugs)
Corticosteroids
Azathioprine
Cyclosporine

Short-term Immunotherapies
Plasmapheresis (removes antibodies; benefit is transient)
Immunoglobulins

A. **Management of anesthesia** includes consideration of altered responses to muscle relaxants and the possibility that antagonism with anticholinesterase drugs may be inadequate.

B. The potential presence of myasthenic syndrome and the need to decrease the doses of muscle relaxants should be considered in patients with known cancer or those undergoing operations to determine the presence of cancer.

XXI. RHEUMATOID ARTHRITIS

Rheumatoid arthritis is the most common chronic inflammatory arthritis, affecting about 1% of adults (females > males). The disease is characterized by symmetrical polyarthropathy and significant systemic involvement. Morning stiffness and involvement of the wrists and metacarpophalangeal joints helps distinguish rheumatoid arthritis from

▬ **Table 26–18** • Management of Anesthesia for Patients with Myasthenia Gravis

Preoperative Medication
Avoid opioids
Advise patient may awaken with a tracheal tube in place
Muscle Relaxants
Anticipate altered responses based on disease and/or drugs used for treatment
Initial dose titrated based on response evoked by peripheral nerve stimulator (consider monitoring at orbicularis oculi muscle)
Short-acting nondepolarizing muscle relaxants may be an alternative to succinylcholine when rapid onset on neuromuscular blockade is warranted
Induction of Anesthesia
Short-acting intravenous drugs
Consider tracheal intubation without skeletal muscle paralysis provided by muscle relaxants
Decrease initial dose of nondepolarizing muscle relaxants if these drugs are selected
Maintenance of Anesthesia
Nitrous oxide plus volatile drugs (decrease doses of muscle relaxants needed)
Short- or intermediate-acting muscle relaxants (decrease initial dose one-half to two-thirds)
Postoperative Care
Recognize that skeletal muscle strength may decrease abruptly
Anticipate need for continued support of ventilation in some patients

osteoarthritis, which typically affects weight-bearing joints and the distal interphalangeal joints. The course of the disease is characterized by exacerbations and remissions.

    A. Signs and symptoms. See Table 26–20.
    B. Treatment. See Table 26–21.
    C. Management of anesthesia. Multiple organ system involvement and side effects of drugs (coagulation, adrenal gland suppression) used to treat rheumatoid arthritis must be appreciated when planning the management of anesthesia (Table 26–21). Preoperatively, patients should be evaluated for airway problems due to the disease process (cervical spine, temporomandibular joints, cricoarytenoid joints) (Table 26–22). Preoperative pulmonary function studies and mea-

Table 26–19 • Comparison of Myasthenic Syndrome and Myasthenia Gravis

Parameter	Myasthenic Syndrome	Myasthenia Gravis
Manifestations	Proximal limb weakness (arms > legs)	Extraocular, bulbar, and facial muscle weakness
	Exercise improves strength	Fatigue with exercise
	Muscle pain common	Muscle pain uncommon
	Reflexes absent or decreased	Reflexes normal
Gender	Males > females	Females > males
Co-existing pathology	Small cell lung cancer	Thymoma
Response to muscle relaxants	Sensitive to succinylcholine	Resistant to succinylcholine
	Sensitive to nondepolarizing muscle relaxants	Sensitive to nondepolarizing muscle relaxants
	Poor response to anticholinesterases	Good response to anticholinesterases

Table 26–20 • Signs and Symptoms of Rheumatoid Arthritis

Joint Involvement
Hands, wrists, and knees (morning stiffness)
Temporomandibular joint
Cervical spine (atlantoaxial subluxation; odontoid process may compress the spinal cord)
Cricoarytenoid (hoarseness)
Systemic Involvement
Cardiovascular (pericardial effusion, pericarditis, myocarditis, coronary artery arteritis, cardiac valve fibrosis, rheumatoid nodules in cardiac conduction system)
Lungs (pleural effusion, interstitial inflammation and fibrosis, restrictive changes with decreased lung volumes and vital capacity)
Neuromuscular (entrapment neuropathies)
Blood (mild anemia)
Eyes (keratoconjunctivitis sicca)

≡ **Table 26–21 • Treatment of Rheumatoid Arthritis**

Drug Therapy
Aspirin and nonsteroidal antiinflammatory drugs (COX-2 evoke fewer gastrointestinal side effects and do not interfere with platelet function)
Methotrexate (bone marrow suppression and hepatic cirrhosis)
Anticytokine therapy (tumor necrosis factor inhibition)
Corticosteroids (osteoporosis, infection, myopathy, poor wound healing)
Immunosuppressive drugs (cyclophosphamide, azathioprine)
Surgery (intractable pain and impaired function)
Joint stabilization
Joint replacement

surement of arterial blood gases and pH may be indicated. The need for postoperative ventilatory support should be anticipated if severe restrictive lung disease is present preoperatively. Postextubation laryngeal obstruction may occur in patients with cricoarytenoid arthritis.

≡ **Table 26–22 • Evaluation and Management of the Airway in Patients with Rheumatoid Arthritis**

Flexion deformity of cervical spine may lead to airway obstruction with induction of anesthesia
Atlantoaxial subluxation (radiologic confirmation) may increase the risk of cervical spinal cord compression or interference with vertebral artery blood flow; avoid excessive movements of neck during laryngoscopy; determine head positions awake that can be tolerated
Limitation of temporomandibular joint mobility plus cervical spine immobility may limit visualization for direct laryngoscopy (consider awake fiberoptic intubation)
Cricoarytenoid arthritis and associated inflammation may make identification of glottic opening difficult

XXII. SPONDYLARTHROPATHIES

Spondylarthropathies are a group of nonrheumatic arthropathies that include ankylosing spondylitis (Marie-Strumpell disease), Reiter's disease, juvenile chronic polyarthropathy, and enteropathic arthropathies. These diseases are characterized by involvement of the sacroiliac joints, peripheral inflammatory arthropathy, and the absence of rheumatic nodules or detectable circulating rheumatoid factor.

A. **Ankylosing spondylitis** is a chronic, usually progressive inflammatory disease involving the articulations of the entire spine and adjacent soft tissues. Cardiomegaly, aortic regurgitation, cardiac conduction abnormalities, and pulmonary fibrosis may be present.

   1. **Treatment** includes administration of antiinflammatory drugs such as indomethacin and phenylbutazone. Bone marrow depression is a potential adverse effect of these drugs.

   2. **Management of anesthesia** in patients with ankylosing spondylitis is influenced by the magnitude of upper airway involvement by the disease, the presence of restrictive patterns of breathing, and the degree of cardiac involvement. Awake fiberoptic tracheal intubation is performed if spinal column deformity is extensive. Regional anesthesia is acceptable but may be technically difficult.

B. **Reiter's disease** consists of nonspecific urethritis, uveitis, and arthritis (cricoarytenoid involvement possible). Symptomatic management is with indomethacin or phenylbutazone.

C. **Juvenile chronic polyarthropathy** is similar to adult rheumatoid arthritis, but cardiac involvement is unusual. An acute form of polyarthritis that presents as fever, rash, lymphadenopathy, and splenomegaly in young children who are negative for rheumatoid factor and HLA-B27 is designated *Still's disease.*

D. **Enteropathic arthropathies** that manifest as an acute migratory inflammatory polyarthritis, most often involving the large joints of the lower extremities, may develop in patients with ileocolitis or ulcerative colitis. Inflammatory bowel disease may be associated with sacroiliitis and occasionally with severe ankylosing spondylitis.

XXIII. OSTEOARTHRITIS

Osteoarthritis is a degenerative process that often affects the articular cartilage of the knees and hips (see Chapter 33). The process differs from rheumatoid arthritis in that there is minimal inflammatory reaction.

A. Degenerative changes are most significant in the middle to lower cervical spine and in the lower lumbar area (associated protrusion of the nucleus pulposus can result in nerve root compression).

B. Treatment of osteoarthritis includes aspirin and reconstructive joint surgery. Corticosteroids are not recommended.

XXIV. PAGET'S DISEASE

Paget's disease of bone is characterized by excessive osteoblastic activity resulting in abnormally thickened but weak bone. Bone pain is the most common symptom.

A. Complications of Paget's disease include fractures, neoplastic degeneration, arthritis, nerve compression, paraplegia, and hypercalcemia.

B. Treatment of Paget's disease is with calcitonin and bisphosphanates.

XXV. MARFAN SYNDROME

Marfan syndrome is an inherited disorder of connective tissue with associated skeletal and cardiovascular abnormalities (Table 26–23).

A. Management of anesthesia. Preoperative evaluation of patients with Marfan syndrome should concentrate on cardiopulmonary abnormalities (Table 26–23).

B. Temporomandibular joint dislocation is a risk during direct laryngoscopy. Sustained increases in systemic blood pressure may be a risk to patients with weakened thoracic aortas. Pneumothorax may develop intraoperatively.

XXVI. KYPHOSCOLIOSIS

Kyphoscoliosis is a deformity of the costovertebral skeletal structures, characterized by anterior flexion (kyphosis) and lateral curvature (scoliosis) of the patient's vertebral column.

≡ Table 26–23 • Abnormalities Associated with Marfan Syndrome

Skeletal
Long tubular bones ("Abe Lincoln appearance")
High arched palate
Pectus excavatum
Kyphoscoliosis
Hyerextensibility of joints
Pulmonary
Pulmonary emphysema
Restrictive lung disease (kyphoscoliosis)
Spontaneous pneumothorax
Ocular
Lens dislocation
Myopia
Retinal detachment
Cardiovascular
Aortic dissection (defective tensile strength; prophylactic
  β-adrenergic blocker therapy, pregnancy increases risk)
Mitral regurgitation (mitral valve prolapse as detected by
  echocardiography)
Cardiac conduction abnormalities

A. **Signs and symptoms.** Restrictive lung disease and pulmonary hypertension progressing to cor pulmonale are the principal causes of mortality in patients with kyphoscoliosis.

B. **Management of anesthesia.** See Table 26–24.

XXVII. ACHONDROPLASIA

Achondroplasia is the most common cause of disproportionate dwarfism (predicted height in males 132 cm and females 122 cm).

A. Central sleep apnea experienced by achondroplastic dwarfs may be a function of brain stem compression due to foramen magnum stenosis. Pulmonary hypertension leading to cor pulmonale is the most common cardiovascular disturbance that develops in dwarfs.

B. **Management of anesthesia** in achondroplastic dwarfs may be influenced by difficulty with airway management, cervical spine instability, and the potential for spinal cord trauma with neck extension. Pituitary

---

≡ Table 26–24 • Management of Anesthesia for
Patients with Kyphoscoliosis

Preoperative
Pulmonary function tests (vital capacity, forced exhaled volume in
  1 second)
Arterial blood gases and pH
Avoid depressant drugs in the preoperative medication
Intraoperative
Confirm adequacy of ventilation and oxygenation
Consider possible adverse effects of nitrous oxide on pulmonary
  vascular resistance (central venous pressure monitoring)
Possible malignant hyperthermia susceptibility
Surgical Correction of Spine Curvature
Minimize blood loss (controlled hypotension)
Detect surgically induced spinal cord damage ("wake-up test"
  and/or somatosensory evoked potential monitoring)
Volatile anesthetics may interfere with evoked potential
  monitoring (use continuous infusions of opioids and/or propofol)
Postoperative paralysis may still occur despite evoked potential
  monitoring (reflects inability of sensory evoked potentials to
  monitor the motor integrity of the spinal cord; reason to utilize
  the wake-up test)
Anticipate need for postoperative support of ventilation

---

dwarfism is more likely to be associated with propor-
tionately smaller airways.

1. A preoperative history of obstructive sleep apnea
   may predispose to the development of upper airway
   obstruction after sedation or induction of anesthesia.
2. Hyperextension of the patient's neck during direct
   laryngoscopy for tracheal intubation should be
   avoided, if possible, considering the likely presence
   of foramen magnum stenosis. Weight rather than
   age is the best guide for predicting the proper size
   of the endotracheal tube for these patients.
3. Regional anesthesia in achondroplastic dwarfs may
   be considered for cesarean section.

C. **Russell-Silver syndrome** is a form of dwarfism characterized by dysmorphic facial features, congenital heart
   defects, and endocrine abnormalities (hypoglycemia).
   1. **Management of anesthesia.** Preoperative evaluation
      considers glucose status (intravenous infusions con-
      taining glucose may be indicated preoperatively).

2. Facial manifestations of this syndrome may make direct laryngoscopy and exposure of the glottic opening difficult. Tracheal tubes smaller than the predicted size may be needed.

XXVIII. BACK PAIN

Back pain is the most common musculoskeletal complaint requiring medical attention (Table 26–25).

A. **Acute back pain** improves within 30 days in 90% of patients. Pain arising from inflammation initiated by mechanical or chemical insult to the surrounding nerve root may be responsive to epidural administration of corticosteroids. A herniated lumbar disc (L4-5, L5-S1) producing radiating pain down the leg may be confirmed by magnetic resonance imaging.

B. **Lumbar spinal stenosis** usually reflects extensive degenerative disc disease and osteophyte formation, most often in elderly patients with chronic back pain and associated sciatica (see Chapter 33). Diagnosis is confirmed by magnetic resonance imaging. Surgical decompression by multilevel laminectomy and fusion are considered for patients with progressive functional deterioration.

XXIX. OTHER MUSCULOSKELETAL SYNDROMES

A. **Rotator cuff tear** is the most common pathologic entity involving the shoulders (estimated to be present in about 50% of individuals more than 55 years of age).
   1. **Treatment** may include corticosteroid injections, arthroscopic release, and total shoulder replacement.
   2. **Management of anesthesia.** Brachial plexus anesthesia utilizing the interscalene approach and continuous infusion of local anesthetic solutions provides anesthesia for shoulder procedures as well as postoperative analgesia.

B. **Floppy infant syndrome** is a term used to describe infants who have weak, hypotonic skeletal muscles owing to neuromuscular or nonneuromuscular causes (diminished cough reflex, aspiration, pneumonia, kyphoscoliosis).
   1. **Management of anesthesia** may be associated with increased sensitivity to nondepolarizing muscle relaxants, hyperkalemia after succinylcholine, and car-

▬ Table 26–25 • Differential Diagnosis of Low Back Pain

Mechanical or Low Back or Leg Pain (97%)
Idiopathic low back pain (lumbar sprain or strain) (70%)
Degenerative processes of discs and facets (age-related) (10%)
Herniated disc (4%)
Spinal stenosis (3%)
Osteoporotic compression fractures (4%)
Spondylolisthesis (2%)
Traumatic fracture ($< 1\%$)
Congenital disease ($< 1\%$)
    Severe kyphosis
    Severe scoliosis
Spondylolysis
Nonmechanical Spinal Conditions (1%)
Cancer (0.7%)
    Multiple myeloma
    Metastatic cancer
    Lymphoma and leukemia
    Spinal cord tumors
    Retroperitoneal tumors
    Primary vertebral tumors
Infection (0.01%)
    Osteomyelitis
    Paraspinal abscess
    Epidural abscess
Inflammatory arthritis
    Ankylosing spondylitis
    Psoriatic spondylitis
    Reiter syndrome
    Inflammatory bowel syndrome
Visceral Disease (2%)
Disease of pelvic organs
    Prostatitis
    Endometriosis
    Pelvic inflammatory disease
Renal disease
    Nephrolithiasis
    Pyelonephritis
    Perinephric abscess
Aortic aneurysm
Gastrointestinal disease
    Pancreatitis
    Cholecystitis
    Penetrating ulcer

Percentages indicate the estimated incidence of these conditions among adult patients.
Adapted from: Deyo RO, Weinstein JN. Low back pain. N Engl J Med 2001;344:363–70.

diac arrest. Malignant hyperthermia susceptibility is a consideration.

2. Ketamine is useful for providing surgical anesthesia without depression of ventilation and avoiding muscle relaxants and other potentially triggering drugs for malignant hyperthermia.

C. **Hyperekplexia** ("stiff baby syndrome") is a rare genetic syndrome characterized by intense skeletal muscle rigidity manifesting immediately after birth and gradually disappearing during the first years of life.

D. **Tracheomegaly** is characterized by marked dilation of the trachea and bronchi, which is due to congenital defects of elastic and smooth muscle fibers of the tracheobronchial tree.

E. **Alcoholic myopathy,** manifesting as proximal skeletal muscle weakness, occurs frequently in alcoholic patients (alcoholic neuropathy affects distal skeletal muscles).

F. **Freeman-Sheldon syndrome** ("whistling face syndrome") is a rare congenital entity characterized by microstomia, camptodactyly, and talipes equinovarus.

1. Patients with this syndrome frequently present for surgical correction of musculoskeletal or facial abnormalities.

2. **Management of anesthesia.** Anesthetic challenges include difficult airway management, risk of developing malignant hyperthermia, and postoperative pulmonary complications.

G. **Prader-Willi syndrome** manifests at birth as skeletal muscle hypotonia, which may be associated with weak swallowing and cough reflexes and upper airway obstruction.

1. The syndrome, which progresses during childhood, is characterized by hyperphagia leading to obesity (pickwickian syndrome possible), plus endocrine abnormalities including hypogonadism and diabetes mellitus.

2. **Management of anesthesia.** The principal concerns for management of anesthesia in these patients are skeletal muscle hypotonia and altered metabolism of carbohydrates (hypoglycemia) and fats. Dental caries are common. Disturbances in thermoregulation may resemble malignant hyperthermia.

H. **Prune-belly syndrome** is characterized by congenital agenesis of the lower central abdominal musculature and by the presence of urinary tract anomalies.

I. **Hallermann-Streiff syndrome** is characterized by oculomandibulodyscephaly and dwarfism.

J. **Dutch-Kentucky syndrome** is a rare inherited disorder characterized by decreased ability to open the mouth due to trismus (fiberoptic laryngoscopy).

K. **Williams-Beuren syndrome** is a rare entity characterized by mental retardation, hypercalcemia, kyphoscoliosis, and skeletal muscle hypotonia. Aortic regurgitation is often present.

L. **Arthrogryposis multiplex congenita** is a rare syndrome characterized by joint contractures and multiple organ system congenital abnormalities (aortic stenosis, coarctation of the aorta, cyanotic heart disease, micrognathia).

M. **Smith-Lemli-Opitz syndrome** is characterized by mental, motor, and growth retardation, with death usually due to pulmonary infections or congenital heart defects.

N. **Multiple pterygium syndrome** is a rare disorder that involves webbing of the skin across joints, which may also involve the airway.

O. **Holt-Oram syndrome** (heart-hand syndrome) is characterized by anomalies of the upper limbs (hypoplastic thumbs) and heart (cyanotic congenital heart disease, cardiac rhythm disturbances, sudden death).

P. **Poland syndrome** is a rare anomaly characterized by congenital absence of the pectoralis minor muscle and its nerve supply (lung herniation may occur).

Q. **Mitochondrial myopathies** are a heterogeneous group of disorders of skeletal muscle energy metabolism.

  1. **Kearns-Sayre syndrome** is a rare mitochondrial myopathy accompanied by heart block (dilated cardiomyopathy and congestive heart failure may be present).

  2. **MELAS syndrome** is a multisystem disorder characterized by stroke-like episodes, evidence of mitochondrial dysfunction in the form of lactic acidosis, seizures, and dementia.

R. **Multicore myopathy** is a heterogeneous group of diseases characterized by proximal skeletal muscle weakness and musculoskeletal abnormalities (scoliosis, high arched palate). Cardiomyopathy may accompany this myopathy.

S. **Spasmodic dysphonia** is a laryngeal disorder characterized by adductor or abductor spasms of the vocal cords.

T. **Erythromelalgia** manifests as painful, swollen, erythematous extremities. Intravascular platelet aggregation may be prominent.

U. **McCune-Albright syndrome** consists of a triad of osseous lesions, melanotic cutaneous macules, and sexual precocity. In addition, conductive and neural hearing loss may occur, and endocrine abnormalities (hyperthyroidism) may be present. Tracheal intubation may be difficult because of airway distortion associated with acromegaly or hypertrophy of soft tissue in the upper airway.

V. **Klippel-Feil syndrome** is characterized by shortness of the neck, resulting from reduction in the number of cervical vertebrae or fusion of several vertebrae into an osseous mass. Movement of the neck is limited, and associated skeletal abnormalities include spinal canal stenosis or kyphoscoliosis.

W. **Osteogenesis imperfecta** is a rare inherited disease of connective tissues that affects bones, sclera, and the inner ear. Bones are extremely brittle because of defective collagen production.

1. Impaired platelet function is likely, and increased serum thyroxine concentrations are common.

2. **Management of anesthesia.** See Table 26–26.

≡ Table 26–26 • Management of Anesthesia in Patients with Osteogenesis Imperfecta

---

Tracheal intubation accomplished with minimal manipulation (cervical and mandibular fractures may occur)
Consider awake fiberoptic tracheal intubation
Succinylcholine-induced fasciculations may induce fractures
Kyphoscoliosis and pectus excavatum may interfere with arterial oxygenation
Automated blood pressure cuffs may produce fractures
Regional anesthesia is acceptable (evaluate coagulation status before proceeding; desmopressin may restore platelet function)
Potential for increased body temperature

X. **Fibrodysplasia ossificans** is a rare inherited disease characterized by interstitial myositis and proliferation of connective tissues. Cervical spine involvement is common (fusion, atlantoaxial subluxation), and temporomandibular joint alterations may have implications for tracheal intubation.

Y. **Deformities of the sternum.** Pectus carinatum (outward protuberance) and pectus excavatum (inward concavity) produce psychological problems, but functional consequences are rare. Obstructive sleep apnea may be more common in children with pectus excavatum.

Z. **Macroglossia** is an infrequent but potentially lethal postoperative complication that most often follows posterior fossa craniotomies performed in the head-down or sitting position (presumed to reflect obstruction to venous outflow from prolonged neck flexion or head-down position). When the onset of macroglossia is immediate it is easily recognized, and airway obstruction does not occur as tracheal extubation is delayed. In some patients, however, the onset of macroglossia is delayed (30 minutes or longer) with the risk of complete upper airway obstruction occurring at an unexpected time during the postoperative period.

27

Infectious Diseases

Infectious diseases, although rarely the indication for surgery, may influence the management of anesthesia (disposable equipment, handling of blood and body fluids) (Stoelting RK, Dierdorf SF. Infectious diseases. In: Anesthesia and Co-Existing Disease, 4th ed. New York, Churchill Livingstone, 2002;551–584). Infection is the most common cause of fever. In children it may cause seizures; and in elderly patients or those with cardiopulmonary disease, increases in body temperature can precipitate cardiac dysrhythmias, myocardial ischemia, and congestive heart failure.

I. PROPHYLACTIC ANTIBIOTICS

Prophylactic antibiotics are used for many of the commonly performed surgical procedures. Because of their broad antimicrobial spectrum and low toxicity, cephalosporins are likely choices for preoperative prophylaxis when the most common pathogens are normal skin, gastrointestinal, and genitourinary flora. Timing of antibiotic administration should coincide with bacterial inoculation, emphasizing that prophylactic drugs need not be routinely administered before the induction of anesthesia. Prolongation of antibiotic therapy beyond the first postoperative day probably affords no additional protection.

A. The incidence of allergic reactions to cephalosporins is low, and administration of these antibiotics to patients with histories of allergies to penicillin is controversial.

B. Vancomycin, when utilized as a prophylactic antibiotic, is administered as a continuous intravenous infusion over 15 to 30 minutes to minimize the risk of drug-induced histamine release and associated hypotension.

II. INFECTIONS DUE TO GRAM-POSITIVE BACTERIA

See Table 27–1.

≡ **Table 27–1 • Infections Due to Gram-Positive Bacteria**

Pneumococci
Bacterial pneumonia
Acute otitis media
Penicillin or antibiotic with similar spectrum
Streptococci
Group A
  Acute pharyngitis and tonsillitis (untreated may lead to rheumatic fever)
  Impetigo
  Cellulitis
  Streptococcal toxic shock syndrome (necrotizing fasciitis or myositis and pneumonia; requires extensive soft tissue débridement; disseminated intravascular coagulation and respiratory failure are common; high doses of penicillin plus clindamycin)
Group B
  Neonatal sepsis
Group D
  Urinary tract infections
  Endocarditis
Staphylococci
Staphylococcus aureus
  Asymptomatic carriers
  Paronychia
  Surgical incision
  Contaminated food
  Staphylococcal toxic shock syndrome (associated with tampon use; multiple organ system involvement)
Staphylococcus epidermidis
  Skin contaminants
  Bacteremia (intravenous catheters, prosthetic heart valves)

III. INFECTIONS DUE TO GRAM-NEGATIVE BACTERIA

See Table 27–2.

IV. INFECTIONS DUE TO SPORE-FORMING ANAEROBES

A. **Clostridial myonecrosis** ("gas gangrene") is a life-threatening infection that may be complicated by hypotension and renal failure.

☰ Table 27–2 • Infections Due to Gram-Negative Bacteria

Escherichia coli-induced diarrhea
Salmonellosis
   Contaminated food
   Bacteremia (typhoid fever)
Shigellosis
   Diarrhea
   Dysentery
Cholera (hypotension and metabolic acidosis owing to large fluid
   and electrolyte losses)

    1. **Treatment** consists of appropriate antibiotics and sur-
       gical débridement of infected tissues.
    2. **Management of anesthesia.** See Table 27–3.
  B. **Tetanus** reflects elaboration of a neurotoxin that inhibits
     the release of acetylcholine at the neuromuscular junction
     while suppressing inhibitory internuncial neurons in the
     central nervous system.
    1. **Signs and symptoms.** See Table 27–4.
    2. **Treatment.** See Table 27–5.
    3. **Management of anesthesia** often includes invasive
       monitoring and control of excessive sympathetic ner-
       vous system activity (volatile anesthetics, β-adrenergic
       antagonists, lidocaine, nitroprusside).
  C. **Botulism** is characterized by acute, symmetrical paralysis
     due to elaboration of a neurotoxin that interferes with
     presynaptic release of acetylcholine.

☰ Table 27–3 • Management of Anesthesia in the Presence of Clostridial Myonecrosis

Consider multiple physiologic derangements
   Hypovolemia
   Anemia
   Renal failure
Theoretical concerns about use of nitrous oxide and
   succinylcholine are unsubstantiated
Electrocautery may be avoided (hydrogen gas)
Cross-infection is unlikely

▬ Table 27–4 • Signs and Symptoms of Tetanus

Trismus (especially of masseter muscles)
Laryngospasm
Inadequate ventilation due to spasm of intercostal muscles and
  diaphragm
Hyperthermia
Increased sympathetic nervous system activity (tachycardia,
  systemic hypertension)

V. INFECTIONS DUE TO SPIROCHETES

  A. **Syphilis** in its tertiary stage is characterized by destructive lesions in the nervous system (tabes dorsalis) and cardiovascular system (aortic regurgitation, ascending aortic aneurysm).
  B. **Lyme disease** is characterized by multisystem involvement (cutaneous, fatigue, encephalopathy, neuropathy, heart block, arthritis) that undergoes exacerbations and remissions.

VI. INFECTIONS DUE TO MYCOBACTERIA

  A. **Tuberculosis** is caused by *Myobacterium tuberculosis,* an obligate aerobe surviving in tissues with high oxygen concentrations, as are present at the apices of the lungs.
    1. **Epidemiology.** Most cases of tuberculosis occur in intravenous drug abusers and those with acquired immunodeficiency syndrome (AIDS). The appearance of multidrug resistant strains of *Myobacterium tuberculosis* has been the reason for the resurgence of tuberculosis worldwide.

▬ Table 27–5 • Treatment of Tetanus

Control of skeletal muscle spasms (diazepam, nondepolarizing
  muscle relaxants)
Prevention of sympathetic nervous system hyperactivity (β-
  adrenergic antagonists)
Support of ventilation of the lungs
Neutralization of circulating exotoxins (penicillin)
Surgical débridement

---

2. **Transmission.** Almost all infections with *Myobacterium tuberculosis* result from aerosol (droplet) inhalation.

3. **Diagnosis** of tuberculosis is based on the presence of clinical symptoms, the epidemiologic likelihood of infections, and the results of diagnostic tests (chest radiographs, sputum smears).

4. **Risk to health care workers.** Health care workers are at increased risk for occupational acquisition of tuberculosis.

   a. **Implications for anesthesiologists.** Anesthesiologists are at increased risk for nosocomial tuberculosis by virtue of events surrounding induction and maintenance of anesthesia that may induce coughing. Bronchoscopy is a high risk procedure associated with the conversion of tuberculin skin tests in anesthesiologists.

   b. Anesthesia personnel should participate in annual tuberculin screening such that any conversion can be promptly treated with chemotherapy.

5. **Treatment** of tuberculosis is with isoniazid (toxic to the peripheral nervous system, liver, kidneys), streptomycin, and rifampin.

6. **Management of anesthesia.** See Table 27–6.

B. **Leprosy** is a highly infectious chronic granulomatous infection caused by *Myobacterium leprae* affecting princi-

---

Table 27–6 • Management of Anesthesia in Patients with Tuberculosis

Universal precautions (AIDS, hepatitis B)

Delay elective surgical procedures until no longer considered infectious (antituberculous chemotherapy, improving clinically, three consecutive negative sputum smears)

Perform tracheal intubation in a negative pressure environment if possible

Place a high efficiency particulate air filter between the Y-connector and mask or tracheal tube

Place bacterial filters on the exhalation limb of the anesthesia delivery circuit

Use a dedicated mechanical ventilator

Postoperative care in an isolation room

AIDS, acquired immunodeficiency syndrome.

pally the skin, mucosa of the upper respiratory tract (nose, uvula, larynx), peripheral nerves (motor paralysis and sensory loss), and cardiovascular system.

VII. SYSTEMIC MYCOTIC INFECTIONS

Systemic mycotic infections (blastomycosis, coccidioidomycosis, histoplasmosis) are fungal infections characterized by pulmonary cavitary lesions that resemble tuberculosis. Amphotericin B administered intravenously is the recommended treatment (renal and hematologic toxicity).

VIII. INFECTIONS DUE TO *MYCOPLASMA*

Infections due to *Mycoplasma* manifest as a nonproductive cough and pharyngitis (primary atypical pneumonia). Treatment is with erythromycin or tetracyclines.

IX. INFECTIONS DUE TO RICKETTSIAL ORGANISMS

Infections due to rickettsial organisms manifest as Rocky Mountain spotted fever (rash, thrombocytopenia, abdominal pain, nonspecific ST changes on the electrocardiogram) or Q fever (hepatosplenomegaly).

X. VIRAL INFECTIONS OF THE UPPER RESPIRATORY TRACT

See Table 27–7.

A. **Management of anesthesia.** Despite some disagreement in the literature, it appears prudent to avoid anesthesia that requires tracheal intubation in patients with or recovering from viral upper respiratory tract infections. Evidence of an increased incidence of complications when anesthesia is administered to at-risk patients includes an increased incidence of intraoperative bronchospasm and laryngospasm in asymptomatic patients with a recent history of viral upper respiratory tract infections.

1. The greatest risk of airway complications when anesthesia is administered in the presence of a viral upper respiratory tract infection seems to be in children < 1 year of age, whereas the risk is much less in children > 5 years of age, presumably because of the presence of anatomically larger airways.
2. When anesthesia cannot be delayed in patients with viral upper respiratory tract infections, it is helpful to

≡ Table 27–7 • Viral Infections of the Upper Respiratory Tract

Influenza Virus
Spread is via nasopharyngeal secretions of infected patients
Self-limited unless complicated by bacterial infection or co-existing chronic pulmonary disease
Prophylaxis provided by polyvalent vaccine
Antiviral drugs (amantadine, rimantadine) specifically inhibit influenza A virus
Rhinovirus
Acute coryza (common cold)
Spread by contact with contaminated environmental surfaces or from skin of infected individuals
Adenovirus
Pharyngitis
Conjunctivitis
Respiratory Syncytial Virus
Infant pneumonia and bronchiolitis
Spread by contaminated secretions on hands and clothes
Ribavirin may be effective
Parainfluenza Virus
Laryngotracheobronchitis
Transmission by person-to-person contact or droplets

consider potential problems (airway hyperreactivity, arterial hypoxemia, postoperative laryngeal edema). Increased airway responsiveness suggests the need to establish suppressant concentrations of volatile anesthetics before tracheal intubation and during surgery.

B. **Human papilloma virus** is responsible for recurrent respiratory papillomatosis. Papillomas are typically located near the vocal cords. Laser ablation is the accepted treatment.

XI. INFECTIONS DUE TO HERPES VIRUS

See Table 27–8.

XII. ACQUIRED IMMUNODEFICIENCY SYNDROME

AIDS describes the occurrence of life-threatening opportunistic infections and/or Kaposi's sarcoma in patients who manifest profound immunosuppression unrelated to drug therapy or known co-existing diseases. The syndrome is initi-

≡ Table 27–8 • Infections Due to Herpes Viruses

Herpes Simplex Virus Type 1
Keratitis
Whitlow
Spread by oral secretions
Acyclovir is treatment
Herpes Simplex Virus Type 2
Genital transmission
Varicella-Zoster Virus
Herpes zoster follows endogenous reactivation
Incidence increased in immunosuppressed patients (forerunner of impending AIDS)
Cytomegalovirus
Heterophile-negative mononucleosis
Transmission by contact with infected secretions in leukocyte-containing blood products
Epstein-Barr Virus
Heterophile-positive (infectious) mononucleosis
Cancer (nasopharyngeal, Burkitt's lymphoma, Hodgkin's disease, lymphoproliferative disease, AIDS)

ated by a human T lymphotropic retrovirus [human immunodeficiency virus (HIV) type 1]. As the virus replicates, T lymphocytes are damaged or destroyed, leading to cell-mediated immunodeficiency and leaving the host unable to cope with a variety of infectious diseases and cancers. Despite the immunosuppression, the infected host is able to mount an immune response to the virus after infection. These antibodies form the basis for most of the diagnostic tests for AIDS but offer little protection against development of the disease.

A. **Transmission** of HIV-1 is by intimate sexual contact or blood-borne contamination (risk very low). Administration of zidovudine (AZT) during the perinatal period greatly decreases maternal transmission of HIV-1 to the newborn.

B. **Natural history.** AIDS is the last stage of a disease process that has an average course of 10 years. Death is usually the result of malnutrition, opportunistic infections, or cancer.

C. **Diagnosis** of AIDS is made when the CD4$^+$ T cell count is < 200 cells/mm^3 or when patients experience the first AIDS-defining opportunistic infections (*Pneumocystis car-*

inii pneumonia most common, cryptococcosis, cytomegalovirus infections, myobacterium infections) or cancer (Kaposi's sarcoma, B cell lymphoma).

1. **Serologic tests** are highly sensitive and specific for HIV-1.
2. Serologic testing is repeated at 6, 12, and 24 weeks after an initial potential exposure to allow sufficient time for possible seroconversion.

D. **Treatment.** See Table 27–9.

E. **Prevention of nosocomial transmission of HIV-1**

1. It is important for health care workers to implement universal blood and body fluid precautions when contact with blood and body fluids is unavoidable (Table 27–10).
2. The risk of acquiring HIV-1 is stratified on the basis of the injury. For all significant exposures, prompt chemoprophylaxis is administered consisting of at least two drugs to which the virus is unlikely to be resistant (Table 27–11).

≡ **Table 27–9** • Treatment of Human Immunodeficiency Virus Infection

---

Antiretroviral Chemotherapy (combination drug therapy)
Nucleoside analogue reverse transcriptase inhibitors
    AZT (suppression of myelopoiesis and erythropoiesis)
    Didanosine (pancreatitis and peripheral neuropathy)
    Zalcitabine (peripheral neuropathy)
    Stavudine (peripheral neuropathy)
    Lamivudine (suppression of myelopoiesis and erythropoiesis)
Protease inhibitor
    Saquinavir
    Ritonavir (gastrointestinal toxicity)
    Indinavir (hyperbilirubinemia, nephrolithiasis)
    Nelfinavir (diarrhea)
Prophylaxis Against Opportunistic Infections
Pneumococcal vaccine
Hepatitis B vaccine
Influenza vaccine
Isoniazid (if positive tuberculin skin tests)
Trimethoprim-sulfamethoxazole

Table 27–10 • Universal Precautions to Prevent Transmission of Human Immunodeficiency Virus

---

Blood and body fluid precautions should be used in all patients, recognizing that it is not possible to identify infected patients reliably

Use barrier precautions to prevent skin and mucous membrane exposure to blood or body fluids that may contain blood

Wear gloves

Wear protective eye shields if droplets likely

Take care to prevent injury when handling sharp devices (do not recap needles)

Health care workers with exudative skin lesions should refrain from direct patient care

Use equipment for cardiopulmonary resuscitation that obviates the need for mouth-to-mouth resuscitation

---

Adapted from: Recommendations for prevention of HIV transmission in health-care setting. MMWR Morb Mortal Wkly Rep 1987;36:629–33.

F. **Management of anesthesia** assumes that all patients are potentially HIV-positive or infected with other blood-borne pathogens (Table 27–10). Lack of evidence of spread of HIV-1 by airborne routes does not eliminate the concern regarding anesthesia equipment, as airway secretions can be mixed with blood (use disposable equipment when possible; for nondisposable items wash with detergent and gas- or steam-sterilize).

1. **Choice of anesthetic drugs and techniques** is influenced by accompanying systemic manifestations of AIDS and any associated opportunistic infections (pneumonia due to *Pneumocystis carinii*, poor nutrition, hypovolemia). Upper airway obstruction and difficulty placing a tracheal tube may accompany supraglottic Kaposi's sarcoma.

2. Postoperatively, these patients are managed in the postanesthesia care unit according to criteria reserved for management of patients with communicable diseases.

XIII. MYOCARDITIS

Myocarditis is a major cause of sudden death in adults < 40 years of age.

Table 27–11 • Antiretroviral Chemoprophylaxis of Percutaneous Exposures to HIV-1-Infected Materials

Type of Exposure	Source Material	Antiretroviral Prophylaxis	Antiretroviral Regimen
Percutaneous	Blood		
	Highest risk	Recommended	AZT plus lamivudine plus indinavir
	Increased risk	Recommended	AZT plus lamivudine with or without indinavir
	No increased risk	Offer	AZT plus lamivudine
	Fluid containing visible blood or other potentially infectious fluid (semen, vaginal secretions, CSF, amniotic fluid) or tissue	Offer	AZT plus lamivudine
	Other body fluids (urine)	Do not offer	
Mucous membranes	Blood	Offer	AZT plus lamivudine with or without indinavir
	Fluid containing visible blood or other potentially infectious fluid (semen, vaginal secretions, CSF, amniotic fluid) or tissue	Offer	AZT with or without lamivudine
	Other body fluids (urine)	Do not offer	

Table continued on following page

Table 27–11 • Antiretroviral Chemoprophylaxis of Percutaneous Exposures to HIV-1-Infected Materials *Continued*

Type of Exposure	Source Material	Antiretroviral Prophylaxis	Antiretroviral Regimen
Skin (increased risk)*	Blood	Offer	AZT plus lamivudine with or without indinavir
	Fluid containing visible blood or other potentially infectious fluid (semen, vaginal secretions, CSF, amniotic fluid) or tissue	Offer	AZT with or without lamivudine
	Other body fluids (urine)	Do not offer	

AZT, zidovudine; CSF, cerebrospinal fluid; HIV-1, human immunodeficiency virus type 1.
* Risk is considered to be increased with exposure to high titers of HIV-1, prolonged skin contact, an extensive area of skin contact, or an area in which skin integrity is visibly compromised. For skin exposures without increased risk, the risk of drug toxicity exceeds the possible benefits.
Adapted from: Schooley RT. Acquired immunodeficiency syndrome. Sci Am Med 1998;1–14.

A. **Causes.** The cause of myocarditis often remains unknown, but a large variety of infections (viral), systemic diseases, drugs (doxorubicin, cocaine), and toxins have been implicated.

B. **Diagnosis.** Endomyocardial biopsy remains the best method for the definitive diagnosis of myocarditis.

XIV. NOSOCOMIAL INFECTIONS

Nosocomial infections are those that occur during the course of a hospital stay (pneumonia, surgical wound infection).

A. **Anesthesia equipment** as a source of cross-contamination between patients is cited as a reason to use disposable anesthetic equipment (validity of this recommendation is unproven).

B. **Gram-negative bacteremia** often reflects a nosocomial infection.

C. **Regional anesthesia and bacteremia.** Performance of epidural or spinal anesthesia in patients with evidence of a systemic infection is an acceptable consideration, provided appropriate antibiotic therapy has been initiated and the patient has shown a positive response to therapy, as evidenced by decreased fever.

XV. SEPSIS AND SEPTIC SHOCK

Sepsis is an infection-induced syndrome defined as the presence of two or more manifestations of a systemic inflammatory response (systemic inflammatory response syndrome) (Table 27–12).

A. **Pathogenesis.** The host response is probably as important as the site of infection or the types of microorganisms in sepsis. Normally, an immunologic cascade ensures a prompt protective response to microbial invasion in

---

≡ Table 27–12 • Identification of Systemic Inflammatory Response Syndrome

Body temperature $> 38°C$ or $< 36°C$
Heart rate > 90 beats/min
Respiratory rate > 32 breaths/min or $PaCO_2 < 32$ mmHg
Leukocytosis or leukopenia

humans. An impaired immunologic response may permit infections to become established, whereas a poorly regulated immunologic response may harm patients by release of endogenously generated inflammatory substances.

1. **Site of infection.** The lungs are the most common sites of infection followed by the abdomen and urinary tract.

2. Positive blood cultures are the accepted proof of infection, but blood cultures are positive in only approximately 30% of patients. Patients with negative blood cultures but presumed to be infected and patients with serious inflammatory conditions not caused by infections (pancreatitis) have clinical signs and symptoms as well as physiologic changes similar to those with documented infections.

3. In patients with confirmed infections, no single pathogen predominates, suggesting that the host response is more important for the outcome of sepsis.

B. **Organ system failure.** Effective treatment of organ system failure is critically important, as the cumulative burden of organ system failure is responsible for the mortality associated with sepsis (average risk of death increases by 15% to 20% for each additional organ system that fails).

1. **Pulmonary dysfunction.** Sepsis places extreme demands on the lungs, and nearly 85% of patients require mechanical support of ventilation.

2. **Cardiovascular dysfunction.** Shock is considered present when the systolic blood pressure is < 90 mmHg and is unresponsive to intravenous fluids or requires support with vasoactive drugs. Septic shock is initially characterized by low cardiac filling pressures (pulmonary capillary wedge pressure < 8 mmHg), low cardiac output, and normal to increased systemic vascular resistance, especially before intravascular fluid volume repletion. A high cardiac output and decreased systemic vascular resistance typically follow intravascular fluid volume repletion.

   a. **Persistent systemic hypotension.** Systemic hypotension that persists after intravascular fluid volume repletion is often the result of low systemic vascular resistance, occasionally combined with impaired myocardial contractility (myocardial depressant factors) and low cardiac output.

    b. Lactic acidosis may reflect global tissue ischemia due to inadequate oxygen delivery or regional (organ-specific) ischemia. It is common practice to treat systemic acidosis (pH < 7.2) with intravenous administration of sodium bicarbonate (correction of the derangement causing anaerobic metabolism is more beneficial).

3. **Central nervous system dysfunction** (septic encephalitis) is often an early symptom of sepsis, particularly in elderly patients.

4. **Renal dysfunction.** Transient oliguria is common and temporally related to hypotension (correction of intravascular fluid volume deficits usually reverses oliguria).

5. **Gastrointestinal dysfunction.** The liver is a mechanical and immunologic filter for portal vein blood and may be a major source of cytokines that cause lung injury. Septic shock usually causes ileus.

6. **Coagulation dysfunction.** Prolongation of the prothrombin time (vitamin K deficiency due to poor dietary intake, liver dysfunction, impaired absorption, antibiotic-induced inhibition of gastrointestinal flora), thrombocytopenia, and disseminated intravascular coagulation may accompany sepsis.

C. **Treatment** of patients with sepsis, especially those manifesting evidence of septic shock includes identification and eradication of the infection utilizing appropriate antibiotics and/or surgical drainage, plus supportive therapy (fluid replacement, nutrition) (Table 27–13).

D. **Management of anesthesia** for patients with sepsis is influenced by the status of the intravascular fluid volume (heart rate, urine output, mentation) and cardiovascular function (Table 27–14).

XVI. INFECTIVE ENDOCARDITIS

Infective endocarditis is a microbial infection (most often streptococcal) that implants on heart valves or on the walls of the endocardium.

A. **Predisposing factors.** See Table 27–15.

B. **Antibiotic prophylaxis** is recommended in susceptible patients when surgical procedures associated with bac-

Table 27–13 • Guidelines for Treatment of Patients with Septic Shock

Abnormality	Intervention	Therapeutic Goals
Infection	Antibiotics	Eradication of infection
	Surgical drainage	
Cardiovascular dysfunction		
Hypotension	Intravascular volume repletion	Mean arterial pressure at least 60 mmHg
	Vasopressors	Pulmonary capillary wedge pressure at least 14–18 mmHg
Tissue hypoperfusion	Intravascular volume repletion	Hemoglobin at least 10 g/dl
	Vasopressors	Oxygen saturation > 88%
	Inotropes	Cardiac index > 4 L/min/m²
		Normalize blood lactate concentrations
Pulmonary dysfunction	Mechanical ventilation	Oxygen saturation > 88%
	Supplemental oxygen	Minimize alveolar-arterial oxygen gradient
Renal dysfunction	Intravascular volume repletion	Normalize serum creatinine concentrations
	Vasopressors	Adequate urine output
	Inotropes	
Liver dysfunction	Intravascular volume repletion	Normalize serum aminotransferase concentrations
	Vasopressors	

Adapted from: Parrillo JE. Pathogenic mechanisms of septic shock. N Engl J Med 1993;328:1471–7.

☰ Table 27–14 • Management of Anesthesia in Patients with Sepsis

Aspiration risk due to possible presence of ileus

Preoperative arterial blood gases (likely need for postoperative ventilation)

Hypoglycemia a risk if total parenteral nutrition infusions are interrupted

Intra-arterial monitoring of systemic blood pressure

Consider placing a central venous or pulmonary artery catheter (alternatively transesophageal echocardiography) for assessing intravascular fluid volume status and myocardial contractility

Avoid sudden decreases in systemic vascular resistance (ketamine)

Ready availability of blood products, inotropes, and vasopressors

Continue monitoring and anticipate the need for mechanical support of ventilation during the postoperative period

---

teremia are planned (Table 27–16). Prophylactic antibiotic therapy must be initiated before surgery, as the drug needs to be present in tissues, as well as in the blood, to provide protection. Furthermore, antibiotic therapy must be continued for 48 to 72 hours after surgery. The specific antibiotic regimen selected should consider the type of bacteria likely to enter the systemic circulation during the operative procedure (Table 27–17).

C. **Signs and symptoms.** Infective endocarditis is considered in patients with heart murmurs, anemia, and fever, particularly if there is a history of co-existing cardiac disease or recent surgical procedure. Evidence of systemic embolization may be present. Congestive heart failure is the most frequent cardiac complication.

XVII. CENTRAL NERVOUS SYSTEM INFECTIONS

Central nervous system infections are often confirmed by computed tomography or magnetic resonance imaging and examination of the cerebrospinal fluid (Table 27–18).

XVIII. BACTERIAL INFECTIONS OF THE UPPER RESPIRATORY TRACT

See Table 27–19.

Table 27–15 • Estimated Risk of Infective Endocarditis Associated with Co-Existing Cardiac Disorders

High Risk
Prosthetic heart valves
Previous infective endocarditis
Cyanotic congenital heart disease
Patent ductus arteriosus
Aortic regurgitation
Aortic stenosis
Mitral regurgitation
Mitral stenosis and regurgitation
Ventricular septal defect
Coarctation of the aorta
Surgically repaired intracardiac lesions with residual hemodynamic abnormalities

Intermediate Risk
Mitral valve prolapse with regurgitation
Pure mitral stenosis
Tricuspid valve disease
Pulmonary stenosis
Asymmetrical septal hypertrophy
Bicuspid aortic valve or calcific aortic stenosis with minimal hemodynamic abnormality
Degenerative valvular disease in elderly patients
Surgically repaired intracardiac lesions with minimal to no hemodynamic abnormality < 6 months after operation

Low Risk
Mitral valve prolapse without regurgitation
Trivial valvular regurgitation on echocardiography without structural abnormality
Isolated atrial septal defect
Arteriosclerotic plaques
Coronary artery disease
Cardiac pacemaker
Surgically repaired intracardiac lesions with minimal to no hemodynamic abnormality > 6 months after operation

Adapted from: Durack DT. Prevention of infective endocarditis. N Engl J Med 1995;332:38–44.

≡ Table 27–16 • Recommendations for Prophylaxis During Various Surgical Procedures that May Cause Bacteremia

Prophylaxis Recommended
Dental operations associated with gingival or mucosal bleeding (includes professional cleaning)
Tonsillectomy or adenoidectomy
Surgery involving the gastrointestinal or respiratory mucosa
Bronchoscopy with a rigid bronchoscope
Sclerotherapy for esophageal varices
Esophageal dilation
Gallbladder surgery
Cystoscopy and urethral dilation
Urethral catheterization if urinary infection present
Urinary tract surgery (prostatic surgery)
Incision and drainage of infected tissues
Vaginal hysterectomy
Vaginal delivery complicated by infection
Prophylaxis Not Recommended
Dental procedures not likely to cause bleeding (adjustment of orthodontic appliances, fillings above the gum line)
Intraoral injection of local anesthetic
Shedding of primary teeth
Tympanoplasty-tube insertion
Tracheal intubation
Bronchoscopy with flexible fiberoptic bronchoscope (with or without biopsy)
Cardiac catheterization
Gastrointestinal endoscopy (with or without biopsy)
Cesarean section
Procedures performed in the absence of infection (urethral catheterization, dilation and curettage, uncomplicated vaginal delivery, therapeutic abortion, insertion or removal of intrauterine devices, sterilization procedures, laparoscopy)

Adapted from: Durack DT. Prevention of infective endocarditis. N Engl J Med 1995;332:38–44.

Table 27-17 • Infective Endocarditis Prophylaxis Based on Likely Invading Organism

Procedure	Organism	Antibiotic Selection		
		Routine	Allergic to Penicillin	Prosthetic Heart Valve
Dental treatment Tonsillectomy Adenoidectomy Nasotracheal intubation Bronchoscopy	α-Hemolytic streptococcus	Penicillin Amoxicillin	Vancomycin or erythromycin	Penicillin plus streptomycin
Hepatobiliary tract	Enterococcus	Penicillin or ampicillin plus gentamicin or streptomycin	Vancomycin	As for routine
Cardiac surgery	Staphylococcus	Penicillinase-resistant penicillins or cephalosporins	As for routine	As for routine

≡ Table 27–18 • Central Nervous System Infections

Meningitis
Fever, headache, vomiting, nuchal rigidity, and obtundation
Seizures if increased intracranial pressure
Coagulopathies
Haemophilus influenzae most common pathogen
Antibiotics with bactericidal effects in cerebrospinal fluid
Brain Abscess
Extension of contiguous infections (paranasal sinuses)
Retrograde venous spread (otitis media)
Hematogenous spread (lung, right-to-left intracardiac shunts)
Obtundation, headache, focal neurologic signs, and seizures
  (increased intracranial pressure)
Antibiotics and/or surgical decompression
Epidural Abscess
Severe backache, local tenderness, paraspinal muscle spasm and
  fever 24–72 hours following performance of block
Flaccid motor paralysis but sensation intact
Magnetic resonance imaging is diagnostic
Laminectomy to minimize likelihood of permanent neurologic
  deficits

XIX. PULMONARY PARENCHYMAL INFECTIONS

Pulmonary parenchymal infections typically develop after an event that impairs normal host defense mechanisms, such as viral infections that alter the physical and chemical characteristics of the normally protective mucous secretions in the airway.

A. **Bacterial pneumonia** is most often caused by inhalation of oropharyngeal secretions containing pneumococci (alcoholism, drug abuse, neurologic disorders).

1. **Diagnosis and treatment.** Bacterial pneumonia is characterized by an initial chill followed by abrupt onset of fever and copious sputum production. Classic radiographic findings may be absent. Polymorphonuclear leukocytosis is typical, and arterial hypoxemia may occur.

2. **Acute bronchitis versus pneumonia.** The distinction is anatomic, as the same organisms cause both diseases.

3. **Legionnaires' disease** is caused by a gram-negative bacillus. Treatment is with erythromycin.

≡ Table 27–19 • Bacterial Infections of the Upper Respiratory Tract

Acute Sinusitis

Common consequence of upper respiratory tract infections

Nasal discharge, fever, leukocytosis, facial pain (increases when lean forward)

Consider when fever develops in presence of a nasotracheal tube

Treat with decongestants and analgesics

Nitrous oxide a theoretical concern

Chronic Sinusitis

Affects an estimated 14% of the population

Invariable feature of cystic fibrosis

Acute Otitis Media

Pain, fever, and hearing loss

Bulging tympanic membrane

Treat with decongestants, analgesics, and antibiotics

Nitrous oxide may increase middle ear pressures if decompression through the eustachian tubes is not possible

Pharyngitis

Viruses are the most common causes (group A streptococcus more likely to cause tonsillitis)

Throat cultures necessary to distinguish between viral and streptococcal pharyngitis

Penicillin or erythromycin for prevention of rheumatic fever

Peritonsillar Abscess

Complication of streptococcal tonsillitis

Dysphagia, muffled voice, and trismus

Antibiotics and needle aspiration

Retropharyngeal Infections

Fever, dysphagia, respiratory stridor, and bulging of the posterior wall of the pharynx

Lateral radiographs of the neck

Penicillin

Fiberoptic laryngoscopy

Ludwig's Angina

Cellulitis of the submandibular, sublingual, and submental regions

Fever and rapidly progressive edema of the anterior neck and floor of the mouth

Upper airway obstruction possible

Tracheostomy

Antibiotics and surgical decompression

Acute Epiglottitis (Supraglottitis)

Young adults with diseases associated with immunosuppression

Prophylactic tracheal intubation probably not necessary if observation facilities and personnel skilled in airway management are available

4. **Aspiration pneumonia.** Aspiration is probably responsible for most bacterial (mixed flora) pneumonias. Risk factors include depressed consciousness (alcohol abuse, drug abuse, trauma, seizures, neurologic disorders), administration of sedatives, abnormalities of deglutition (presence of nasogastric tubes, bowel obstruction), and induction and recovery from anesthesia.

   a. **Signs and symptoms.** Clinical manifestations (airway obstruction, atelectasis, arterial hypoxemia) of pulmonary aspiration depend in large part on the nature (solids, acidic fluids) and volume of aspirated material.

   b. **Treatment.** Penicillin-sensitive anaerobes are the most likely cause of aspiration pneumonia.

5. **Bacterial versus viral etiology.** Nonbacterial pneumonia (*Mycoplasma pneumoniae*) occurs in previously healthy, young patients. It is characterized by nonproductive cough and absence of leukocytosis. Interstitial infiltrates on the chest radiograph suggest a nonbacterial etiology.

B. **Lung abscess** is most likely to develop after pneumonia (alcohol abuse, poor dental hygiene, septic embolization in drug abusers). Chest radiography is needed to establish the presence of a lung abscess.

XX. INTRA-ABDOMINAL INFECTIONS

Intra-abdominal infections may manifest as *peritonitis* or *subphrenic abscess* (unexplained fever in patients who have recently undergone intra-abdominal surgery).

XXI. URINARY TRACT INFECTIONS

Urinary tract infections are the most common of all bacterial infections affecting humans. They typically manifest as dysuria and frequency.

XXII. OSTEOMYELITIS

Osteomyelitis is a difficult to treat infection characterized by progressive inflammatory destruction of bone.

A. **Antibiotic prophylaxis during bone surgery.** In patients undergoing bone surgery, antibiotics should be administered intravenously 30 minutes before incision of the skin and for no longer than 24 hours after surgery.

B. Patients receiving prosthetic orthopedic devices have a high susceptibility to infection when only a few microorganisms of low pathogenicity, such as *Staphylococcus epidermidis* are present.

XXIII. FEVER OF UNDETERMINED ORIGIN

Fever of undetermined origin (> 38.3°C on several occasions during a 21-day period) is usually due to infection, cancer, or a connective tissue disorder. Ultrasonography and computed tomography are useful for detecting hidden sites of infection.

XXIV. INFECTIONS IN IMMUNOSUPPRESSED HOSTS

Infections in immunosuppressed hosts may be the principal cause of morbidity, rather than the primary illness. Neutropenia is the most important factor predisposing to bacterial infections in the presence of cancer or after organ transplantation.

A. **Pneumonia** is the most common infectious cause of death in immunosuppressed hosts.

1. *Pneumocystis carinii* **pneumonia** is a common opportunistic cause of interstitial pneumonia in immunosuppressed hosts, especially those with AIDS.

2. This pneumonia typically manifests as a sudden onset of fever, nonproductive cough, tachypnea, and progressive dyspnea. The degree of arterial hypoxemia and extent of infiltrate on chest radiographs (diffuse, bilateral symmetrical interstitial and alveolar infiltrative patterns that are predominantly perihilar) correlates best with the breathing rate.

B. High inspired concentrations of oxygen with or without positive end-expiratory pressure may be needed during anesthesia.

28

Cancer

Cancer is the second most frequent cause of death in the United States, exceeded only by heart disease (Stoelting RK, Dierdorf SF. Cancer. In: Anesthesia and Co-Existing Disease, 4th ed. New York, Churchill Livingstone, 2002;585–610).

I. MECHANISM

Cancer results from an accumulation of mutations in genes (oncogenes) that regulate cellular proliferation. Stimulation of oncogene formation by carcinogens (tobacco, alcohol, sunlight) is estimated to be responsible for 80% of cancers in the United States. In support of a protective role of the immune system is the increased incidence of cancer in immunosuppressed patients, such as those with acquired immunodeficiency syndrome (AIDS) and those receiving organ transplants.

II. DIAGNOSIS

See Table 28–1.

III. TREATMENT

See Table 28–2.

IV. IMMUNOLOGY OF CANCER CELLS

Tumor cells are antigenically different from normal cells and may therefore elicit immune reactions similar to those that cause rejection of histoincompatible allografts. Antigens that are present in cancer cells but not in normal cells are designated tumor-specific antigens. Antigens that are present in cancer cells and in normal cells (concentrations higher in tumor cells) are designated tumor-associated antigens. Antibodies to tumor-associated antigens can be used for the immunodiagnosis of cancer. Most spontaneously occurring tumors appear to be weakly antigenic.

≡ Table 28–1 • Diagnosis of Cancer

Interference with organ function due to tumor bulk
Aspiration cytology
Biopsy (needle, incisional, excisional)
Monoclonal antibodies (recognize antigens for specific cancers, such as prostate, lungs, breasts, ovaries)
Imaging techniques (computed tomography, magnetic resonance imaging)

V. PARANEOPLASTIC SYNDROMES

Paraneoplastic syndromes manifest as pathophysiologic disturbances that may accompany cancer (Table 28–3).

A. **Neuromuscular abnormalities** manifesting as skeletal muscle weakness (myasthenic syndrome) may be associated with prolonged responses to muscle relaxants.

B. **Ectopic hormone production** by tumors results in predictable physiologic effects (Table 28–4).

C. **Hypercalcemia** in hospitalized patients is most often due to cancer, reflecting local osteolytic activity from bone metastases (especially breast cancer) or ectopic hormonal activity associated with tumors that arise from the kidneys, lungs, pancreas, or ovaries. The rapid onset of hypercalce-

---

≡ Table 28–2 • Treatment of Cancer

Chemotherapy (side effects may influence management of anesthesia; see Table 28–8)
Irradiation
Surgery (removal of the entire tumor or to decrease tumor mass)
Angiogenesis inhibitors
Acute and chronic pain management
  Nonsteroidal antiinflammatory drugs (mild to moderate pain)
  Opioids (severe pain; consider alternative routes of administration including transdermal, transmucosal, intravenous, neuraxial)
  Tricyclic antidepressant drugs
  Anticonvulsant drugs (chronic neuropathic pain)
  Corticosteroids (lower pain perception, improve mood and appetite)
  Neurolytic procedures (celiac plexus block for pancreatic cancer, cordotomy, dorsal rhizotomy, dorsal column stimulators)

≡ Table 28–3 • Pathophysiologic Manifestations of Paraneoplastic Syndromes

Manifestation	Syndrome
Fever	Tumor lysis syndrome
Anorexia	Adrenal insufficiency
Weight loss	Nephrotic syndrome
Anemia	Ureteral obstruction
Thrombocytopenia	Pulmonary osteoarthropathy
Coagulopathies	Pericardial effusion
Neuromuscular abnormalities	Pericardial tamponade
Ectopic hormone production	Superior vena cava obstruction
Hypercalcemia	Spinal cord compression
Hyperuricemia	Brain metastasis

≡ Table 28–4 • Ectopic Hormone Production

Hormone	Associated Cancer	Manifestations
Corticotropin	Lung (small cell) Thyroid (medullary) Thymoma Carcinoid Non-beta islet cell of pancreas	Cushing syndrome
Antidiuretic hormone	Lung (small cell) Pancreas Lymphomas	Water intoxication
Gonadotropin	Lung (large cell) Ovary Adrenal	Gynecomastia Precocious puberty
Melanocyte-stimulating hormone	Lung (small cell)	Hyperpigmentation
Parathyroid hormone	Renal Lung (squamous) Pancreas Ovary	Hyperthyroidism
Thyrotropin	Choriocarcinoma Testicular (embryonal)	Hyperthyroidism
Thyrocalcitonin	Thyroid (medullary)	Hypocalcemia
Insulin	Retroperitoneal tumors	Hypoglycemia

Table 28–5 • Signs and Symptoms
of Bleomycin-Induced
Interstitial Pneumonitis

Nonproductive cough
Dyspnea
Tachypnea
Fever
Altered diffusion capacity for carbon monoxide
Increased alveolar-to-arterial difference for oxygen
Radiographic evidence of diffuse pulmonary infiltrates

---

mia that occurs in patients with cancer may manifest as
lethargy, coma, and polyuria.
  D. Acute respiratory complications. The acute onset of dyspnea may reflect extension of the tumor or the effects of
  chemotherapy. Bleomycin-induced interstitial pneumonitis and fibrosis is the most commonly encountered pulmonary complication of chemotherapy (Table 28–5).
  E. Acute cardiac complications. See Table 28–6.
  F. Superior vena cava obstruction. See Table 28–7. Treatment
  consists of prompt irradiation or chemotherapy to reduce
  the size of the tumor, thereby relieving venous and airway
  obstruction. Bronchoscopy and mediastinoscopy to obtain
  a tissue diagnosis can be hazardous, especially in the presence of co-existing airway obstruction and increased pressure in the mediastinal veins.
  G. Spinal cord compression. Pain, skeletal muscle weakness,
  sensory loss, and autonomic nervous system dysfunction

Table 28–6 • Cardiac Complications Related
to Cancer

Pericardial effusions (most common cause of electrical alternans)
Cardiac tamponade (most likely in association with pericardial
  effusion due to carcinoma of the lung)
Atrial fibrillation
Cardiomyopathy (patients treated with doxorubicin or
  daunorubicin)
  Refractory congestive heart failure
  Cardiomegaly

Table 28–7 • Signs and Symptoms of the Superior Vena Cava Syndrome

Venous engorgement (especially jugular veins and leg veins)
Dyspnea
Airway obstruction
Hoarseness (edema of vocal cords)
Increased intracranial pressure

reflect the presence of metastatic lesions in the epidural space. Once total paralysis has developed, results of surgical laminectomy or irradiation to decompress the spinal cord are equally poor.

VI. MANAGEMENT OF ANESTHESIA

A. **Side effects of chemotherapy.** Preoperative evaluation of patients with cancer includes consideration of possible pathophysiologic side effects of the disease and recognition of the potential adverse side effects that may be associated with cancer chemotherapeutic drugs (Table 28–8). Preoperative clinical tests to detect side effects related to treatment with chemotherapeutic drugs may be useful (Table 28–9).

1. **Pulmonary and cardiac toxicity.** The preoperative history of drug-induced pulmonary fibrosis (dyspnea, nonproductive cough) or congestive heart failure may influence the subsequent conduct of anesthesia. Bleomycin-treated patients may be vulnerable to interstitial pulmonary edema, presumably due to impaired lymphatic drainage owing to drug-induced pulmonary fibrosis (titrate intravascular fluid replacement). Depressant effects of anesthetic drugs on myocardial contractility may be enhanced in patients with drug-induced cardiac toxicity.

2. **Neurotoxicity.** See Table 28–10.

B. **Preoperative preparation.** Preoperatively, correction of nutrient deficiencies, anemia, coagulopathy, and electrolyte abnormalities may be needed. The presence of hepatic or renal dysfunction may influence the choice of anesthetic drugs and muscle relaxants. Attention to aseptic techniques is important, as immunosuppression occurs with most chemotherapeutic drugs.

Table 28–8 • Adverse Side Effects Produced by Cancer Chemotherapeutic Drugs

	Immuno-suppression	Thrombo-cytopenia	Leuko-penia	Anemia	Cardiac Toxicity	Pulmonary Toxicity	Renal Toxicity
Alkylating agents							
Bulsulfan (Myleran)	+	+++	+++	+++		++	++
Chlorambucil (Leukeran)	+	++	++	++		+	
Cyclophosphamide (Cytoxan)	++++	+	++	+		+	+
Melphalan (Alkeran)	+	++	++	++		+	
Thiotepa (Thiotepa)	+	+++	+++	+++		+	
Antimetabolites							
Methotrexate (Methotrexate)	+++	+++	+++	+++		+	++
6-Mercaptopurine (Purinethol)	+++	++	++	++			++
Thioguanine (Thioguanine)	+++	+	++	++			
5-Fluorouracil (Fluorouracil)	++++	+++	+++	+++			
Plant alkaloids							
Vinblastine (Velban)	++	+	+++	+			
Vincristine (Oncovin)	++	+	++	+			+
Antibiotics							
Doxorubicin (Adriamycin)		+	+++	++	+++		
Daunorubicin (Daunomycin)	+	++	+++	++	+++		

Hepatic Toxicity	CNS Toxicity	Peripheral Nervous System Toxicity	Autonomic Nervous System Toxicity	Stomatitis	Plasma Cholinesterase Inhibition	Other
			+		+	Adrenocortical-like effect (+)
						Hemolytic anemia (++)
+	+				+	Hemolytic anemia (++)
+				+	++	Hemolytic anemia (++)
						Hemorrhagic cystitis (+++)
					+	Inappropriate ADH secretion (+)
					++	Hemolytic anemia (++)
						Hemolytic anemia (++)
+				+++		
+++				+		
+++				+		
	+			+++		
		+	+	+		Inappropriate ADH secretion (+)
	+	++	++			
+				++		Red urine (+)
				++		Red urine (+)

Table continued on following page

≡ **Table 28–8 •** Adverse Side Effects Produced by
Cancer Chemotherapeutic Drugs (Continued)

	Immuno-suppression	Thrombo-cytopenia	Leuko-penia	Anemia	Cardiac Toxicity	Pulmo-nary Toxicity	Renal Toxicity
Antibiotics *(Cont'd)*							
Bleomycin (Blenoxane)		+	+	+		+++	
Mithramycin (Mithracin)	+	++++	++++	+++			++
Nitrosoureas							
Carmustine (BiCNU)		++	++	++		+	+
Lomustine (CeeNU)		+++	+++	++			
Enzymes							
L-Asparaginase (Elspar)	++	+	+	+			+

ADH, antidiuretic hormone; +, minimal; ++, mild; +++, moderate; ++++, marked.
Adapted from Selvin BL. Cancer chemotherapy: Implications for the anesthesiologist. Anesth Analg 1981;60:425–34, with permission.

    C. **Postoperative considerations.** Postoperative mechanical support of the patient's ventilation is often required, particularly following invasive or prolonged operations and in patients with preoperative drug-induced pulmonary fibrosis.

VII. COMMON CANCERS ENCOUNTERED IN CLINICAL PRACTICE

    A. **Lung cancer,** the leading cause of cancer death among men and women, accounts for nearly one-third of all cancer deaths in the United States. It is largely a preventable disease as more than 90% of lung cancer deaths are related to cigarette smoking.

       1. **Signs and symptoms.** Patients with lung cancer present with features related to the extent of the disease including regional manifestations, signs and symptoms of metastatic disease, and various paraneoplastic syndromes related indirectly to the cancer (Table 28–3).

Hepatic Toxicity	CNS Toxicity	Peripheral Nervous System Toxicity	Autonomic Nervous System Toxicity	Stomatitis	Plasma Cholinesterase Inhibition	Other
				+++		
++	+			+++		Coagulation defects (+++) Hypocalcemia (+) Hypokalemia (+)
			+			
+			+			
+++	+		+			Hemorrhagic pancreatitis (+) Coagulation defects (+)

≡ **Table 28–9 • Preoperative Tests in Patients with Cancer**

Hematocrit
Platelet count
White blood cell count
Prothrombin time
Electrolytes
Liver function tests
Renal function tests
Blood glucose concentrations
Arterial blood gases
Chest radiograph
Electrocardiogram

≡ Table 28–10 • Neurotoxicity Associated with Chemotherapy

Peripheral Neuropathy
Vincristine (sensorimotor peripheral neuropathy, autonomic nervous system neuropathy)
Cisplatin (damages dorsal root ganglia)
Paclitaxel (sensory ataxia, proximal skeletal muscle weakness)
Corticosteroids (myopathy)
Encephalopathy
Cyclophosphamide (acute delirium)
Cytarabine (acute delirium, cerebellar degeneration)
Methotrexate (dementia)

---

2. **Histologic subtypes.** See Table 28–11.
3. **Diagnosis.** Cytologic analysis of sputum is often sufficient for the diagnosis of lung cancer. Flexible fiberoptic bronchoscopy, in combination with a biopsy, brushings, or washings is a standard procedure during the initial evaluation of lung cancer. Video-assisted thoracoscopic surgery is useful for diagnosing peripheral lung lesions and pleura-based tumors, and it is an alternative to anterior mediastinoscopy.
4. **Treatment.** Surgical resection (lobectomy, pneumonectomy) is the most effective treatment for lung cancer. Surgery has little effect on survival when disease has spread to unilateral mediastinal lymph nodes.
5. **Management of anesthesia** in patients with lung cancer includes preoperative consideration of tumor-induced effects that may manifest as malnutrition, pneumonia, pain, and ectopic endocrine effects, such as hyponatremia. The propensity of lung cancer to metastasize to the brain and bones may be of possible significance. When resection of lung tissue is planned, it is important to evaluate underlying pulmonary and cardiac function, especially for the presence of pulmonary hypertension.
   a. **Mediastinoscopy.** Hemorrhage and pneumothorax are the most frequently encountered complications of mediastinoscopy.
   b. Compression of the right subclavian artery may cause loss of distal pulses (erroneous diagnosis of cardiac arrest). Unrecognized compression of the

Table 28–11 • Clinical and Pathologic Features of Lung Cancer

| | | 5-Year Survival (%) | | |
Histologic Subtype	Incidence (%)	All Cases	Resectable Cases	Associated Symptoms
Squamous	25–40	11	40	Hypercalcemia
Adenocarcinoma	30–50	5	30	Hypercoagulability
				Osteoarthropathy
Large cell	10	4	30	Gynecomastia
				Galactorrhea
Small cell	15–24	2	5–10	Inappropriate ADH secretion
				Ectopic corticotropin secretion
				Eaton-Lambert syndrome

ADH, antidiuretic hormone.
Adapted from: Skarin AT. Lung cancer. Sci Am Med 1997;1–20.

right carotid artery by the mediastinoscope may manifest as a postoperative neurologic deficit.

B. Colorectal cancer. Colon cancer is second only to lung cancer as a cause of cancer death in the United States.

1. **Etiology.** Most colorectal tumors arise from premalignant adenomatous polyps.

2. **Diagnosis.** The rationale for colorectal cancer screening (digital rectal examination, fecal occult blood testing, colonoscopy) is that earlier detection increases the surgical cure rate.

3. **Signs and symptoms** of colorectal cancers reflect the anatomic location of the cancer, ranging from anemia and fatigue (ascending colon) to abdominal cramping and obstruction (transverse colon). Colorectal cancers initially spread to regional lymph nodes and then through the portal venous circulation to the liver, which represents the most common visceral site of metastases.

4. **Treatment.** Radical surgical resection (lymph nodes draining the involved bowel and blood vessels) offers the best potential for cure in patients with invasive colorectal cancers.

5. **Management of anesthesia** for surgical resection of colorectal cancer may be influenced by disease-induced anemia and the effects of any metastases present in the liver or lungs. Chronic large bowel obstruction probably does not increase the risk of aspiration on induction of anesthesia, although extreme abdominal distension could interfere with adequate ventilation and oxygenation. Immunosuppression produced by transfused blood may be undesirable, emphasizing the importance of considering the risk and benefits of blood transfusions administered to these patients.

C. Prostate cancer is the second leading cause of cancer death among men.

1. **Diagnosis.** Use of prostate-specific antigen (PSA) testing has changed the way prostate cancer is diagnosed (level > 10 ng/ml suggests the presence of prostate cancer regardless of the findings on the rectal examination. The rectal examination can only evaluate the posterior and lateral aspects of the prostate. Transrectal ultrasonography is utilized regardless of the PSA level.

2. **Treatment.** Focal, well differentiated prostate cancer is usually cured by transurethral resection. If lymph nodes are involved, radical prostatectomy or definitive radia-

tion therapy is often recommended. Hormonal ablative therapy is indicated for management of metastatic prostate cancer because this cancer is under the trophic influence of androgen hormones.

D. **Breast cancer.** Women in the United States have a 12.6% lifetime risk of developing breast cancer.

1. **Risk factors.** The principal risk factors for the development of breast cancer are increasing age and family history.

2. **Screening.** Recommended screening strategies for breast cancer include the triad of breast self-examination, clinical breast examination by a professional, and screening mammography.

3. **Prognosis.** Axillary node status and tumor size are the two most important determinants of outcome in patients with early breast cancer.

4. **Treatment.** Breast conservation therapy (lumpectomy with radiotherapy) and modified radical mastectomy (including axillary nodes) provide similar survival rates. Distant micrometastatic spread is correlated with the number of lymph nodes, thus providing useful prognostic information. Morbidity of breast cancer surgery is largely related to side effects of lymph node dissection (lymphedema and restricted arm motion).

   a. **Systemic treatment.** The recognition that many women with early-stage breast cancer already have distant micrometastases at the time of diagnosis is the rationale for systemic therapy [ovarian ablation, tamoxifen therapy (temperature disturbances, increased risk of uterine cancer), chemotherapy (bone marrow suppression, leukemia, doxorubicin-induced cardiac impairment manifesting as congestive heart failure)].

   b. High-dose irradiation may be associated with plexopathy or nerve damage, pneumonitis, pulmonary fibrosis, and cardiac damage.

5. **Management of anesthesia.** Preoperative evaluation of patients for side effects related to chemotherapy is recommended. Placing intravenous catheters in the ipsilateral arm is avoided as exacerbation of lymphedema and the susceptibility to infection are considerations (also avoid compression and heat). Injection of isosulfan blue dye for sentinel lymph node mapping may cause transient decreases in the SpO_2 readings from the pulse

oximeter. The presence of bone pain and pathologic fractures is considered when selecting regional anesthesia and positioning patients during surgery.

VIII. LESS COMMON CANCERS ENCOUNTERED IN CLINICAL PRACTICE

See Table 28–12.

IX. LYMPHOMAS AND LEUKEMIAS

A. **Hodgkin's disease** is a lymphoma with an infective (Epstein-Barr) and genetic association. Impaired immunity, as present in patients with an organ transplant or AIDS, appears to predispose to the development of lymphoma.

1. **Signs and symptoms.** Typically, a painless enlarging mass appears in the patient's neck. Cyclic increases in body temperature and unexplained weight loss may

---

≡ Table 28–12 • Less Common Cancers Encountered in Clinical Practice

Cardiac Tumors
Cardiac myxomas (most often occur in the left atrium)
  Signs and symptoms include interference with filling and emptying of the involved cardiac chamber and release of emboli from the myxoma)
  Diagnosis is with echocardiography
  Treatment is surgical resection
  Management of anesthesia considers possible presence of low cardiac output and arterial hypoxemia due to obstruction at the tricuspid valve (exacerbated by changes in body position), avoid placement of right atrial catheters if myxoma is in right atrium
Metastatic cardiac tumors (lung, breast, Kaposi's sarcoma, leukemia)
  Malignant pericardial effusion and cardiac tamponade
  Echocardiography useful for diagnosis
Primary malignant tumors (sudden onset and progression of refractory congestive heart failure)
Head and Neck Cancers
History of alcohol abuse and cigarette smoking
Bone metastases (hypercalcemia)
Preoperative nutritional therapy
Surgical treatment often utilizes laser

≡ Table 28–12 • Less Common Cancers Encountered in Clinical Practice *Continued*

Thyroid Cancer
Pheochromocytomas (multiple endocrine neoplasia type 2)
Esophageal Cancer
History of alcohol abuse and cigarette smoking
Malnutrition (hypovolemia and hypotension on induction of anesthesia)
Consider possible presence of liver disease and chronic obstructive pulmonary disease
Gastric Cancer (usually far advanced when discovered)
Weight loss and ascites
Liver Cancer (males with cirrhosis caused by hepatitis B)
Gallbladder Cancer (discovered unexpectedly at cholecystectomy)
Pancreatic Cancer
Total pancreatectomy or pancreatoduodenectomy (Whipple procedure)
Celiac plexus block for management of pain (hypotension)
Renal Cell Cancer
High-output congestive heart failure if arteriovenous fistulas present
Bladder Cancer
Testicular Cancer (curable even when distant metastases present)
Uterine Cervix Cancer (in situ treated with a cone biopsy)
Uterine Cancer (vaginal bleeding)
Ovarian Cancer
Cutaneous Melanoma
Sunlight (ultraviolet light)
Change in color, size, shape, or surface of a mole
Metastases to lymph nodes, brain, liver, lungs, bones
Bone Cancer
Multiple Myeloma
  Painful pathologic fractures (vertebral collapse)
  Anemia
  Thrombocytopenia
  Hypercalcemia
  Renal failure
  Recurrent infections (bone marrow suppression)
  Spinal cord compression
Osteosarcoma (long bones)
  Increased plasma concentrations of alkaline phosphatase
  Lung metastases
Ewing's Tumor (pelvis, femur, tibia)
Chondrosarcoma (pelvis, ribs, upper end of femur or humerus)

≡ Table 28–13 • Lymphocytic and Myeloid Leukemias

Acute Lymphoblastic Leukemia
Central nervous system complications
Opportunistic infections (*Pneumocystis carinii* and
  cytomegalovirus)
Chemotherapy
Chronic Lymphocytic Leukemia
Common in adults and rare in children
Anemia
Hypersplenism (pancytopenia, thrombocytopenia)
Chemotherapy with alkylating drugs
Adult T Cell Leukemia
Rapidly fatal (leukocytosis, hepatosplenomegaly, hypercalcemia)
Opportunistic infections (*Pneumocystis carinii* and
  cytomegalovirus)
Acute Myeloid Leukemia
Granulocytopenia
Thrombocytopenia
Anemia
Chemotherapy with daunorubicin and cytarabine
Bone marrow transplantation
Chronic Myeloid Leukemia
Massive hepatosplenomegaly
Hyperuricemia (treat with allopurinol)
Busulfan
Bone marrow transplantation

---

occur. Moderately severe anemia is often present. Peripheral neuropathies and spinal cord compression may
occur as a direct result of tumor growth.

2. **Treatment** includes surgical exploration for classifying
   the disease in preparation for selecting appropriate therapy (radiotherapy, chemotherapy).

**≡ Table 28–14 • Chemotherapy for Treatment
of Leukemia**

Administer chemotherapeutic drugs that depress bone marrow
  activity (risks are hemorrhage and infection)
Destruction of tumor cells produces a uric acid load (urate
  nephropathy and gouty arthritis)
Nutritional support to prevent hypoalbuminemia and loss of
  immunocompetence

B. **Leukemia** is the uncontrolled production of leukocytes owing to cancerous mutation of lymphogenous or myelogenous cells. Lymphatic leukemias begin in lymph nodes, whereas myeloid leukemias begin in the bone marrow (Table 28–13). An expanding mass of cells that infiltrate the bone marrow renders patients functionally aplastic (anemia, thrombocytopenia, hemorrhage, infections).

1. **Chemotherapy for treatment of leukemia.** Chemotherapy is intended to decrease the number of tumor cells, so organomegaly regresses and the function of the bone marrow improves (Table 28–14).

2. **Bone marrow transplantation for treatment of leukemia.** Regardless of the type of bone marrow transplantation (autologous or allogeneic), recipients must undergo preoperative regimens designed to achieve bone marrow ablation produced by combinations of total body irradiation and chemotherapy. Bone marrow is usually harvested by repeated aspiration from the donor's pos-

---

≡ Table 28–15 • Complications of Bone Marrow Transplantation

Graft-Versus-Host Disease
Pancytopenia and immunodeficiency
Oral ulceration and mucositis
Esophageal ulceration
Diarrhea with fluid and electrolyte loss
Hepatitis with coagulopathy
Bronchiolitis obliterans
Interstitial pneumonitis
Pulmonary fibrosis
Renal failure
Graft Rejection
Minimize likelihood by maximum immunosuppression
Pulmonary Complications
Interstitial pneumonitis (fever, arterial hypoxemia, acute respiratory failure)
Often due to cytomegalovirus
High-dose corticosteroids may be effective
Veno-occlusive Disease of the Liver
Jaundice
Hepatomegaly
Ascites
Progressive hepatic and renal failure

terior iliac crest. The time for bone marrow engraftment is usually 10 to 28 days.

   a. Anesthesia for bone marrow transplantation. General anesthesia or regional anesthesia is needed for aspiration of bone marrow from the donor's iliac crest. Nitrous oxide may be avoided in the donor because of potential bone marrow depression associated with use of this drug (no evidence that nitrous oxide adversely affects bone marrow engraftment).

   b. Brief heparinization before removal of bone marrow may influence the selection of spinal or epidural anesthesia.

   c. Complications of bone marrow transplantation. See Table 28–15.

29

Diseases Related to Immune System Dysfunction

The immune system, which consists of a number of lymphoid organs (thymus, lymph nodes, tonsils, spleen) is responsible for protecting the host against infections and recognizing foreign substances (Stoelting RK, Dierdorf SF. Disorders related to immune system dysfunction. In: Anesthesia and Co-Existing Disease, 4th ed. New York, Churchill Livingstone, 2002;611–628). Immunologically active cells of the immune system are lymphocytes characterized as B lymphocytes and T lymphocytes (Fig. 29–1). Humoral immunity is mediated by B lymphocytes that differentiate into antibody-producing plasma cells when stimulated by antigens. Antibodies are secreted by plasma cells as a heterogeneous group of plasma proteins designated immunoglobulins (Ig) (Table 29–1). Most antibodies are IgG, and antigens that preferentially induce IgE antibodies are designated allergens. Cellular immunity that may result in rejection of transplanted foreign tissues is mediated by T lymphocytes. The complement system serves as the principal humoral effector of immunologically induced inflammation (Fig. 29–2).

I. ALLERGIC REACTIONS

Allergic reactions may be due to antigen-antibody interactions (anaphylaxis, immune-mediated hypersensitivity), release of chemical mediators (histamine) in response to certain drugs (first-time exposure) that occurs in the absence of antigen-antibody interactions (anaphylactoid), and activation of the complement pathway.

A. Anaphylaxis is a life-threatening manifestation of antigen-antibody interactions in which prior exposure of the host to specific antigens (foods, drugs) has evoked production of antigen-specific IgE antibodies, rendering the host sensitized. Vasoactive mediators released by degranulation of mast cells and basophils are responsible for clinical manifestations of anaphylaxis (Table 29–2).

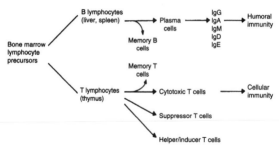

Fig. 29–1 • Immune system.

1. **Diagnosis** of anaphylaxis is suggested by the dramatic nature of the clinical manifestations in close temporal relation to exposure to antigens (may mimic pulmonary embolism, myocardial infarction, aspiration, vasovagal reaction).

   a. Hypotension and cardiovascular collapse may be the only manifestations of anaphylaxis in patients rendered unconscious by general anesthesia.

   b. The initial in vivo response of plasma IgE concentrations is a decrease, reflecting the complexing of antibodies with newly injected antigens. After this initial decrease, there is often an overshoot of IgE concentrations. Biochemical proof of anaphylaxis (degranulation) is also provided by increases in plasma tryptase concentrations in blood samples collected 1 to 2 hours after the suspected allergic drug reaction.

   c. Identification of the offending antigens is provided by positive intradermal tests (alternatively, commercially available antigens utilizing the radioallergosorbent test and enzyme-linked immunosorbent assay).

2. **Treatment.** The three immediate goals in the treatment of anaphylaxis are reversal of arterial hypoxemia, replacement of intravascular fluid volume, and inhibition of further cellular degranulation with release of vasoactive mediators (Table 29–3).

B. **Allergic rhinitis** is an IgE-mediated inflammatory disease involving the nasal mucous membranes [symptoms are often seasonal when pollens (antigens) come into direct contact with the respiratory mucosa].

   1. Viral upper respiratory tract infections may mimic allergic rhinitis; but in contrast to allergic rhinitis, symptoms of

Table 29-1 • Properties of Human Immunoglobulins

Property	IgG	IgA	IgM	IgD	IgE
Location	Plasma, amniotic fluid	Plasma, saliva, tears	Plasma	Plasma	Plasma
Plasma concentration (mg/dl)	550–1900	60–333	45–145	0.3–30.0	Trace
Half-time (days)	23	6	5	3	2.5
Function	Immunity; defense against infections	Topical defense against infections	Lysis of bacterial cell walls	Not known	Anaphylaxis

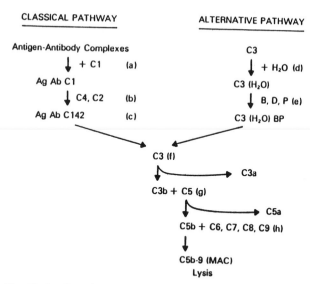

Fig. 29–2 • Complement system consists of the classic pathway and alternative pathway. (From Frank MM. Complement in the pathophysiology of human disease. N Engl J Med 1987;316: 1525–30, with permission.)

viral respiratory tract infections are usually short-lived (< 7 days) and include fever.

2. **Treatment** of allergic rhinitis includes avoidance of offending allergens, the use of antihistamines (terfenadine), and administration of allergen-specific immunotherapy.

C. **Allergic conjunctivitis** is the ocular equivalent of allergic rhinitis (pruritus is prominent).

D. **Allergic asthma** manifests as reversible airway obstruction and bronchospasm accompanied by inflammation of the airways and increased bronchial smooth muscle reactivity triggered by specific allergens. Sodium metabisulfite as utilized as a preservative for certain drugs could evoke bronchospasm.

E. **Food allergy** results from antibody-mediated degranulation of gastrointestinal tract mast cells when exposed to specific antigens.

Table 29–2 • Vasoactive Mediators Released During Antigen/Antibody-Induced Degranulation

Vasoactive Mediator	Physiologic Effect
Histamine	Increased capillary permeability
	Peripheral vasodilation
	Bronchoconstriction
Leukotrienes	Increased capillary permeability
	Intense bronchoconstriction
	Negative inotropy
	Coronary artery vasoconstriction
Prostaglandins	Bronchoconstriction
Eosinophil chemotactic factor	Attraction of eosinophils
Neutrophil chemotactic factor	Attraction of neutrophils
Platelet-activating factor	Platelet aggregation and release of vasoactive amines

F. **Drug allergy.** Allergic reactions to drugs may reflect anaphylaxis, drug-induced release of histamine (anaphylactoid reactions), or activation of the complement system. Regardless of the mechanism responsible for life-threatening drug reactions, manifestations and treatment are the same (Table 29–3). The magnitude of histamine release produced on reexposure to drugs that previously resulted in anaphylactoid reactions can be decreased by reducing the dose of drug and slowing its rate of infusion. Allergic drug reactions must be

Table 29–3 • Treatment of Anaphylactic Reactions

Supplemental oxygen
Balanced salt solutions (may need 1–4 L)
Epinephrine (10–100 μg IV)
Diphenhydramine (50–100 mg IV)
β_2-Agonists (albuterol by inhaler)
Corticosteroids (cortisol or methylprednisolone)

distinguished from drug intolerance, idiosyncratic reactions, and drug toxicity (Table 29–4). Evidence of histamine release along veins into which drugs are injected reflects localized and nonimmunologic release of histamine insufficient to evoke anaphylactoid reactions (these patients should not be labeled as allergic).

1. **Perioperative period.** Allergic reactions have been reported with virtually all drugs that may be injected during the administration of anesthesia (exceptions may be ketamine and benzodiazepines) (Table 29–5).

2. Cardiovascular collapse is the predominant manifestation of life-threatening allergic drug reactions in anesthetized patients.

3. It is important to consider the possible role of latex sensitivity when presumed allergic reactions to drugs occur (it is estimated that as many as 15% of allergic reactions during anesthesia are due to latex).

4. Most drug-induced allergic reactions manifest within 10 minutes of intravenous injection of the offending drug (exception is latex, which is typically delayed as long as 30 minutes). Allergic reactions should be considered whenever there are abrupt decreases in systemic blood

---

≡ **Table 29–4 • Differential Diagnosis of Drug Allergy versus Drug Toxicity**

Parameter	Drug Allergy	Drug Toxicity
Mechanisms	Antigen-antibody interactions	Dependent on chemical properties of drug
Manifestations	Hypotension Bronchospasm Urticaria	Variable for each drug
Predictability	Poor	Good based on animal and human studies
Prior exposure	Required	Not required
Dose-related	No	Yes
Onset	Usually within 10 minutes	Usually delayed
Incidence	Low	High, especially if dose is sufficient

☰ Table 29–5 • Causes of Allergic Reactions During the Perioperative Period

Muscle Relaxants

Responsible for more than 60% of perioperative drug-induced allergic reactions

Cross-sensitivity exists between muscle relaxants (antigenic quaternary ammonium groups)

Induction Drugs

Barbiturates (rare but likely to be life-threatening)

Propofol (bronchospasm more common than with other allergic drug reactions)

Local Anesthetics

Estimated that only 1% of all local anesthetic reactions are allergic reactions (more often systemic reactions)

Ester local anesthetics (metabolized to paraaminobenzoic acid) are more likely to evoke allergic reactions than amides

Consider role of preservatives

Cross-sensitivity does not exist between ester and amide local anesthetics

Opioids

Morphine but not fentanyl may evoke histamine release in susceptible patients

Volatile Anesthetics

Cross-sensitivity exists between volatile anesthetics (halothane, enflurane, isoflurane, desflurane) that are metabolized to oxidative halide metabolites

Sevoflurane is not metabolized to oxidative halide metabolites

Protamine

May be more likely in patients allergic to seafoods

Therapeutic dilemma when known to be allergic and neutralization of heparin is needed

Antibiotics

Cross-sensitivity between cephalosporins and penicillin appears to be low

Vancomycin may evoke significant histamine release especially with rapid intravenous injection

Blood and Plasma Volume Expanders

Allergic reactions to properly cross-matched blood occur in about 3% of patients (pruritus, urticaria, fever)

Dextran can activate complement system

Intravascular Contrast Media

Vascular Graft Material

Latex-Containing Medical Devices

pressure and increases in heart rate that exceed 30% of the control value.

5. **Latex-containing medical devices.** Cardiovascular collapse during anesthesia and surgery has been attributed to anaphylaxis triggered by latex. A feature that appears to distinguish latex-induced allergic reactions from drug-induced allergic reactions is the delayed onset (typically > 30 minutes versus < 10 minutes for drug reactions). Contact with latex at mucosal surfaces is probably the most significant route of latex exposure (inhalation may sensitize health care workers).

   a. **Diagnosis.** Sensitized patients develop IgE antibodies directed against latex antigens (skin prick testing, radioallergosorbent tests, enzyme-linked assays). Operating room personnel and patients with spina bifida have an increased incidence of latex allergy (most often manifests as cutaneous sensitivity). Health care workers are at increased risk for developing severe latex allergic reactions should they become patients and undergo surgical procedures.

   b. **Management of anesthesia.** See Table 29–6.

≡ **Table 29–6 •** Management of Anesthesia in Patients with Known or Suspected Latex Allergy

---

Questions as to symptoms related to latex exposure (especially high risk patients including those with spina bifida, multiple prior operations, health care workers, atopic individuals, history of fruit allergies)

Consider preoperative antihistamines and corticosteroids (not reliably protective)

Provide "latex-free environment" intraoperatively

    Nonlatex gloves

    Multidose bottles with latex caps not used

    Do not inject through latex ports

    Select anesthesia equipment (delivery tubing, ventilator bellows, blood pressure cuffs, pulse oximeter probes, electrocardiogram leads, syringes) on the basis of being latex-free

---

II. ANESTHESIA AND IMMUNOCOMPETENCE

A. Resistance to infection. Effects of anesthetics on resistance to infection are transient, reversible, and of minor importance compared with the prolonged immunosuppressive effects of cortisol and catecholamines released as part of the hormonal response to surgery. There is no evidence that the incidence of postoperative infections can be altered by the depth of anesthesia or by the techniques selected to produce anesthesia.

B. Resistance to cancer. There is no evidence that short-term effects of anesthetic drugs are of any significance in the resistance of the host to cancer. As with infection, the most important concern is immunosuppression produced by the hormonal response to surgical stimulation.

III. DISORDERS OF IMMUNOGLOBULINS

See Tables 29–7, 29–8, and 29–9.

IV. DISORDERS OF THE COMPLEMENT SYSTEM

A. Hereditary angioedema is a rare autosomal dominant disorder due to decreased functional activity of the plasma complement protein known as *C1 esterase inhibitor* manifesting as episodic and sometimes life-threatening airway edema (Fig. 29–2). In the absence of C1 esterase inhibitor, the initial activation of the complement pathway is not regulated, leading to the release of vasoactive mediators that increase vascu-

---

≡ Table 29–7 • Disorders of the Immunoglobulins

X-Linked Agammaglobulinemia
Recurrent bacterial infections in affected males
Treat with gamma globulin plus antibiotics when infection occurs
Acquired Hypogammoglobulinemia
Resembles X-linked agammaglobulinemia but does not appear to be genetically determined
Selective Immunoglobulin A Deficiency
Recurrent sinus and pulmonary infections
Often remains undetected until screened as potential blood donors

Table continued on following page

≡ **Table 29–7** • Disorders of the Immunoglobulins
Continued

Selective Immunoglobulin A Deficiency (Continued)
May develop anti-IgA antibodies and experience life-threatening
anaphylactic reactions should they be transfused with blood
containing IgA
Cold Autoimmune Diseases (see Table 29–8)
Cryoglobulinemia
   Abnormal proteins (cryoglobulins) precipitate on exposure to
   cold (usually blood temperatures < 33°C)
   During anesthesia it is important to maintain body temperature
   above the thermal reactivity of cryoglobulins (increase
   ambient temperature of the operating room, warm and
   humidify inhaled gases, warm intravenous fluids)
   Hypothermic cardiopulmonary bypass and use of cold
   cardioplegia solutions may not be possible
Cold hemagglutinin disease
   IgM autoantibodies in plasma react with antigens on the
   patient's erythrocytes in the presence of decreased body
   temperatures
   Hemolytic anemia and signs of vascular occlusion (acrocyanosis,
   Raynaud's phenomenon)
   Avoid cold environments
   Cyclophosphamide may be effective in suppressing
   IgM-producing cells
   During anesthesia (often for splenectomy) avoid exposure to
   cold operating room environments
Multiple Myeloma
Waldenström's Macroglobulinemia
Neoplastic proliferation of IgM-secreting plasma cells that infiltrate
bone marrow
Plasmapheresis to remove abnormal proteins and decrease
viscosity of the plasma
Amyloidosis
Accumulation of insoluble fibrillar proteins (amyloid) in various
tissues (see Table 29–9)
Sudden death
Hyperimmunoglobulinemia E Syndrome
Recurrent bacterial infections (consider risk of epidural abscesses
if an epidural or spinal anesthetic is selected)
Wiskott-Aldrich Syndrome
X-linked recessive disease manifesting as thrombocytopenia,
eczema, and increased susceptibility to infections
Ataxia Telangiectasia
Progressive cerebellar ataxia, recurrent sinus and bacterial
infections and development of telangiectasia of the bulbar
conjunctivae

Table 29-8 • Cold Autoimmune Diseases

Disease	Thermal Reactivity (°C)	Associated Conditions	Response to Cold Exposure
Cryoglobulins	17–33	Macroglobulinemia	Hyperviscosity Platelet aggregation Renal failure
Cold hemagglutinin disease	15–32	None	Acrocyanosis Hemolysis Raynaud's phenomenon
Paroxysmal cold hemoglobinuria	10–15	Syphilis	Hemolysis Jaundice Renal failure
Acquired cold autoimmune disease	4–25	*Mycoplasma* infection Mononucleosis Leukemia	Acrocyanosis Hyperviscosity Hemolysis

▆ Table 29–9 • Signs of Amyloid Accumulation

Macroglossia (contributes to airway obstruction and interferes with direct laryngoscopy)
Salivary glands (mimics angioneurotic edema)
Heart (heart block)
Kidneys (nephrotic syndrome)
Gastrointestinal tract (malabsorption, ileus, obstruction)
Peripheral nerves (carpal tunnel syndrome)
Autonomic nervous system (delayed gastric emptying, orthostatic hypotension)
Joints (pain, limited motion)

lar permeability. Attacks may occur spontaneously or be triggered by trauma (dental procedures, direct laryngoscopy) or emotional stress.

1. **Diagnosis** is on the basis of family history, prior attacks of angioedema, and documentation of low or absent levels of C1 esterase inhibitor.

2. **Signs and symptoms.** Hereditary angioedema is characterized by episodic and painless edema (increased vascular permeability) of the skin (face and extremities) and mucous membranes (respiratory and gastrointestinal tract). Laryngeal edema is the most dangerous manifestation and can lead to airway obstruction and asphyxiation.

▆ Table 29–10 • Treatment of Hereditary Angioedema

Long-Term Prophylaxis
Anabolic steroids (stanozolol, danazol)
Antifibrinolytics (aminocaproic acid, tranexamic acid)
Short-Term Prophylaxis
Indicated for patients who are not receiving long-term prophylaxis but who are scheduled for dental or surgical procedures that require tracheal intubation
Anabolic steroids for 5–7 days before surgery or intravenous administration of C1 esterase inhibitor or fresh frozen plasma immediately before surgery
Acute Attack
Intravenous administration of C1 esterase inhibitor (response within 60 minutes)
Tracheal intubation if airway obstruction

≡ Table 29–11 • Management of Anesthesia in Patients with Hereditary Angioedema

Pretreatment with anabolic steroids (stanozolol) and intravenous administration of C1 esterase inhibitor or fresh frozen plasma

Minimize incidental trauma to the oropharynx (suctioning)

Intramuscular injections acceptable

Regional anesthesia acceptable

Do not avoid tracheal intubation if it can contribute to safe conduct of the anesthesia

Laryngeal distortion from edema may render laryngeal mask airways ineffective

3. **Treatment.** See Table 29–10.
4. **Management of anesthesia.** See Table 29–11.
5. **Emergency airway management** during an acute attack includes administration of supplemental oxygen and consideration of emergency tracheal intubation (presence of airway edema limits the usefulness of fiberoptic laryngoscopy). Personnel and equipment are available to perform an emergency tracheostomy.

≡ Table 29–12 • Examples of Autoimmune Diseases

Organ-Specific Diseases	*Systemic Diseases*
Insulin-dependent diabetes mellitus	Rheumatic fever
Myasthenia gravis	Rheumatoid arthritis
Graves' disease	Ankylosing spondylitis
Thyroiditis	Systemic lupus erythematosus
Addison's disease	Scleroderma
Pernicious anemia	Polymyositis
Male infertility	Goodpasture syndrome
Primary biliary cirrhosis	Chronic graft-versus-host disease
Chronic active hepatitis	Hypereosinophilic syndrome
Crohn's disease	Lyme disease
Autoimmune hemolytic anemia	Kawasaki disease
Psoriasis	Immunoglobulin A deficiency
	Hereditary complement deficiency
	Vasculitis
	Sarcoidosis

B. **Complement protein C2 deficiency** may be present in patients with systemic lupus erythematosus or related disorders such as Schönlein-Henoch purpura.

C. **Complement protein C3 deficiency** is associated with increased susceptibility to life-threatening bacterial infections.

V. AUTOIMMUNE DISEASES

Autoimmune diseases occur when the host's own tissues act as self-antigens to evoke the production of autoantibodies resulting in tissue injury (Table 29–12).

30

Psychiatric Diseases and Substance Abuse

The prevalence of psychiatric illnesses increases the likelihood of such diseases presenting as co-existing diseases in patients undergoing anesthesia and surgery (Stoelting RK, Dierdorf SF. Psychiatric diseases and substance abuse. In: Anesthesia and Co-Existing Disease, 4th ed. New York, Churchill Livingstone, 2002;629–654). Important considerations are the potential drug interactions introduced by medications used to treat psychiatricillnesses. Substance abuse and suicide represent significant occupational hazards for anesthesiologists compared with other nonoperating-room physicians.

I. MENTAL DEPRESSION

Mental depression is the most common psychiatric disease (affects 2% to 4% of the population). It is distinguished from normal sadness and grief by the severity and duration of the mood disturbances and the presence of fatigue, loss of appetite, and insomnia.

A. **Diagnosis** of major mental depression is based on the presence of at least five characteristics and the exclusion of organic causes or a normal reaction to the death of a loved one (Table 30–1). Alcoholism and major depression often occur together. Mental depression and dementia may be difficult to distinguish in elderly patients. All patients with depression should be evaluated for the potential to commit suicide. In the United States, suicide is the tenth leading cause of death, and for physicians under 40 years of age it ranks first.

B. **Treatment** of mental depression is with antidepressant drugs and/or electroconvulsive therapy (ECT). At least 70% to 80% of patients respond to pharmacologic therapy, and at least 50% who do not respond to antidepressants do respond favorably to ECT.

▬ Table 30–1 • Characteristics of Severe Mental Depression

Depressed mood
Decreased interest in daily activities and physical appearance
Fluctuations in body weight
Insomnia or hypersomnia
Fatigue
Decreased ability to concentrate
Recurrent thoughts of suicide

1. **Selective serotonin reuptake inhibitors** (SSRIs) are the most broadly prescribed class of antidepressants and are the drugs of choice for treating mild to moderate mental depression. Unlike tricyclic antidepressants, SSRIs lack anticholinergic effects and do not cause postural hypotension or delayed conduction of cardiac impulses. They also do not appear to have an effect on seizure thresholds (Table 30–2).

   a. Among the SSRIs, fluoxetine is a potent inhibitor of certain hepatic cytochrome P_{450} enzymes. As a result, this drug may increase plasma concentrations of drugs that depend on hepatic metabolism for clearance. The addition of fluoxetine to treatment with tricyclic antidepressant drugs may result in a two- to fivefold increase in the plasma concentrations of the tricyclic drug. Cardiac antidysrhythmia drugs and some β-adrenergic antagonists may be metabolized by the same enzyme systems that are inhibited by fluoxetine, resulting in potentiation of their effects.

   b. Monoamine oxidase inhibitors (MAOIs) combined with fluoxetine may cause the development of a serotonin syndrome (anxiety, chills, ataxia, insomnia).

2. **Other second-generation antidepressants** include drugs unrelated to SSRIs, tricyclic antidepressants, and MAOIs (Table 30–2).

3. **Tricyclic antidepressants.** Side effects of antidepressant drugs influence drug choice because all of these drugs are equally effective if administered in equivalent doses (Table 30–2).

   a. **Management of anesthesia.** Treatment with tricyclic antidepressants need not be discontinued before ad-

Table 30–2 • Antidepressant Drugs Used to Treat Psychiatric Diseases

Drug	Sedative Potency	Anticholinergic Potency	Orthostatic Hypotension	Cardiac Dysrhythmia Potential
Selective Serotonin Uptake Inhibitors				
Fluoxetine	+	+	+	0
Paroxetine	+	+	+	0
Sertaline	+	+	+	0
Fluvoxamine	+	+	+	0
Other Second-Generation Antidepressants				
Bupropion	+	+	+	0
Venlafaxine	+	+	*	0
Trazodone	+++	+	+++	0
Nefazodone	++	+	++	0
Tricyclic Antidepressants				
Amitriptyline	+++	++++	+++	++
Amoxapine	+	++	++	++
Clomipramine	+++	+++	+++	++

Table continued on following page

Table 30-2 • Antidepressant Drugs Used to Treat Psychiatric Diseases *Continued*

Drug	Sedative Potency	Anticholinergic Potency	Orthostatic Hypotension	Cardiac Dysrhythmia Potential
Tricyclic Antidepressants (Continued)				
Desipramine	+	+	+++	++
Doxepin	+++	++	+++	++
Imipramine	++	++	+++	+++
Nortriptyline	+	+	+	+++
Protriptyline	+	+++	+	+++
Trimipramine	+++	++	++	++
Related Polycyclics				
Anixaoube	+	+	++	++
Malprotiline	++	+	++	++

* May cause systemic hypertension.
0, none; +, mild; ++, moderate; +++, marked; ++++, greatest.

ministration of anesthesia for elective operations. Alterations in responses to drugs administered during the perioperative period, however, should be anticipated in treated patients (increased anesthetic requirements, exaggerated systemic blood pressure responses following administration of indirect-acting vasopressors, such as ephedrine).

b. The potential for hypertensive crises is greatest during acute treatment (first 14 to 21 days) with tricyclic antidepressants, whereas chronic treatment is associated with down-regulation of receptors and a decreased likelihood of exaggerated systemic blood pressure responses following administration of sympathomimetic drugs.

4. **Monoamine oxidase inhibitors.** Patients who do not respond to antidepressants may benefit from treatment with MAOIs (phenelzine, isocarboxazid, tranylcypromine). These drugs have negligible anticholinergic effects and do not sensitize the heart to cardiac dysrhythmogenic effects of epinephrine. The principal clinical problems associated with use of these drugs is the possible occurrence of severe systemic hypertension if treated patients ingest foods that contain tyramine (cheese, wines) or receive drugs characterized as sympathomimetics. Systemic hypertension, hypotension, hyperthermia, depression of ventilation, seizures, and coma may follow administration of opioids to patients being treated with MAOIs.

a. **Management of anesthesia.** Anesthesia can be safely conducted in patients being chronically treated with MAOIs (Table 30–3).

b. **Postoperative care.** Provision of analgesia during the postoperative period is influenced by the potential adverse interactions between opioids and MAOIs (decreased doses of morphine or fentanyl are recommended if opioids are necessary to achieve analgesia).

5. **Electroconvulsive therapy** is indicated for treatment of severe mental depression in patients who are unresponsive to drugs or those who become acutely suicidal. Increased intracranial pressure is a contraindication to ECT. Typically, about eight treatments are necessary with more than 75% of treated patients showing a favorable response.

a. **Side effects.** See Table 30–4.

b. **Management of anesthesia.** See Table 30–5.

≡ **Table 30-3 •** Management of Anesthesia in Patients Treated Chronically with Monoamine Oxidase Inhibitors

Avoid opioids in the preoperative medication

Benzodiazepines acceptable to treat preoperative anxiety

Induction of anesthesia with intravenous drugs (ketamine an unlikely selection) recognizing that depression of ventilation may be exaggerated

Maintenance of anesthesia with nitrous oxide and volatile anesthetics (fentanyl has been utilized without apparent adverse effects)

Nondepolarizing muscle relaxants acceptable (pancuronium an unlikely selection)

Regional anesthesia acceptable but risk of hypotension and need for vasopressor therapy must be considered (avoid adding epinephrine to local anesthetic solutions)

Select phenylephrine in decreased doses if a vasopressor is needed [potential for hypertensive crises is greatest during acute treatment (first 14–21 days)]

≡ **Table 30-4 •** Side Effects of Electroconvulsive Therapy

Parasympathetic nervous system stimulation
    Bradycardia
    Hypotension
Sympathetic nervous system stimulation
    Tachycardia
    Hypertension
    Cardiac dysrhythmias
Increased cerebral blood flow
Increased intracranial pressure
Increased intraocular pressure
Increased intragastric pressure
Hypoventilation

≡ **Table 30–5 • Management of Anesthesia for Electroconvulsive Therapy**

Patients are fasted but preanesthetic medication is not recommended as drug-produced sedation could prolong the recovery period

Atropine or glycopyrrolate is commonly administered intravenously 1–2 minutes before induction of anesthesia and delivery of the electrical current to decrease the likelihood of bradycardia

Methohexital 0.5–1.0 mg/kg IV (alternatively propofol 1.5 mg/kg IV) for induction of anesthesia

Succinylcholine 0.3–0.5 mg/kg IV to attenuate contraction of skeletal muscles but still permit visual confirmation of seizure activity

Preoxygenation and support of ventilation with supplemental oxygen

Monitors include pulse oximetry and the electrocardiogram

II. MANIA

Mania is an autosomal dominant disease manifesting clinically as sustained periods of mood elevation and in severe cases delusions and hallucinations.

A. **Treatment** is with lithium (requires about 14 days for a response), and in severe cases combination therapy with an antipsychotic drug (haloperidol) is utilized.

1. **Lithium** is efficiently absorbed after oral administration. Therapeutic serum concentrations for acute mania are 1.0–1.2 mEq/L and for prophylaxis 0.6–0.8 mEq/L. Monitoring serum lithium concentrations is recommended to decrease the likelihood of toxicity.

   a. **Toxicity** is likely when the serum lithium concentrations are > 2 mEq/L (Table 30–6). Loop diuretics or thiazide diuretics increase renal tubular resorption of lithium and may increase serum lithium concentrations by as much as 50%.

   b. Administration of sodium-containing solutions or osmotic diuretics favors renal excretion of lithium in patients who exhibit evidence of lithium toxicity.

2. **Carbamazepine,** is an anticonvulsant that is useful for treating patients who are unresponsive to lithium. Side effects may include leukopenia, aplastic anemia, and hepatotoxicity.

☰ Table 30-6 • Manifestations of
Lithium Toxicity

Skeletal muscle weakness
Ataxia
Sedation
Widening of the QRS complex and heart block
Hypotension
Seizures
Hypothyroidism
Leukocytosis

B. **Management of anesthesia** includes evaluation for lithium toxicity and recognition that stimulation of urine output with loop or thiazide diuretics could adversely increase serum lithium concentrations. The response to muscle relaxants could be prolonged and co-existing sedation could manifest as decreased anesthetic requirements.

III. SCHIZOPHRENIA

Schizophrenia is the most common psychotic disorder, accounting for about 20% of all patients treated for mental illness.
   A. **Treatment.** See Table 30-7.
      1. **Side effects.** See Table 30-8.
      2. **Neuroleptic malignant syndrome** is a rare potentially fatal complication of antipsychotic drug therapy. It manifests as fever, skeletal muscle rigidity (may be so severe that mechanical support of ventilation becomes necessary), autonomic nervous system instability (tachycardia, labile systemic blood pressure, cardiac dysrhythmias), altered consciousness, and increased serum creatine kinase concentrations reflecting skeletal muscle damage.
         a. **Treatment** of neuroleptic malignant syndrome includes discontinuation of antipsychotic drug therapy and administration of bromocriptine (dopamine agonist) or dantrolene in an attempt to decrease skeletal muscle rigidity.
         b. **Relation to malignant hyperthermia.** Despite the similarities, there is no evidence of a pathophysiologic link between these two syndromes.

Table 30-7 • Drugs Used to Treat Schizophrenia

Phenothiazines
  Chlorpromazine
  Thioridazine
  Prochlorperazine
  Perphenazine
  Triflupromazine
  Fluphenazine
Thioxanthenes
  Chlorprothixene
  Thiothixene
Butyrophenones
  Haloperidol
Dibenzoxazepines
  Loxapine
Dihydroindolones
  Molindone
Dibenzodiazepines
  Clozapine
Benzisoxazoles
  Risperidone
Long-acting injectable preparations

Adapted from: Kane JM. Schizophrenia. N Engl J Med 1996;334:34–41.

IV. ANXIETY DISORDERS

Anxiety disorders can be responses to exogenous stimuli (situational anxiety, pain, angina pectoris) or endogenous stimuli (Table 30–9). A single dose of benzodiazepine may be useful for treating specific phobias (fear of flying), whereas performance anxiety ("stage fright") is treated with β-antagonists that do not produce sedation.

  A. Panic disorders appear to be inherited and are characterized as discrete periods of intense fear that are not triggered by a severe anxiogenic stimulus (often accompanied by dyspnea, tachycardia, chest pain, and fear of dying).

  B. Tricyclic antidepressants and MAOIs are effective treatments for panic attacks.

V. AUTISM

Autism is a developmental disorder characterized by disturbances in the rate of development of physical, social, and language skills.

☰ Table 30–8 • Side Effects of Antipsychotic Drugs

Central Nervous System
Extrapyramidal symptoms (present in 50%–70% of patients)
  Acute dystonia (treat with diphenhydramine 25–50 mg IV)
  Akathisia
  Parkinsonism
  Tardive dyskinesia (choreoathetoid movements)
Sedation (possible decreased anesthetic requirements)
Cognitive impairment
Dysregulation of body temperature control
Seizures
Toxic psychosis
Autonomic nervous system dysfunction
  Hypotension (α-adrenergic blockade)
  Tachycardia
  Dry mouth
  Blurred vision
  Urinary retention
Neuroleptic malignant syndrome
Cardiovascular System
Prolonged QT interval
Torsade de pointes
Respiratory Tract
Pharyngeal and laryngeal dysfunction
Respiratory dyskinesia
Endocrine System
Amenorrhea
Galactorrhea
Weight gain
Hematologic Problems
Leukopenia
Agranulocytosis
Gastrointestinal Tract
Decreased bowel motility
Cholestatic jaundice
Ophthalmic Problems
Increased intraocular pressure
Opacities of lens and cornea

Adapted from: Kane JM. Schizophrenia. N Engl J Med 1996;334:34–41.

≡ Table 30–9 • Manifestations of
Anxiety Disorders

Tremor
Dyspnea
Tachycardia
Diaphoresis
Insomnia
Irritability
Polyuria
Fatigue
Diarrhea
Skeletal muscle tension

VI. SUBSTANCE ABUSE AND DRUG OVERDOSE

See Table 30–10.

A. **Diagnosis.** Substance abuse is often first suspected or recognized during the medical management of another disorder [hepatitis, acquired immunodeficiency syndrome (AIDS), pregnancy, chronic pain, personality disorders]. Drug overdose is the leading cause of unconsciousness observed in patients admitted to emergency departments (often more than one class of drugs as well as alcohol have been ingested)

≡ Table 30–10 • Characteristic Symptoms for
Psychoactive Drug Dependence

Drugs taken in greater doses for longer periods of time than
  intended
Unsuccessful attempts to decrease use of drug
Increased time spent obtaining the drug
Frequent intoxication or withdrawal symptoms
Restricted social or work activities because of drug use
Continued drug use despite social or physical problems related to
  drug use
Evidence of tolerance to effects of the drug
Characteristic withdrawal symptoms
Drug use to avoid withdrawal symptoms

≡ Table 30–11 • Evaluation of Depth of Central Nervous System Depression in the Presence of Drug Overdose

---

Response to painful stimulation
Activity of gag reflex
Presence or absence of hypotension
Breathing rate
Size and responsiveness of the pupils

(Table 30–11). Conditions other than drug overdose may result in unconsciousness, emphasizing the importance of laboratory tests (electrolytes, blood glucose concentrations, arterial blood gases, renal and liver function tests) for confirming the diagnosis.

B. Treatment. See Table 30–12.
C. Alcoholism. See Table 30–13.
  1. Treatment of alcoholism is total abstinence from alcohol ingestion.
  2. Overdose is treated by maintenance of ventilation (alcohol blood concentrations > 500 mg/dl) and a high index of suspicion of hypoglycemia.
  3. Withdrawal syndrome. See Table 30–14.
  4. Wernicke-Korsakoff syndrome [loss of neurons in the cerebellum (Wernicke's encephalopathy) and loss of memory (Korsakoff's psychosis)] is not an alcohol withdrawal syndrome, but its occurrence establishes that these patients are or have been physically dependent on alcohol. Treatment is intravenous administration of thiamine.

≡ Table 30–12 • Treatment of Drug Overdose

Secure airway (absence of gag reflex confirms that protective laryngeal reflexes are dangerously depressed and there is need to place a cuffed tracheal tube)
Support ventilation
Support circulation
Monitor body temperature (hypothermia common)
Consider methods to remove ingested substances (gastric lavage, charcoal, forced diuresis, hemodialysis)

☰ Table 30–13 • Medical Problems Related to Alcoholism

Central Nervous System Effects
Psychiatric disorders (depression, antisocial behavior)
Nutritional disorders (Wernicke-Korsakoff)
Withdrawal syndrome
Cerebellar degeneration
Cerebral atrophy
Cardiovascular Effects
Dilated cardiomyopathy
Cardiac dysrhythmias
Systemic hypertension
Gastrointestinal Disturbances
Esophagitis
Gastritis
Pancreatitis
Hepatic cirrhosis (portal hypertension manifesting as esophageal varices or hemorrhoids)
Skin and Musculoskeletal Effects
Spider angiomas
Myopathy
Osteoporosis
Endocrine and Metabolic Effects
Decreased serum testosterone concentrations (impotence)
Decreased gluconeogenesis (hypoglycemia)
Ketoacidosis
Hypoalbuminemia
Hypomagnesemia
Hematologic Effects
Thrombocytopenia
Leukopenia
Anemia

5. **Alcohol and pregnancy.** Alcohol crosses the placenta and may result in fetal alcohol syndrome (craniofacial dysmorphology, growth retardation, mental retardation, congenital heart disease).

6. **Management of anesthesia.** (See Chapter 18.) The potential presence of disulfiram-induced sedation and hepatotoxicity should be suspected in alcoholic patients being treated with this drug. Disulfiram may be associated with hypotension during general anesthesia, whereas drug-induced polyneuropathy may influence the selection of regional anesthesia.

☰ Table 30–14 • Alcohol Withdrawal Syndrome

Early Manifestations (6–8 hours after decreases in the blood alcohol level)
Generalized tremor
Autonomic nervous system hyperactivity
Insomnia
Agitation
Delirium Tremens (2–4 days after cessation of alcohol ingestion; develops in 5% of patients and is life-threatening)
Hallucinations
Combativeness
Hyperthermia
Tachycardia
Hypotension/hypertension
Seizures
Treatment
Diazepam (5–10 mg IV every 5 minutes until patient becomes calm)
Esmolol until heart rate < 100 beats/min
Correction of electrolyte (magnesium) and metabolic (thiamine) derangements
Lidocaine
Physical restraint

D. **Cocaine**
 1. **Side effects.** See Table 30–15. Cocaine overdose evokes overwhelming sympathetic nervous system stimulation of the cardiovascular system.
 2. **Treatment** of cocaine overdose includes administration of nitroglycerin for management of myocardial ischemia. β-Adrenergic blockade (esmolol) may accentuate cocaine-induced coronary artery vasospasm. α-Adrenergic blockade may be effective treatment for coronary vasoconstriction due to cocaine, but its use in the presence of systemic hypotension is questionable. Benzodiazepines are effective in the treatment of seizures. Active cooling procedures may be necessary if hyperthermia accompanies cocaine overdose.
 3. **Management of anesthesia** in patients acutely intoxicated with cocaine must consider the vulnerability of these patients to myocardial ischemia and cardiac dysrhythmias (avoid drugs that stimulate the sympathetic nervous system). Thrombocytopenia associated with co-

---

≡ Table 30–15 • Signs and Symptoms of Cocaine Abuse

Coronary vasospasm
Myocardial ischemia
Myocardial infarction
Ventricular cardiac dysrhythmias (ventricular fibrillation)
Systemic hypertension
Tachycardia
Spontaneous abortions
Fetal malformation
Hyperpyrexia (seizures)
Cerebrovascular accidents
Nasal septal atrophy
Paranoid thinking
Withdrawal syndrome (fatigue, mental depression, increased appetite)
Death

---

caine abuse may influence the selection of regional anesthesia. In the absence of acute intoxication, chronic abuse of cocaine has not been shown to be predictably associated with adverse anesthetic interactions, although the possibility of cardiac dysrhythmias remains a constant concern.

E. **Opioids.** Opioid dependence rarely develops from the use of these drugs to treat acute postoperative pain. It is possible to become addicted to opioids within less than 14 days if the drug is administered daily in ever-increasing doses. Numerous medical problems, which should be evaluated preoperatively, are likely to be encountered in opioid addicts (Table 30–16).

   1. **Overdose.** See Table 30–17.
   2. **Withdrawal syndrome** from opioids is unpleasant but is rarely life-threatening (Table 30–18).
   3. **Rapid opioid detoxification** utilizing high doses of opioid antagonists (nalmefene) administered to patients during general anesthesia followed by naltrexone maintenance avoids the unpleasant aspects of opioid withdrawal during the awake state.

      a. **Anesthetic considerations** include the possible increase in serum catecholamine concentrations (changes in systemic blood pressure and tachycardia)

≡ Table 30–16 • Medical Problems Associated with Chronic Opioid Abuse

Acquired immunodeficiency syndrome (AIDS)
Hepatitis
Cellulitis
Superficial skin abscesses
Septic thrombophlebitis
Tetanus
Endocarditis with or without pulmonary emboli
Systemic septic emboli and infarctions
Aspiration pneumonitis
Adrenal gland dysfunction
Malaria
Malnutrition
Positive and false-positive serologies
Transverse myelitis

during anesthesia-assisted opioid detoxification (consider preoperative treatment with clonidine and administration of β-antagonists during anesthesia).

   b. Deep general anesthesia with skeletal muscle paralysis and controlled ventilation of the lungs may be recommended.

   4. **Management of anesthesia.** See Table 30–19.

F. **Barbiturates.** Chronic barbiturate abuse is not associated with pathophysiologic changes (most commonly abused orally for insomnia and to antagonize stimulant effects of other drugs). In contrast to opioids, lethal doses of barbitu-

≡ Table 30–17 • Signs and Symptoms of Opioid Overdose

Slow breathing rate (administer naloxone until > 12 breaths/min)
Normal to increased tidal volume
Miotic pupils
Unconsciousness
Seizures
Pulmonary edema
Arterial hypoxemia
Gastric atony

≡ Table 30–18 • Time Course of Opioid Withdrawal Syndrome

Drug	Onset	Peak Intensity	Duration
Meperidine Dihydromorphine	2–6 hours	8–12 hours	4–5 days
Codeine Morphine Heroin	6–18 hours	36–72 hours	7–10 days
Methadone	24–48 hours	3–21 days	6–7 weeks

rates do not increase at the same rate as tolerance to sedative and euphoric effects.

1. **Overdose** is associated with central nervous system depression, hypoventilation, and hypotension.
2. **Withdrawal syndrome.** In contrast to opioid withdrawal, the abrupt cessation of excessive barbiturate ingestion is associated with potentially life-threatening responses (cardiovascular collapse, seizures).
3. **Management of anesthesia** is most likely to be influenced by cross-tolerance with depressant effects of anesthetic drugs.

G. **Benzodiazepines,** when ingested in excess, produce tolerance and dependence. The combination of benzodiazepines with other depressants (alcohol) may produce exaggerated effects. Treatment of an overdose is supportive, with administration of a specific benzodiazepine antagonist (flumazenil) if central nervous system depression is profound.

≡ Table 30–19 • Management of Anesthesia in the Presence of Opioid Addiction

Current Opioid Abuse
Maintain opioid (methadone)
Volatile anesthetics selected
Anticipate perioperative hypotension
Rehabilitated Opioid Addict
Volatile anesthetics selected
Anticipate exaggerated postoperative pain (methadone has minimal analgesic activity)

H. Amphetamines stimulate the release of catecholamines, resulting in increased cortical alertness with associated appetite suppression and decreased need for sleep. Approved uses of amphetamines are treatment of narcolepsy, attention-deficit disorders, and hyperactivity associated with minimal brain dysfunction.

   1. Physiologic dependence is profound, and chronic abuse results in depletion of body stores of catecholamines.
   2. **Overdose** causes anxiety, psychotic states, progressive central nervous system irritability, and cardiovascular stimulation.
   3. **Withdrawal syndrome** is characterized by extreme lethargy and mental depression.
   4. **Management of anesthesia.** See Table 30–20.

I. Hallucinogens produce psychological dependence, but there is no evidence of physical dependence or withdrawal symptoms.

   1. **Overdose** is usually not life-threatening. Treatment is symptomatic (calm and quiet environment with minimal external stimuli).
   2. **Management of anesthesia** may be complicated by acute panic responses (treat with diazepam).

J. Marijuana abuse is associated with sedation, tachycardia, orthostatic hypotension, and bronchitis, which are considerations in the management of anesthesia in these patients.

K. Tricyclic antidepressant overdose is the most common cause of death from drug ingestion (potential lethal dose may only be 5 to 10 times the daily therapeutic dose).

≡ Table 30–20 • Management of Anesthesia in the Presence of Amphetamine Abuse

Acute Amphetamine Intoxication
Systemic hypertension
Tachycardia
Hyperthermia
Increased anesthetic requirements
Exaggerated responses to vasopressors
Chronic Amphetamine Intoxication
Decreased response to vasopressors
Decreased anesthetic requirements

Table 30–21 • Signs and Symptoms of Tricyclic Antidepressant Drug Overdose

Seizures
Coma (lasts 24–72 hours)
Intense anticholinergic effects
Tachycardia
Mydriasis
Urinary retention
Delayed gastric emptying

1. An overdose principally affects the central nervous system, parasympathetic nervous system, and cardiovascular system (Table 30–21).
2. **Treatment** of tricyclic antidepressant overdose in the presence of protective upper airway reflexes consists of induced emesis and/or gastric lavage plus pharmacologic treatment of specific symptoms (Table 30–22).

L. **Salicyclic acid overdose.** See Table 30–23.

M. **Acetaminophen overdose** manifests as vomiting, abdominal pain, and life-threatening centrilobular hepatic necrosis (treat with acetylcysteine).

N. **Methyl alcohol ingestion** results in metabolic acidosis, reflecting its metabolism to formaldehyde and formic acid.
   1. A toxic effect of these metabolites on the optic nerve is associated with blindness.

Table 30–22 • Pharmacologic Treatment of Tricyclic Antidepressant Overdose

Side Effect	Treatment
Seizures	Diazepam
	Phenytoin
Cardiac dysrhythmias	Lidocaine
	Phenytoin
Heart block	Isoproterenol
Hypotension	Crystalloid or colloid solutions
	Sympathomimetics
	Inotropes

▀ Table 30–23 • Salicylic Acid Overdose

Symptoms parallel salicylate blood levels (> 85 m/dl in severe overdoses)
Hyperventilation (resulting alkalosis favors renal excretion of salicylic acid; maintain pH > 7.4)
Hypoglycemia
Noncardiogenic pulmonary edema
Hyperthermia
Seizures

---

2. **Treatment** consists of intravenous administration of alcohol, which competes with methyl alcohol for the enzyme alcohol dehydrogenase (same treatment for ethylene glycol).

O. **Petroleum product ingestion** results in hydrocarbon pneumonitis secondary to pulmonary aspiration. Sudden death may reflect cardiac dysrhythmias.

P. **Organophosphate overdose** leads to excessive accumulation of acetylcholine at nicotinic (neuromuscular junctions) and cholinergic receptor sites (Table 30–24). Pharmacologic

---

▀ Table 30–24 • Symptoms of Organophosphate (Insecticide) Overdose

Nicotinic Effects (neuromuscular junctions)
Skeletal muscle fasciculations
Skeletal muscle weakness
Skeletal muscle paralysis (apnea)
Muscarinic Effects
Salivation
Lacrimation
Miosis
Diaphoresis
Bronchospasm
Bradycardia
Hyperperistalsis (diarrhea, urination)
Central Nervous System Effects
Grand mal seizures
Unconsciousness
Apnea
Hyperthermia

≡ Table 30–25 • Treatment of Organophosphate (Insecticide) Overdose

Drug	Dose
Atropine	2 mg IV until ventilation improves Usual dose for severe toxicity is 15–20 mg during the first 3 hours
Pralidoxime	600 mg IV
Diazepam	5–10 mg IV; repeat until seizures are controlled

treatment is necessary to prevent death, which is usually due to apnea (Table 30–25).

Q. **Carbon monoxide poisoning** may be accidental (fire-related smoke inhalation, poorly functioning heating systems, motor vehicle exhaust fumes, tobacco smoke) or intentional. Intraoperative increases in carboxyhemoglobin concentrations may reflect carbon monoxide formation as a result of degradation of volatile anesthetics (exception sevoflurane) by the strong bases present in some but not all carbon dioxide absorbents. Blood carboxyhemoglobin concentrations commonly reach levels of 10% in smokers compared with 1% to 3% in nonsmokers.

1. **Pathophysiology.** Carbon monoxide toxicity appears to result from a combination of tissue hypoxia and direct carbon monoxide-mediated damage at the cellular level. Carbon monoxide competes with oxygen for binding to hemoglobin (affinity of hemoglobin for carbon monoxide is 200 to 250 times greater than its affinity for oxygen).

≡ Table 30–26 • Signs and Symptoms of Carbon Monoxide Poisoning

Mimic nonspecific viral illness (headache, nausea, vomiting, weakness)
Difficulty concentrating
Syncope and seizures (cerebral vasodilation, which can lead to cerebral edema)
Angina pectoris
Cardiac dysrhythmias
Pulmonary edema
Carboxyhemoglobin levels (may not parallel severity of symptoms)

≡ Table 30–27 • Diagnosis of Carbon Monoxide Poisoning

High index of suspicion as no pathognomonic signs or symptoms

Increased plasma concentrations of carboxyhemoglobin (severe poisoning when blood carboxyhemoglobin concentrations > 40%)

Pulse oximetry cannot distinguish carboxyhemoglobin from oxyhemoglobin [SpO_2 values may be unchanged or falsely increased, whereas unexplained decreases may trigger measurement of arterial blood gases (calculation of SaO_2 from a nomogram based on measured PaO_2 results in erroneous conclusions)]

The consequence of this competitive binding is a shift of the oxygen-hemoglobin dissociation curve to the left.

2. **Signs and symptoms.** See Table 30–26.

   a. **Delayed neuropsychiatric syndrome.** Cognitive dysfunction, personality changes, parkinsonism, dementia, and psychosis occur in 10% to 30% of individuals following apparent recovery from carbon monoxide intoxication.

   b. Delayed neuropsychiatric sequelae due to intraoperative exposure to carbon monoxide have been described as late as 21 days after anesthesia.

3. **Diagnosis.** See Table 30–27.

4. **Treatment** is removing the individual from the source of carbon monoxide production and administering 100% oxygen (shortens the half-time of carbon monoxide by competing at the binding sites for hemoglobin and improves tissue oxygenation). Hyperbaric oxygen therapy is a consideration in the presence of coma and carboxyhemoglobin concentrations > 40%.

31

Diseases Associated with Pregnancy

Pregnancy and subsequent labor and delivery are accompanied by unique physiologic changes that may be further altered by co-existing diseases (Stoelting RK, Dierdorf SF. Diseases associated with pregnancy. In: Anesthesia and Co-Existing Disease, 4th ed. New York, Churchill Livingstone, 2002;655–685).

I. PHYSIOLOGIC CHANGES ASSOCIATED WITH PREGNANCY

A. Changes in the cardiovascular system during pregnancy provide for the needs of the developing fetus and prepare the mother for those events that accompany labor and delivery (Table 31–1).

1. Decreased venous return due to obstruction of the inferior vena cava by the gravid uterus, when the parturient assumes the supine position, results in *supine hypotension syndrome* in about 10% of parturients as they approach term.

2. Capillary engorgement of the mucosal lining of the upper respiratory tract emphasizes the need for gentleness during instrumentation of the upper airway.

3. Induction of anesthesia, emergence from anesthesia, and changes in the depth of anesthesia are notably faster in parturients (combination of increased minute ventilation and decreased functional residual capacity), and dose requirements for volatile anesthetic drugs may be decreased (makes parturients susceptible to anesthetic overdoses). Induction of anesthesia in parturients may be associated with marked decreases in arterial oxygenation if apnea is prolonged, as during tracheal intubation, reflecting decreased oxygen reserves secondary to decreases in functional residual capacity (potential value of preoxygenation).

≡ **Table 31–1 •** Physiologic Changes
Accompanying Pregnancy

Physiologic Parameter	Average Change from Nonpregnant Value
Intravascular fluid volume	+35%
Plasma volume	+45%
Erythrocyte volume	+20%
Cardiac output	+40%
Stroke volume	+30%
Heart rate	+15%
Peripheral circulation	
Systolic blood pressure	No change
Systemic vascular resistance	−15%
Diastolic blood pressure	−15%
Central venous pressure	No change
Femoral venous pressure	+15%
Minute ventilation	+50%
Tidal volume	+40%
Breathing rate	+10%
PaO_2	+10 mmHg
$PaCO_2$	−10 mmHg
pHa	No change
Total lung capacity	No change
Vital capacity	No change
Functional residual capacity	−20%
Expiratory reserve volume	−20%
Residual volume	−20%
Airway resistance	−35%
Oxygen consumption	+20%
Renal blood flow and glomerular filtration rate	−50%
Serum cholinesterase activity	−25%

    4. Gastrointestinal changes during pregnancy (enlarged uterus interferes with gastric emptying, and progesterone prolongs gastric emptying time) make parturients vulnerable to aspiration of gastric contents. Parturients tend to develop hypoglycemia more readily than nonpregnant females.

  B. Regional anesthetic techniques in parturients require an understanding of the neuronal pathways responsible for transmission of pain during labor and delivery (Fig. 31–1).

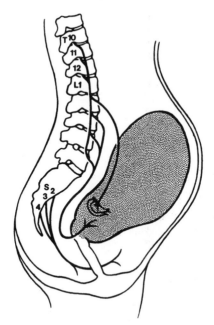

Fig. 31–1 • Pain pathways during parturition. Afferent pain impulses from the cervix and uterus are carried by nerves that accompany sympathetic nervous system fibers and enter the spinal cord at T10-L1. Pain pathways from the perineum travel to S2-4 through the pudendal nerves.

1. **Lumbar epidural.** When performing lumbar epidural techniques for provision of analgesia during labor and delivery or anesthesia for cesarean section, it is important to confirm the absence of intravascular placement of the epidural catheter ("test dose" of solutions containing local anesthetic and epinephrine, 10 to 15 μg). This test dose may be unreliable in parturients because of maternal heart rate variability (injection immediately after a uterine contraction decreases the likelihood of confusing epinephrine-induced tachycardia with pain-induced tachycardia). Hypotension caused by regional anesthesia administered to parturients during labor and

delivery may require administration of small doses of ephedrine, 5 to 10 mg IV (parturients with uteroplacental insufficiency) or phenylephrine, 20 to 100 μg IV.

2. **Combined spinal-epidural** technique provides a more rapid onset of analgesia than the lumbar epidural approach, and production of minimal motor block may permit parturients to ambulate during early labor.

II. PREGNANCY-INDUCED HYPERTENSION

Pregnancy-induced hypertension (PIH) encompasses a range of disorders collectively and formerly known as toxemia of pregnancy. It includes isolated systemic hypertension (nonproteinuric hypertension), preeclampsia (proteinuric hypertension), and eclampsia (Fig. 31–2).

A. **Gestational hypertension** is characterized by the onset of systemic hypertension, without proteinuria or edema, during the last few weeks of gestation or during the immediate postpartum period.

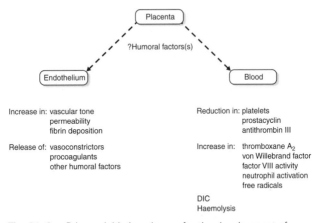

Fig. 31–2 • Primary initiating change for the development of pregnancy-induced hypertension (preeclampsia) may be placental ischemia. DIC, disseminated intravascular coagulation. (From Mushambi MC, Halligan AW, Williamson K. Recent developments in the pathophysiology of pre-eclampsia. Br J Anaesth 1996;76: 133–48. © The Board of Management and Trustees of the British Journal of Anaesthesia. Reproduced by permission of Oxford University Press/British Journal of Anaesthesia.)

B. **Preeclampsia** is a syndrome exhibited after 20 weeks of gestation manifesting as systemic hypertension, proteinuria, and generalized edema (Table 31–2).

  1. **HEELP syndrome.** Hemolysis (H), elevated liver transaminase enzymes (EL), and low platelet counts (LP) represents a severe form of preeclampsia.

     a. **Treatment** of HEELP syndrome may include urgent delivery of the fetus by cesarean section.

     b. **Management of anesthesia** and choice of regional anesthesia may be influenced by the presence of thrombocytopenia.

  2. **Pathophysiology.** Preeclampsia is a syndrome that affects virtually all maternal organ systems (Figs. 31–2, 31–3).

C. **Eclampsia** is present when seizures are superimposed on preeclampsia.

D. **Treatment** of PIH is delivery of the fetus and placenta. Until delivery is possible, treatment is based on managing

---

☰ Table 31–2 • Manifestations and Complications of Preeclampsia

Systemic hypertension (> 140/90 mmHg)
Congestive heart failure
Decreased colloid oncotic pressure
Pulmonary edema
Arterial hypoxemia
Laryngeal edema
Cerebral edema (headaches, visual disturbances, changes in level of consciousness)
Grand mal seizures
Cerebral hemorrhage
Hypovolemia
HEELP syndrome
Disseminated intravascular coagulation
Proteinuria (> 2 g daily)
Oliguria
Acute tubular necrosis
Epigastric pain
Decreased uterine blood flow
Intrauterine growth retardation
Premature labor and delivery
Abruptio placentae

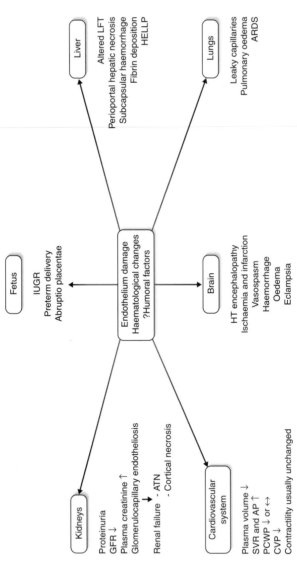

Liver

Altered LFT
Periportal hepatic necrosis
Subcapsular haemorrhage
Fibrin deposition
HELLP

Lungs

Leaky capillaries
Pulmonary oedema
ARDS

Fetus

IUGR
Preterm delivery
Abruptio placentae

Endothelium damage
Haematological changes
?Humoral factors

Brain

HT encephalopathy
Ischaemia and infarction
Vasospasm
Haemorrhage
Oedema
Eclampsia

Kidneys

Proteinuria
GFR ↓
Plasma creatinine ↑
Glomerulocapillary endotheliosis
Renal failure - ATN
                - Cortical necrosis

Cardiovascular system

Plasma volume ↓
SVR and AP ↑
PCWP ↓ or ↔
CVP ↓
Contractility usually unchanged

Fig. 31-3 • *See legend on opposite page*

≡ Table 31-3 • Treatment of Systemic Hypertension Associated with Preeclampsia

Maintain Diastolic Blood Pressure < 110 mmHg
Hydralazine 5–10 mg IV every 20–30 minutes
Hydralazine 5–20 mg/hr IV as a continuous infusion following administration of 5 mg IV
Labetalol 50 mg IV or 100 mg PO
Labetalol 20–160 mg/hr IV as a continuous infusion
Nitroglycerin 10 μg/min IV titrated to response
Nitroprusside 0.25 μg/kg/min IV titrated to response
Prevent Seizures
Magnesium 4–6 g IV followed by 1–2 g/hr IV as a continuous infusion (goal is to maintain serum concentrations of 2.0–3.5 mEq/L)
Toxicity
    4.0–6.5 mEq/L associated with nausea, vomiting, diplopia, somnolence, loss of patellar reflexes
    6.5.–7.5 mEq/L associated with skeletal muscle paralysis, apnea
    10 mEq/L or higher associated with cardiac arrest

the signs and symptoms of the secondary effects of pre-eclampsia (Table 31–3).

1. **Systemic hypertension.** Cerebral hemorrhage is a major cause of maternal death from preeclampsia and eclampsia. It may be recommended that maternal systemic blood pressure be maintained at < 170/110 mmHg and > 130/90 mmHg.

   a. **Acute treatment.** See Table 31–3.

Fig. 31–3 • Multiple organ system function changes accompany preeclampsia. AP, arterial pressure; ARDS, acute respiratory distress syndrome; ATN, acute tubular necrosis; CVP, central venous pressure; GFR, glomerular filtration rate; HEELP, hemolysis, elevated liver enzymes, low platelets; HT, hypertensive; IUGR, intrauterine growth retardation; LFT, liver function tests; PCWP, pulmonary capillary wedge pressure; SVR, systemic vascular resistance. (From Mushambi MC, Halligan AW, Williamson K. Recent developments in the pathophysiology and management of pre-eclampsia. Br J Anaesth 1996;76:133–48. © The Board of Management and Trustees of the British Journal of Anaesthesia. Reproduced by permission of Oxford University Press/British Journal of Anaesthesia.)

b. **Chronic treatment.** Many antihypertensive drugs (methyldopa, β-adrenergic antagonists, nifedipine) have been used for the chronic treatment of systemic hypertension owing to preeclampsia (angiotensin-converting enzyme inhibitors are associated with teratogenic effects on the fetus).

2. **Hypovolemia.** Correction of hypovolemia may be recommended before administration of antihypertensive drugs (crystalloids at 1–2 ml/kg/hr IV with adjustments in the infusion rate based on the patient's clinical condition, urine output, and central venous pressure measurements).

3. **Oliguria.** When oliguria persists, treatment with intravenous fluid challenges of 500 to 1000 ml of crystalloid solutions may be recommended.

4. **Seizures.** See Table 31–3.

   a. **Dose.** Magnesium sulfate is administered intravenously or intramuscularly with the goal of achieving therapeutic concentrations of 2.0 to 3.5 mEq/L (Table 31–3). Serum concentrations > 4 mEq/L may cause toxicity, which is treated with intravenous administration of calcium gluconate.

   b. **Drug interactions.** Potentiation of both depolarizing and nondepolarizing muscle relaxants by magnesium is clinically significant. Doses of sedative and opioids may be decreased, as magnesium can potentiate their effects. Deleterious effects of magnesium do not occur in nonasphyxiated full-term neonates.

E. **Management of anesthesia**

1. **Emergency cesarean section and choice of anesthesia.** The notion that time spent instituting regional anesthesia would be detrimental to the well-being of the fetus is the reason general anesthesia has been advocated for parturients requiring emergency cesarean section for fetal distress. Nevertheless, spinal and even epidural anesthesia may be established in a timely manner and thus avoid the possible depressant effects of general anesthesia drugs on the fetus and the risk of failed or difficult tracheal intubation.

2. **Epidural analgesia.** Management of anesthesia for labor and delivery in volume-repleted preeclamptic parturients is often with continuous lumbar epidural analgesia utilizing combinations of opioids (fentanyl 50 to 100 μg) and local anesthetics (ropivacaine, bupivacaine, lido-

caine) while maintaining left uterine displacement. Thrombocytopenia is common and may influence the selection of regional anesthesia in these parturients, although evidence supporting occurrence of epidural hematomas is not available. Before continuous lumbar epidural anesthesia is instituted, parturients should be hydrated (1–2 L of Ringer's lactate solution). Coagulation studies are performed before placing an epidural catheter, particularly if preeclampsia is severe.

    a. Initially, a segmental band of anesthesia (T10-L1) provides analgesia for uterine contractions.

    b. As the second stage of labor is entered, lumbar epidural analgesia can be extended to provide perineal analgesia.

3. Spinal anesthesia may be discouraged in parturients with preeclampsia because of the risk of severe hypotension (unproven notion and prehydration before performance of spinal anesthesia is desirable).

4. General anesthesia. Risks of general anesthesia in parturients with preeclampsia include potentially difficult tracheal intubation owing to laryngeal edema, potential aspiration of gastric contents, increased sensitivity to nondepolarizing muscle relaxants, exaggerated pressor responses to direct laryngoscopy and tracheal intubation, and impaired placental blood flow.

    a. Induction of anesthesia. Before induction of anesthesia (often thiopental and succinylcholine) attempts are made to restore intravascular fluid volume.

    b. Airway management. Exaggerated edema of the upper airway structures may interfere with visualization of the glottic opening, and laryngeal swelling may result in the need to insert a smaller tracheal tube than anticipated. Short-duration laryngoscopy is the most predictable method for minimizing the magnitude and duration of systemic blood pressure and heart rate responses evoked by tracheal intubation.

    c. Maintenance of anesthesia. Low doses of volatile anesthetics (0.5 to 1.0 MAC) with or without 50% nitrous oxide can be used for maintenance of anesthesia. Determinants of neonatal depression are prolonged uterine incision-to-delivery time (duration of anesthesia only important when prolonged more than 20 minutes prior to delivery). After delivery, anesthesia is typically supplemented with opioids.

III. PREGNANCY AND CO-EXISTING MEDICAL DISEASES

See Table 31–4.

A. **Eisenmenger syndrome** consists of obliterative pulmonary vascular disease with resultant pulmonary hypertension, right-to-left intracardiac shunts, and arterial hypoxemia. Pregnancy is poorly tolerated, and mortality can approach 30%.

   1. The major hazards facing parturients with Eisenmenger syndrome are decreased systemic vascular resistance (may accompany normal pregnancy and result in increased right-to-left intracardiac shunt) and thromboembolism.

   2. **Management of anesthesia.** The principle of any technique of analgesia or anesthesia chosen for patients with Eisenmenger syndrome is to avoid decreases in systemic vascular resistance or in cardiac output. The possibility of paradoxical air embolism is great.

      a. If continuous lumbar epidural techniques are selected for vaginal delivery, it is crucial that decreases in systemic vascular resistance be minimized. Epinephrine probably should not be added to local anesthetic solutions.

      b. Delivery by cesarean section is most often accomplished using general anesthesia, although epidural anesthesia has been successfully utilized. Intravenous drugs may have a more rapid onset of action, whereas the rate of increase in arterial concentrations of inhaled drugs is slowed because of decreased pulmonary blood flow. Positive-pressure ventilation may decrease pulmonary blood flow.

B. **Cocaine abuse** among parturients is associated with multiple organ system involvement, including the cardiovascular (systemic hypertension, cardiac dysrhythmias, sudden death), respiratory (asthma, dyspnea, pulmonary edema), neurologic (cerebral hemorrhage), and hematologic (thrombocytopenia) systems (Fig. 31–4). The incidence of acquired immunodeficiency syndrome (AIDS) and syphilis is increased among cocaine-abusing parturients.

   1. **Obstetric complications.** See Table 31–5.

☰ Table 31–4 • Pregnancy and Co-Existing Medical Diseases

Heart Disease (estimated to be present in 1.6% of all parturients)
Circulatory Changes and Co-Existing Heart Disease
    Increases in cardiac output during pregnancy and following delivery may result in congestive heart failure
    Analgesia provided by continuous lumbar epidural techniques can minimize adverse effects of increased cardiac output due to pain or anxiety
Mitral Stenosis (most common valvular defect)
    Increased incidence of pulmonary edema, atrial fibrillation, and paroxysmal atrial tachycardia
    Continuous lumbar epidural techniques producing segmental analgesia (minimizes undesirable effects produced by pain on heart rate and cardiac output whereas sacral analgesia prevents the parturient's urge to push and the associated adverse effects of Valsalva maneuvers on venous return)
Mitral Regurgitation (usually tolerates pregnancy well)
Aortic Regurgitation (usually develops after child-bearing years)
    Continuous lumbar epidural techniques recommended
Aortic Stenosis (usually develops after child-bearing years)
Tetralogy of Fallot
    Pain during labor and vaginal delivery may increase pulmonary vascular resistance and magnitude of right-to-left shunt
    Regional anesthesia may decrease systemic blood pressure owing to decreased systemic vascular resistance
Eisenmenger Syndrome
Coarctation of the Aorta
Primary Pulmonary Hypertension
Cardiomyopathy of Pregnancy (see Chapter 7)
Dissecting Aneurysm of the Aorta
Prosthetic Valve Replacement
    Coumarin anticoagulant is replaced with heparin
Diabetes Mellitus
Insulin requirements increase during pregnancy
Increased risk of ketoacidosis
Pregnancy-induced hypertension is common
Neonates are often large for gestational age
Regional anesthesia has advantages of avoiding hyperglycemic response to surgery and drug-induced depression of the fetus
Myasthenia Gravis
Neonatal myasthenia gravis develops in 20–30% of babies born to affected mothers
Cocaine Abuse

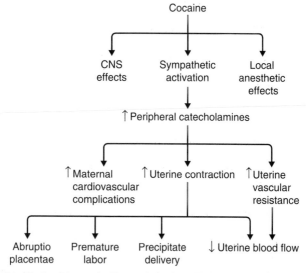

Fig. 31–4 • Maternal effects of cocaine. (From Kain ZN, Rimar S, Barash PG. Cocaine abuse in the parturient and effects on the fetus and neonate. Anesth Analg 1993;77:835–45. © 1993, Lippincott Williams & Wilkins, with permission.)

≡ **Table 31–5 • Obstetric Complications Associated with Cocaine Abuse During Pregnancy**

Spontaneous abortion
Preterm labor
Premature rupture of the membranes
Abruptio placentae
Precipitous labor
Stillbirth
Maternal hypertension
Meconium aspiration
Low Apgar scores at birth

2. **Management of anesthesia.** The single most important predictor of cocaine abuse is the absence of prenatal care. Cocaine-induced thrombocytopenia is considered if regional anesthesia is planned. Body temperature increases and sympathomimetic effects associated with cocaine may mimic malignant hyperthermia.

IV. PREGNANCY AND CO-EXISTING SURGICAL DISEASES

It is estimated that 1% to 2% of parturients in the United States undergo surgical procedures unrelated to pregnancy (pregnancy may be unrecognized at the time of surgery) (Table 31–6; Fig. 31–5).

≡ **Table 31–6** • Objectives for Management of Anesthesia in Parturients Undergoing Nonobstetric Operative Procedures

---

Maternal Safety
Recognize decreased oxygen reserves
Airway management may be difficult
Supine hypotension syndrome
Altered anesthetic requirements
Increased risk for aspiration
Avoidance of Intrauterine Fetal Hypoxia and Acidosis
Minimize maternal hypotension, arterial hypoxemia and excessive changes in $PaCO_2$
Treat hypotension with left uterine displacement, intravenous fluids, leg elevation, and ephedrine
Maternal supplemental oxygen
Avoidance of Teratogenic Drugs
Critical period of organogenesis is between 15 and 56 days
No evidence that inhaled anesthetics (including nitrous oxide), opioids, sedatives, benzodiazepines, or local anesthetics are teratogenic
No evidence that anesthetics adversely affect later mental and neurologic development
Premature Labor
No evidence that anesthetic drugs or techniques predispose to premature labor
Underlying disease and/or the site of surgery determines the likelihood of premature labor
Treatment of Premature Labor
Selective β_2-agonists
Side effects of β_2-agonists include pulmonary edema, cardiac dysrhythmias, and hypokalemia
Fetal effects include tachycardia and hypoglycemia

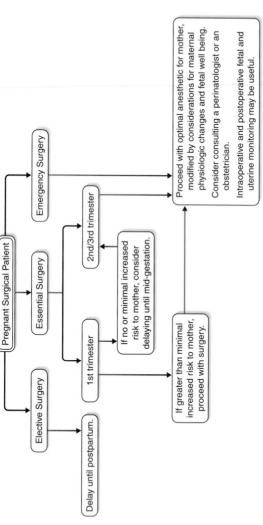

Fig. 31-5 • Recommendations for management of parturients and surgical procedures. (From Rosen MA. Management of anesthesia for the pregnant surgical patient. Anesthesiology 1999;91:1159–63. © 1999, Lippincott Williams & Wilkins, with permission.)

A. **Management of anesthesia.** Women of child-bearing age should be asked about their last menstrual period and pregnancy testing offered to avoid elective surgical procedures during early gestation. Elective surgery other than postpartum tubal ligation is deferred until about 6 weeks after delivery, when the physiologic changes of pregnancy have passed.

1. Perioperative monitoring of fetal heart rate is advocated after about 16 weeks' gestation.

2. Emergency surgery during the first trimester may be performed with regional or general anesthesia. Regardless of the anesthetic technique selected, supplemental oxygen administration is indicated.

B. **Postpartum tubal ligation** may utilize residual anesthesia from delivery (requires a T5 sensory level) thus eliminating concerns about the risk of aspiration and timing of surgery (often delay 8 to 12 hours postpartum before inducing anesthesia, although there is no demonstrable difference in gastric fluid volume and pH when parturients are studied 1 to 8 hours after vaginal delivery).

C. **In vitro fertilization.** It is unclear if nitrous oxide or other anesthetics have undesirable effects on in vitro fertilization and gamete intrafallopian transfer procedures.

V. COMPLICATIONS ASSOCIATED WITH DELIVERY

A. **Abnormal presentations and multiple births.** Description of fetal position is based on the relation of the fetal occiput, chin, or sacrum to the left or right side of the parturient (90% of deliveries are cephalic presentations in the occiput transverse or occiput anterior positions).

1. **Persistent occiput posterior** position occurs when the occiput fails to undergo internal rotation to the occiput anterior position, resulting in prolonged and painful (back pain) labor. Regional anesthetic techniques that relax the maternal perineal muscles are best avoided until spontaneous internal rotation of the fetal head occurs. Analgesia can be provided with segmental (T10-L1) lumbar epidural techniques.

2. **Breech presentation** characterizes about 3.5% of all pregnancies and is associated with increased maternal (cervical lacerations, perineal injury, retained placenta, hemorrhage) and neonatal (arterial hypoxemia, acidosis, prolapsed umbilical cord) morbidity.

    a. Cesarean delivery is often selected for delivery. During regional anesthesia, uterine hypertonus may make it difficult to extract the fetus through the uterine incision (induce general anesthesia followed by tracheal intubation, intravenous nitroglycerin).

    b. Vaginal delivery may utilize intramuscular or intravenous medications, perineal infiltration of local anesthetic solutions, or a pudendal block. Rapid induction of general anesthesia and tracheal intubation may be necessary if perineal muscle relaxation is inadequate for delivery of the after-coming fetal head or if the lower uterine segment contracts and traps the head. Continuous lumbar epidural anesthetic techniques provide analgesia and maximal perineal relaxation for delivery of the fetal head.

3. Multiple gestations. PIH, anemia, premature labor, breech presentations, retained placenta, and hemorrhage are more common with multiple gestations. The second twin is more likely to be depressed, presumably reflecting periods of fetal arterial hypoxemia and acidosis due to contraction of the uterus or premature separation of the placenta.

    a. Management of anesthesia. Considerations for the choice of anesthesia in the presence of multiple gestations are related to the frequent occurrence of prematurity and breech presentations.

    b. Continuous lumbar epidural anesthesia provides good analgesia, and perineal muscle relaxation may be useful for forceps deliveries.

B. Hemorrhage in obstetric patients. See Table 31–7.

C. Uterine rupture occurs in up to 0.1% of full-term pregnancies and may be associated with separation of previous uterine scars, rapid spontaneous delivery, excessive oxytocin stimulation, or multiple parity (more than 80% of uterine ruptures are spontaneous without an obvious explanation).

    1. Signs and symptoms. Severe abdominal pain (often referred to the shoulder owing to subdiaphragmatic irritation by intra-abdominal blood), maternal hypotension, and disappearance of fetal heart tones suggest uterine rupture.

    2. Epidural analgesia produced by dilute concentrations of local anesthetics may be utilized safely in parturients who have delivered previously by cesarean section.

≡ Table 31–7 • Hemorrhage in Obstetric Patients

Cause	Signs and Symptoms	Predisposing Conditions
Placenta previa	Painless vaginal bleeding	Advanced age Multiple parity
Abruptio placentae	Abdominal pain Bleeding partially or wholly concealed Uterine irritability Shock Coagulopathy Acute renal failure Fetal distress	Multiple parity Uterine anomalies Compression of inferior vena cava Chronic systemic hypertension
Uterine atony	Complete atony may result in 2000 ml blood loss in 5 minutes Treatment is intravenous oxytocin	Multiple parity Polyhydramnios Large fetus Retained placenta
Retained placenta	Requires uterine relaxation and manual removal of the placenta	
Asherman syndrome	Hemorrhage Placenta invades the uterine myometrium Emergency hysterectomy	

D. **Amniotic fluid embolism** is a rare catastrophic, life-threatening complication of pregnancy that occurs in the setting of a disrupted barrier between the amniotic fluid and maternal circulation. Multiparous parturients experiencing tumultuous labors are at increased risk for the occurrence of amniotic fluid embolism.

1. **Signs and symptoms.** See Table 31–8.
2. **Diagnosis** is based on clinical signs and symptoms, increased pulmonary artery pressures and decreased cardiac output, and confirmation of amniotic fluid material in the parturient's blood, as aspirated from a central venous or pulmonary artery catheter. Conditions that

---

≡ Table 31–8 • Signs and Symptoms of Amniotic Fluid Embolism

Dyspnea
Arterial hypoxemia
Seizures
Loss of consciousness
Hypotension
Cardiopulmonary arrest
Coagulopathy (resembles disseminated intravascular coagulation and may be only presenting symptom)
Acute cor pulmonale

---

can mimic amniotic fluid embolism include pulmonary aspiration, pulmonary embolism, venous air embolism, local anesthetic toxicity, and high sensory levels produced by spinal or epidural anesthesia (Table 31–9).

3. **Treatment.** See Table 31–10.

VI. DIAGNOSIS AND MANAGEMENT OF FETAL DISTRESS

A. Fetal distress due to intrauterine hypoxia and acidosis is most likely to occur when uterine blood flow decreases with each contraction.

B. **Electronic fetal monitoring** permits evaluation of fetal well-being by following changes in fetal heart rate, as recorded using an external monitor (Doppler) or fetal scalp electrode. Fetal scalp sampling is indicated when abnormal fetal heart rate patterns persist (pH near 7.0 is usually associated with fetal depression).

1. **Beat-to-beat variability.** Fetal heart rate varies 5 to 20 beats/min, with a normal rate of 120 to 160 beats/min. Fetal distress due to arterial hypoxemia, acidosis, or central nervous system damage is associated with minimal to absent beat-to-beat variability.

2. **Early decelerations.** See Figure 31–6.

3. **Late decelerations.** See Figure 31–7.

4. **Variable decelerations.** See Figure 31–8.

Table 31-9 • Differential Diagnosis of Amniotic Fluid Embolism

Signs and Symptoms	Amniotic Fluid Embolism	High Epidural	Total Spinal
Oxygenation	Arterial hypoxemia Not responsive to oxygen	Arterial hypoxemia Responsive to oxygen	Arterial hypoxemia Responsive to oxygen
Ventilation	Hypoventilation Respiratory distress Cough	Hypoventilation Respiratory distress Cannot cough	Hypoventilation Respiratory distress Cannot cough
Onset	Sudden onset Coincident with open uterine veins	Slow onset	Fast onset
Central nervous system	Loss of consciousness Agitation Seizures	Awake Some agitation No seizures	Loss of consciousness No movement No seizures
Cardiovascular system	Profound shock Difficult to resuscitate Cardiac arrest common Pulmonary hypertension Left and right heart failure Increased central venous pressure	Normal to decreased systemic blood pressure Easy to resuscitate Cardiac arrest uncommon Normal pulmonary artery pressures Normal cardiac function Increased central venous pressure	Normal to decreased systemic blood pressure Easy to resuscitate Cardiac arrest uncommon Normal pulmonary artery pressures Normal cardiac function Increased central venous pressure
Coagulation	Disseminated intravascular coagulation	Normal	Normal

Adapted from: Noble WH, St-Amand J. Amniotic fluid embolus. Can J Anaesth 1993;40:971–80.

Table 31–10 • Treatment of Amniotic Fluid Embolism

Tracheal intubation

Mechanical ventilation with 100% oxygen (positive end-expiratory pressure may improve oxygenation)

Inotropic support as guided by central venous pressure monitoring (dopamine, dobutamine, norepinephrine)

Correction of coagulopathy (fresh frozen plasma, cryoprecipitate, platelets)

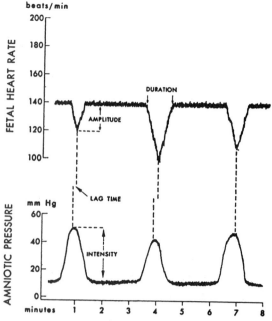

Fig. 31–6 • Early decelerations of the fetal heart rate are characterized by a short lag time between the onset of uterine contractions and the beginning of fetal heart rate slowing. Maximum heart rate slowing is usually < 20 beats/min and occurs at the peak intensity of the contraction. Heart rate returns to normal by the time the contraction has ceased. The most likely explanation for this early deceleration is a vagal reflex response to compression of the fetal head. (From Shnider SM. Diagnosis of fetal distress: fetal heart rate. In: Shnider SM, editor. Obstetric Anesthesia: Current Concepts and Practice. Baltimore, Williams & Wilkins, 1970;197–203, with permission.)

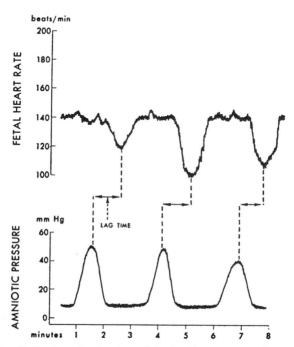

Fig. 31–7 • Late decelerations of the fetal heart rate are characterized by a delay (lag time) between the onset of the uterine contraction and the beginning of fetal heart rate slowing. The fetal heart rate does not return to normal until after the contraction has ceased. A mild late deceleration pattern is present when slowing is < 20 beats/min, profound slowing is present when fetal heart slows > 40 beats/min. Late fetal heart rate decelerations indicate fetal distress owing to uteroplacental insufficiency. (From Shnider SM. Diagnosis of fetal distress: fetal heart rate. In: Shnider SM, editor. Obstetrical Anesthesia: Current Concepts and Practice. Baltimore, Wilkins & Wilkins, 1970;197–203, with permission.)

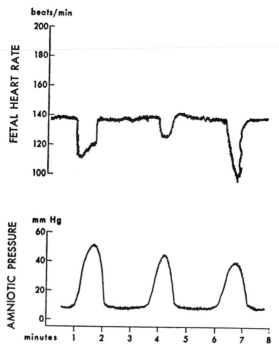

Fig. 31–8 • Variable decelerations of the fetal heart rate are characterized by decreases in the heart rate of varying magnitude and duration that do not show a consistent relation to uterine contractions. This pattern of fetal heart rate slowing is associated with umbilical cord compression. (From Shnider SM. Diagnosis of fetal distress: fetal heart rate. In: Shnider SM, editor. Obstetrical Anesthesia: Current Concepts and Practice. Baltimore, Williams & Wilkins, 1970;197–203, with permission.)

VII. EVALUATION OF THE NEONATE

A. The importance of assessment immediately after birth is to identify promptly any depressed neonate who requires active resuscitation.

B. Apgar score. As a guide to identifying and treating depressed neonates, the Apgar score has not been surpassed (Table 31–11).

VIII. IMMEDIATE NEONATAL PERIOD

See Table 31–12.

Table 31–11 • Evaluation of Neonates Using the Apgar Score

Parameter	0	1	2
Heart rate (beats/min)	Absent	< 100	> 100
Respiratory effort	Absent	Slow Irregular	Crying
Reflex irritability	No response	Grimace	Crying
Muscle tone	Limp	Flexion of extremities	Active
Color	Pale, cyanotic	Body pink, extremities cyanotic	Pink

☰ Table 31–12 • Abnormalities Present at Birth or Manifesting Shortly after Delivery

Meconium Aspiration
Arterial hypoxemia
Pulmonary hypertension
Persistent fetal circulation
Pneumothorax
Treatment is oropharyngeal suctioning at the time of delivery;
  tracheal intubation and suctioning are performed selectively
  (those with Apgar scores > 7 are managed conservatively)
Choanal Stenosis and Atresia
Absent air entry despite breathing efforts
Unable to pass a catheter through each naris
Oral airway may be necessary
Functional atresia is due to blood, mucus, or meconium (treat
  with nasal suctioning)
Heroin may cause congestion of the nasal mucosa
Diaphragmatic Hernia
Respiratory distress at birth, cyanosis, and scaphoid abdomen
Tracheal intubation (attempts to reexpand the ipsilateral lung may
  result in pneumothorax)
Hypovolemia
Mean arterial pressure < 50 mmHg
Hypoglycemia
Hypotension, tremors, seizures
Tracheoesophageal Fistula
Suspect when polyhydramnios is present
Catheter cannot be passed into the stomach
Laryngeal Anomalies
Stridor at birth
Pierre Robin Syndrome
Glossoptosis and micrognathia
Respiratory obstruction when tongue is sucked against the
  posterior pharyngeal wall (insert an oral airway or pull tongue
  forward with a clamp)
Prone position may be helpful
Do not administer muscle relaxants

32

Diseases Presenting in Pediatric Patients

Pediatric patients present unique anatomic, physiologic, and pharmacologic considerations for the management of anesthesia in the presence of disorders that occur exclusively or with increased frequency in this age group (Stoelting RK, Dierdorf SF. Diseases presenting in pediatric patients. In: Anesthesia and Co-Existing Disease, 4th ed New York, Churchill Livingstone, 2001;687–737). Neonates (up to 28 days of age) and infants (1 to 6 months of age) comprise the age groups in which differences from adults are most marked.

I. UNIQUE CONSIDERATIONS IN PEDIATRIC PATIENTS

A. **Airway anatomy.** The large head and tongue, mobile epiglottis, and anterior position of the larynx characteristic of neonates makes tracheal intubation easier with the neonate's head in a neutral or slightly flexed position than with the head extended. The cricoid cartilage is the narrowest portion of the larynx in pediatric patients and necessitates selection of tracheal tubes that minimize the risk of trauma to the airway and subsequent development of subglottic edema.

B. **Physiology.** Physiologic differences between children and adults are important determinants when planning management of anesthesia in pediatric patients.

1. **Respiratory system.** See Table 32–1. The single most important difference that distinguishes pediatric patients physiologically from adult patients is oxygen consumption.

2. **Cardiovascular system.** Neonates are highly dependent on the heart rate for maintenance of cardiac output and systemic blood pressure.

3. **Distribution of body water.** Extracellular fluid volume (ECF) is equivalent to about 40% of body weight in neonates compared with about 20% in adults (similar

▬ Table 32-1 • Mean Pulmonary Function Values

Parameter	Neonates (3 kg)	Adults (70 kg)
Oxygen consumption (ml/kg/min)	6.4	3.5
Alveolar ventilation (ml/kg/min)	130	60
Carbon dioxide production (ml/kg/min)	6	3
Tidal volume (ml/kg)	6	6
Breathing frequency (min)	35	15
Vital capacity (ml/kg)	35	70
Functional residual capacity (ml/kg)	30	35
Tracheal length (cm)	5.5	12
PaO_2 (mmHg)	65–85	85–95
$PaCO_2$ (mmHg)	30–36	36–44
pH	7.34–7.40	7.36–7.44

in children and adults after 18 to 24 months). Intraoperative fluid replacement may be considered as maintenance fluids (often glucose-containing solutions) and replacement fluids (Table 32–2).

4. **Renal function.** Glomerular filtrations rate is greatly decreased in term neonates but increases nearly fourfold by 3 to 5 weeks.

▬ Table 32-2 • Intraoperative Fluid Therapy in Pediatric Patients

Surgical Procedure	5% Glucose in Lactated Ringer's (ml/kg/hr)		
	Maintenance	Replacement	Total
Minor surgery (herniorrhaphy)	4	2	6
Moderate surgery (pyloromyotomy)	4	4	8
Extensive surgery (bowel resection)	4	6	10

   5. **Hematology.** See Table 32–3.
   6. **Thermoregulation.** Neonates and infants are vulnerable to development of hypothermia during the perioperative period. Steps designed to decrease loss of body heat include transporting neonates in heated modules, increasing the ambient temperature of operating rooms, and humidifying and warming inspired gases.
C. **Pharmacology**
   1. **Anesthetic requirements.** See Figure 32–1.
   2. **Muscle relaxants.** Infants may be more sensitive to the effects of nondepolarizing muscle relaxants, but the relatively large volumes of distribution result in calculation of initial doses similar to those for adults. Neonates and infants require more succinylcholine on a body weight basis than do older children to produce comparable degrees of neuromuscular blockade.
D. **Pharmacokinetics.** Uptake of inhaled anesthetics is more rapid in infants than in older children or adults (reflects the infant's high alveolar ventilation relative to their functional residual capacity). More rapid uptake may unmask negative inotropic effects of volatile anesthetics resulting in an increased incidence of hypotension in neonates and infants (decreased margin of safety).
E. **Monitoring.** Decreased cardiovascular reserves, altered anesthetic requirements, and exaggerated hypotensive responses during general anesthesia make monitoring the

≡ **Table 32–3** • Normal Hemogram Values in Neonates, Infants, and Children

Age	Hemoglobin (g/dl)	Hematocrit (%)	Leukocytes (cells/mm³)
1 Day	19.0	61	18,000
2 Weeks	17.3	54	12,000
1 Month	14.2	43	
2 Months	10.7	31	
6 Months	12.3	36	10,000
1 Year	11.6	35	
6 Years	12.7	38	
10–12 Years	13.0	39	8,000

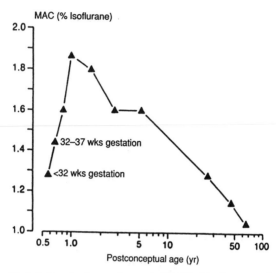

Fig. 32-1 • Anesthetic requirements (MAC) of isoflurane and postconceptual age. [From LeDez KM, Lerman J. The minimum alveolar concentration (MAC) of isoflurane in preterm neonates. Anesthesiology 1987;67:301–7, with permission.]

systemic blood pressure especially important in neonates and infants during the perioperative period. Blood sampled from an artery that arises distal to the ductus arteriosus (left radial artery, umbilical artery, posterior tibial artery) may not accurately reflect the PaO_2 being delivered to the retina or brain in the presence of a patent ductus arteriosus. Monitoring body temperature is useful during the perioperative period to detect the development of hypothermia as well as the rare patient manifesting malignant hyperthermia. Small tidal volumes in neonates and infants may result in dilution of end-tidal carbon dioxide concentrations measured by capnography.

II. NEONATAL MEDICAL DISEASES

See Table 32–4.

A. Respiratory distress syndrome (RDS) is responsible for 50% to 75% of deaths that occur in preterm infants, re-

≡ Table 32–4 • Neonatal Medical Diseases

Respiratory distress syndrome
Bronchopulmonary dysplasia
Intracranial hemorrhage
Retinopathy of prematurity
Apneic spells
Sudden infant death syndrome
Kernicterus
Hypoglycemia
Sepsis

flecting deficiencies in alveoli of surface-active phospholipids known as surfactant. Antenatal corticosteroids may accelerate maturation of the fetal lungs and prevent the development of RDS in preterm neonates.

1. **Management of anesthesia** includes maintenance of oxygenation as confirmed by monitoring the PaO_2 in a preductal artery (pulse oximetry is an alternative).

2. Pneumothorax is an ever-present danger and should be considered if oxygenation deteriorates abruptly in neonates being treated for RDS.

B. **Bronchopulmonary dysplasia** is a chronic pulmonary disorder (increased airway reactivity, decreased pulmonary compliance, ventilation-to-perfusion mismatch) that usually afflicts children with a history of RDS.

1. **Management of anesthesia** includes tracheal intubation, delivery of increased inspired concentrations of oxygen, and mechanical ventilation of the lungs.

2. The possible presence of airway hyperreactivity suggests the need to establish a surgical level of anesthesia before instrumentation of the airway is initiated.

C. **Intracranial hemorrhage**

1. **Periventricular-intraventricular hemorrhage** is a risk in premature newborns. Ultrasonographic scanning and computed tomography are useful for identifying periventricular-intraventricular hemorrhage.

2. **Management of anesthesia** includes avoidance of arterial hypoxemia and hypercapnia and maintenance of systolic blood pressure within the normal range.

D. **Retinopathy of prematurity** is probably due to multiple interacting factors, the most significant being prematurity (weighing < 1500 g). Arterial hyperoxia is an important risk factor, but prematurity must also be present. The risk of retinopathy is negligible in infants > 44 weeks postconceptual age.

   1. **Management of anesthesia** in susceptible infants may include attempts to maintain the PaO_2 between 60 and 80 mmHg (dilute delivered oxygen concentrations with nitrous oxide and/or room air).

   2. Attempts to prevent arterial hyperoxia must be tempered with the realization that arterial hypoxemia can result in irreversible brain damage.

E. **Apnea spells** (cessation of breathing that lasts at least 30 seconds and produces cyanosis and bradycardia) occurs in an estimated 20% to 30% of preterm neonates during the first month of life. Inguinal hernia and incarceration of an inguinal hernia are common in preterm infants.

   1. **Management of anesthesia.** Inhaled and injected anesthetics affect the control of breathing and contribute to upper airway obstruction, thereby increasing the likelihood of apneic spells during the postoperative period, especially in preterm infants < 60 weeks postconceptual age.

   2. Preterm infants with a history of apneic spells are probably not suitable candidates for outpatient surgery.

F. **Sudden infant death syndrome** (SIDS) is the most frequent cause of death in infants 1 to 2 months of age. There is no evidence that general anesthesia triggers SIDS.

G. **Kernicterus** is the term applied to a syndrome caused by the toxic effects of unconjugated bilirubin on the central nervous system (hypertonicity, opisthotonos, spasticity). **Treatment** of hyperbilirubinemia includes phototherapy (converts bilirubin to photobilirubin), exchange blood transfusions, and drugs.

H. **Hypoglycemia.** In contrast to adults, neonates have poorly developed systems for maintaining adequate serum glucose concentrations and therefore are susceptible to the development of hypoglycemia (irritability, seizures, bradycardia, hypotension, apnea). Manifestations of hypoglycemia may be masked by anesthetic drugs.

I. **Hypocalcemia.** Fetal calcium stores are largely achieved during the last trimester of gestation (preterm neonates may be susceptible to hypocalcemia).

J. **Sepsis** in neonates may reflect an immature immune system. Suggestive signs of sepsis in neonates include lethargy, skeletal muscle hypotonia, hypoglycemia, and ventilatory distress. Common sequelae of untreated neonatal sepsis include meningitis and disseminated intravascular coagulation.

III. NEONATAL SURGICAL DISEASES

Neonatal surgical diseases may require life-saving surgery or be best managed by stabilizing the neonate followed by corrective surgery (Table 32–5).

A. **Congenital diaphragmatic hernia** is characterized by pulmonary hypoplasia due to intrauterine compression of the developing lungs by the herniated viscera through incomplete embryologic closure of the diaphragm. Death is most often due to pulmonary hypoplasia or persistent pulmonary hypertension.

1. **Signs and symptoms.** See Table 32–6.
2. **Treatment.** See Table 32–7.
3. **Management of anesthesia.** See Table 32–8.
4. **Postoperative management.** Postoperative ventilation of the lungs is required by almost all neonates with congenital diaphragmatic hernia. The prognosis of these neonates is ultimately determined by the degree of pulmonary hypoplasia. Sudden deterioration with profound arterial hypoxemia and metabolic acidosis may reflect the reappearance of fetal circulation patterns (right-to-left shunting through the foramen ovale and ductus arteriosus).

≡ Table 32–5 • Neonatal Surgical Diseases

Congenital diaphragmatic hernia
Esophageal atresia
Abdominal wall defects
Omphalocele
Gastroschisis
Hirschsprung's disease
Pyloric stenosis
Necrotizing enterocolitis
Congenital hyperinsulinism
Lobar emphysema

≡ **Table 32–6** • Signs and Symptoms of Congenital Diaphragmatic Hernia

Scaphoid abdomen
Barrel-shaped chest
Bowel sounds in chest (auscultation)
Arterial hypoxemia (right-to-left shunting via the ductus arteriosus as a manifestation of persistent fetal circulation)
Loops of intestine in chest (chest radiographs)
Increased incidence of congenital heart disease

B. **Esophageal atresia** affects about 1 in 4000 neonates, with the most common form of the disorder manifesting as a blind upper esophageal pouch and a distal esophagus that forms a tracheoesophageal fistula. About 20% of neonates with esophageal atresia have major co-existing cardiovascular anomalies (ventricular septal defect, tetralogy of Fallot, coarctation of the aorta, atrial septal defect), and 30% to 40% are born preterm.

1. **Signs and symptoms.** Diagnosis of esophageal atresia is usually made soon after birth, when an oral catheter cannot be passed into the stomach or when neonates exhibit cyanosis and coughing during oral feedings (aspiration is common).

2. **Treatment** is ligation of the defect and primary anastomosis of the esophageal segments by an extrapleural approach (may be staged if premature and significant anomalies or pneumonitis are present).

3. **Management of anesthesia.** Proper placement of the tracheal tube above the carina but below the tracheo-

≡ **Table 32–7** • Treatment of Congenital Diaphragmatic Hernia

Decompression of the stomach
Supplemental oxygen (avoid positive-pressure ventilation)
Awake tracheal intubation [avoid excessive airway pressures ($> 25–30$ cmH$_2$O can result in pneumothorax)]
Preoperative stabilization (may include extracorporeal membrane oxygenation, permissive hypercapnia)

▬ Table 32–8 • Management of Anesthesia for Patients with Congenital Diaphragmatic Hernia

Awake tracheal intubation after preoxygenation

Cannulate preductal artery (right radial or temporal artery) for monitoring systemic blood pressure, blood gases, and pH

Nitrous oxide avoided

Opioids plus muscle relaxants may be alternatives to inhaled drugs

Monitor airway pressures (maintained at < 25–30 cmH$_2$O to minimize the risk of pneumothorax)

Attempts to expand the hypoplastic lung following reduction of the hernia may result in damage to the normal lung

Anticipate underdeveloped abdominal cavity (tight abdominal closures may cause cephalad displacement of the diaphragm, decreased functional residual capacity, and compression of the inferior vena cava)

---

esophageal fistual is critical (confirm with a pediatric fiberoptic bronchoscope). If nitrous oxide is not administered, it may be necessary to dilute the concentrations of oxygen delivered to neonates with air to avoid arterial hyperoxia and the risk of retinopathy of prematurity. Decreased tracheal cartilage may manifest as tracheal collapse when tracheal extubation is performed.

C. **Abdominal wall defects**

1. **Omphalocele** manifests as external herniation of abdominal viscera through the base of the umbilical cord (high incidence of prematurity and congenital defects including cardiac anomalies).

2. **Gastroschisis** manifests as external herniation of abdominal viscera through a defect in the anterior abdominal wall (high incidence of prematurity but rarely associated with other congenital anomalies).

3. **Preoperative preparation** includes prevention of infections and minimization of fluid and heat loss from exposed abdominal viscera (hypovolemia is evidenced by hemoconcentration and metabolic acidosis).

4. **Management of anesthesia.** Important aspects of managing anesthesia for treatment of omphalocele and gastroschisis include maintenance of body temperature and

continuation of fluid replacement. Awake tracheal intubation after decompression of the stomach is often recommended. If nitrous oxide is not used, delivered concentrations of oxygen are adjusted by dilution with air, as these often preterm neonates are vulnerable to the development of retinopathy of prematurity. Muscle relaxants are used judiciously, as excessive skeletal muscle relaxation may make it difficult to determine whether primary surgical abdominal wall closure is feasible.

D. **Hirschsprung's disease** is characterized by the absence of ganglion cells in the rectum. Surgical treatment is designed to bring ganglionated bowel down to the anus through a transanal or combined abdominoperoneal approach.

E. **Imperforate anus** is often associated with other congenital anomalies, especially genitourinary abnormalities and a tethered spinal cord.

F. **Pyloric stenosis** generally manifests in male infants 2 to 5 weeks of age.

1. **Signs and symptoms.** Pyloric stenosis is characterized by persistent vomiting, resulting in the loss of hydrogen ions from the stomach (dehydration and hypokalemic, hypochloremic, metabolic alkalosis).

2. **Treatment.** Surgical treatment of pyloric stenosis is not an emergency (treat initially with intravenous fluids to correct electrolyte abnormalities).

3. **Management of anesthesia.** Pulmonary aspiration of gastric fluid is a risk in infants with pyloric stenosis (risk is increased if there was prior radiographic examination of the gastrointestinal tract using barium).

4. **Postoperative management.** Postoperative depression of ventilation often occurs in infants with pyloric stenosis.

G. **Necrotizing enterocolitis** is primarily a disease of small preterm infants. It is characterized by hypoperfusion of the gastrointestinal tract with subsequent mucosal and bowel wall ischemia.

1. **Signs and symptoms.** The most common initial signs of necrotizing enterocolitis are abdominal distension and bloody feces. RDS requiring mechanical ventilation of the neonate's lungs frequently co-exists.

2. **Treatment.** Medical treatment (decompression, intravenous fluids, antibiotics) is often successful, with surgery reserved for neonates in whom sepsis, bowel perforation, and progressive metabolic acidosis occur.

3. **Management of anesthesia.** Neonates with necrotizing enterocolitis are frequently hypovolemic and require vigorous fluid resuscitation with crystalloid and colloid solutions before induction of anesthesia. Volatile anesthetics can produce significant hypotension in these neonates, particularly if hypovolemia is present. Nitrous oxide should be avoided, as it may increase the size of gas bubbles in the mesenteric veins and the portal venous system. Postoperative mechanical ventilation of the neonate's lungs is usually required.

H. **Congenital hyperinsulinism,** characterized by excessive secretion of insulin (diffuse involvement of pancreatic beta cells or focal adenomatous islet cell hyperplasia), is the most common cause of recurrent hypoglycemia in neonates.

I. **Lobar emphysema** may be congenital (hypoplasia of supporting cartilage) or acquired (mucous plugs, vascular compression of bronchi).

1. **Signs and symptoms.** The overdistended lobe produces compression atelectasis of normal lung tissues, mediastinal shift, and impaired venous blood return, with subsequent arterial hypoxemia and hypotension.

2. **Management of anesthesia** for surgical lobectomy in the treatment of lobar emphysema must consider cardiovascular and pulmonary changes that can occur with mechanical ventilation of the lungs (positive-pressure ventilation of the lungs before the chest is open may cause rapid expansion of emphysematous lobes as gas enters but cannot leave, with sudden mediastinal shifts and cardiac arrest).

IV. INTRAUTERINE FETAL SURGERY

Intrauterine fetal surgery may be performed if a congenital malformation is life-threatening (surgical repair of myelomeningocele before 25 weeks of gestation may preserve neurologic function).

V. MINIMALLY INVASIVE SURGERY

Minimally invasive surgery has the advantages of less likelihood of adhesion formation, decreased postoperative pain, more rapid recovery, and shorter hospitalization.

VI. TRAUMA

Trauma is the leading cause of death in children more than 1 year of age (blunt head trauma from motor vehicle accidents).

Most preventable deaths are due to airway obstruction, pneumothorax, intra-abdominal bleeding, or an expanding intracranial hematoma.

VII. NERVOUS SYSTEM

See Table 32–9.

VIII. CRANIOFACIAL ABNORMALITIES

A. **Cleft lip and palate** are often associated with other congenital anomalies (heart disease), deglutition abnormalities (pulmonary aspiration), respiratory tract infections (chronic otitis media), and anemia (poor nutrition).

1. **Treatment** of cleft lip is cheiloplasty at 2 to 3 months of age and for cleft palate is palatoplasty performed at about 18 months of age.

2. **Management of anesthesia.** Induction of anesthesia is influenced by the degree of airway abnormality [intravenous injection of sedative drugs followed by muscle

---

≡ Table 32–9 • Diseases of the Nervous System that Afflict Pediatric Patients

Cerebral palsy [symptom complex rather than a specific disease; describes a group of nonprogressive but often changing motor impairment syndromes (skeletal muscle spasticity); high incidence of epilepsy and cognitive disorders; risk of gastroesophageal reflux and intraoperative hypothermia; succinylcholine does not evoke excessive potassium release]

Hydrocephalus (obstructive or nonobstructive; possibility of increased intracranial pressure; air embolism a risk during shunt insertion)

Myelomeningocele (increased incidence of latex allergy, succinylcholine acceptable)

Craniostenosis (possibility of increased intracranial pressure; blood loss likely with corrective surgery)

Epilepsy (see Chapter 17)

Down syndrome (atlantoaxial instability and congenital heart disease are considerations)

Neurofibromatosis (see Chapter 17)

Reye syndrome (increased intracranial pressure, coagulopathy, liver failure)

relaxants versus administration of volatile anesthetics and tracheal intubation during spontaneous ventilation (Pierre Robin)].

    a. Maintenance of anesthesia is most often accomplished with volatile anesthetics plus nitrous oxide (presence of associated congenital heart disease may influence drug selections). It is likely that the surgical site will be infiltrated with local anesthetic solutions containing epinephrine. A high index of suspicion for accidental dislodgement of the tube from the trachea must be maintained during the operative procedure.

    b. Postoperative care. Postoperative airway problems are common following palatoplasty surgery (edema resulting in upper airway obstruction) and may require tracheal intubation following completion of the surgery.

B. Mandibular hypoplasia is a prominent feature of several syndromes affecting pediatric patients (Pierre-Robin syndrome, Treacher Collins syndrome, Goldenhar syndrome, Nager syndrome) in which the small mandible leaves little room for the tongue and makes the larynx appear to be anterior (upper airway obstruction and difficult tracheal intubation are likely to result).

    1. Preoperative evaluation for children with severe mandibular hypoplasia begins with evaluation of the upper airway and formulation of plans for tracheal intubation. The cardiovascular system is assessed and the hemoglobin concentration measured.

    2. Tracheal intubation. Administration of muscle relaxants to these patients is not recommended until the tracheal tube is in place. Fiberoptic tracheal intubation accomplished after induction of anesthesia with volatile anesthetics (sevoflurane) is acceptable provided a patent upper airway can be maintained. Regardless of the approach selected, alternative methods must be immediately available (cricothyrotomy, tracheostomy). Tracheal extubation following surgery is delayed until these patients are fully awake and alert.

C. Hypertelorism is an increased distance between the eyes and is associated with many craniofacial anomalies (Crouzon's disease, Apert syndrome).

    1. Treatment is surgical (mandibular osteotomies, craniotomy, maxillary osteotomies, rib grafts) and requires several hours for completion.

    2. Management of anesthesia. See Table 32–10.

▬ Table 32–10 • Management of Anesthesia for
Surgical Correction of Hypertelorism

Consider elective tracheostomy
Excessive blood loss (averages 1.2 blood volumes, decrease
  blood loss by placing patient in 15–20 degrees of head-up tilt;
  controlled hypotension utilizing nitroprusside)
Hypothermia (warm blood)
Peripheral nerve injury (especially ulnar neuropathy)
Intracranial hypertension (maintain $PaCO_2$ at 30–35 mmHg;
  consider nitrous oxide and opioids for maintenance of
  anesthesia)
Intra-arterial monitoring of systemic blood pressure
Corneal abrasions (ocular proptosis)
Invasive monitoring
Postoperative mechanical ventilation of the lungs (do not attempt
  to reverse opioids or muscle relaxants)

IX. DISORDERS OF THE UPPER AIRWAY

See Table 32–11.

A. Acute epiglottitis (supraglottitis) is a short-lived disease
that usually presents with characteristic signs and symptoms (Table 32–12). Although children are most often affected, acute epiglottitis may also present in adults.

1. **Diagnosis.** Acute epiglottitis is a medical emergency,
and the diagnosis is based principally on clinical signs.
Attempts to visualize the epiglottis should not be undertaken, as any instrumentation, even a tongue blade,

---

▬ Table 32–11 • Disorders of the
Upper Airway

Acute epiglottitis (supraglottitis)
Laryngotracheobronchitis
Postintubation laryngeal edema
Foreign body aspiration
Laryngeal papillomatosis
Lung abscess

■ Table 32–12 • Clinical Features of Acute Epiglottitis (Supraglottitis) and Laryngotracheobronchitis

Parameter	Acute Epiglottitis	Laryngotracheo-bronchitis
Age group affected	2–8 years (most often in boys)	< 2 years
Incidence	Accounts for 5% of children with stridor	Accounts for about 80% of children with stridor
Etiologic agent	Bacterial (*Haemophilus influenzae*)	Viral
Onset	Rapid over 24 hours	Gradual over 24–72 hours
Signs and symptoms	Inspiratory stridor Pharyngitis Drooling Fever (often > 39°C) Lethargic to restless Insists on sitting up and leaning forward Tachypnea Cyanosis	Inspiratory stridor "Barking" cough Rhinorrhea Fever (rarely > 39°C)
Laboratory results	Neutrophilia	Lymphocytosis
Lateral radiographs of the neck	Swollen epiglottitis	Narrowing of the subglottic area
Treatment	Oxygen Urgent tracheal intubation or tracheostomy during general anesthesia Fluids Antibiotics Corticosteroids (?)	Oxygen Aerosolized racemic epinephrine Humidity Fluids Corticosteroids Tracheal intubation for severe airway obstruction

may provoke laryngospasm. Unless acute respiratory distress is present, a lateral view chest radiograph is obtained.

2. **Treatment.** When airway obstruction is impending, it is common to bring the child to the operating room where preparations are completed for tracheal intubation and possible emergency tracheostomy. Definitive treatment of acute epiglottitis includes administering antibiotics (ampicillin) and establishing a secure airway until inflammation of the epiglottis has subsided. Management of adult acute epiglottitis is similar to that for children, although the routine need for tracheal intubation in adults is unclear.

3. **Management of anesthesia.** See Table 32–13.

B. **Laryngotracheobronchitis** (croup) is a viral infection of the upper respiratory tract that usually presents with characteristic signs and symptoms (Table 32–12).

1. **Treatment** of laryngotracheobronchitis includes administration of supplemental oxygen and racemic epinephrine as well as humidification of inspired gases. Administration of corticosteroids is of unproven efficacy.

2. Tracheal intubation is required if physical exhaustion occurs, as evidenced by increased $PaCO_2$.

C. **Postintubation laryngeal edema** is a potential complication of tracheal intubation in all children, although the incidence is highest in children 1 to 4 years of age.

≡ Table 32–13 • Management of Anesthesia in the Presence of Acute Epiglottitis

Place an intravenous catheter (consider administration of anticholinergic drugs)
Preparation for emergency cricothyrotomy or tracheostomy
Induction of anesthesia with volatile anesthetics (halothane, sevoflurane)
Direct laryngoscopy for tracheal intubation (and confirmation of diagnosis) when adequate depth of anesthesia is achieved
Replace orotracheal tube with a nasotracheal tube
Consider tracheal extubation (in the operating room) when evidence that edema has subsided (air leak around tracheal tube)

1. Predisposing factors include mechanical trauma to the child's upper airway during tracheal intubation and placing a tube that produces a tight fit (no air leak around the tube with the positive airway pressure equivalent to 15 to 25 cmH$_2$O).

2. **Treatment** of postintubation laryngeal edema is with humidification of the inspired gases and hourly administration of aerosolized racemic epinephrine until symptoms subside [0.05 ml/kg (maximum 0.5 ml) in 2.0 ml of saline]. The efficacy of corticosteroids is unproven.

D. **Foreign body aspiration** into the airways, with its resultant airway obstruction, can produce a wide range of responses (asphyxiation to asymptomatic). Children 1 to 3 years of age are most susceptible to foreign body aspiration.

1. **Signs and symptoms** of foreign body aspiration include cough, wheezing, and decreased air entry into the affected lung (may mimic upper respiratory tract infections, asthma, or pneumonia). If the aspirated foreign body is radiolucent, indirect evidence can be obtained by demonstrating hyperinflation of the affected lung with atelectasis distal to the foreign body.

2. **Treatment** for aspirated foreign bodies requires endoscopic removal utilizing fiberoptic bronchoscopy, ideally within 24 hours of aspiration.

3. **Management of anesthesia.** Techniques for induction of anesthesia depend on the severity of airway obstruction. When airway obstruction is present, induction of anesthesia using only volatile anesthetics such as sevoflurane in oxygen is useful. There is no evidence that the method of ventilation (spontaneous versus positive pressure) influences the outcomes during and following bronchial or tracheal foreign body removal. Skeletal muscle paralysis produced with succinylcholine or short-acting nondepolarizing muscle relaxants may be required for removal of the bronchoscope and foreign body if the object is too large to pass through the moving vocal cords.

   a. Complications that may occur during bronchoscopy include airway obstruction, fragmentation of the foreign body, arterial hypoxemia, and hypercapnia. Trauma to the tracheobronchial tree from the foreign body and instrumentation can result in subglottic edema.

    b. Chest radiographs should be obtained after bronchoscopy for detection of atelectasis or pneumothorax.

E. Laryngeal papillomatosis may require surgical therapy with laser coagulation (necessitates skeletal muscle paralysis to produce quiescent vocal cords and precautions against airway fires).

F. Lung abscess may require surgical drainage using an anesthetic technique that incorporates a double-lumen tracheal tube or bronchial blocker.

G. Jeune syndrome is an inherited disorder characterized by deformity of the chest wall leading to ventilatory failure (asphyxiating thoracic dystrophy).

X. MALIGNANT HYPERTHERMIA

Malignant hyperthermia is a pharmacogenetic disease that does not manifest until genetically susceptible patients are exposed to triggering drugs (volatile anesthetics) or stressful environmental factors. It is presumed that a defect in calcium release channels (ryanodine receptors) results in susceptibility to malignant hyperthermia. Malignant hyperthermia has an estimated incidence of 1 in 12,000 pediatric anesthesias and 1 in 40,000 adult anesthesias. Two-thirds of malignant hyperthermia-susceptible patients manifest this syndrome during their first general anesthesia.

A. Signs and symptoms. There are no clinical features specific for malignant hyperthermia. Diagnosis depends on a knowledge of features that can occur during malignant hyperthermia (Table 32–14).

B. Treatment. See Table 32–15.

C. Identification of susceptible patients. Prior anesthetic history is important, although a negative history does not necessarily indicate that patients are not susceptible to malignant hyperthermia. Myopathic syndromes may be associated with an increased risk of malignant hyperthermia. About 70% of patients susceptible to malignant hyperthermia have increased resting plasma concentrations of creatine kinase (not a definitive screening test for malignant hyperthermia).

    1. In vitro skeletal muscle contracture tests. Skeletal muscle biopsies (vastus muscles of the thighs) with in vitro isometer contracture testing (separate exposures to halothane and caffeine) provides definitive confirmation of susceptibility to malignant hyperthermia.

Table 32-14 • Clinical Features of Malignant Hyperthermia

Timing	Clinical Signs	Changes in Monitored Variables	Biochemical Changes
Early	Masseter spasm Tachypnea Rapid exhaustion of soda lime	Increased minute ventilation Increasing end-tidal carbon dioxide concentrations	Increased $PaCO_2$
	Warm soda lime canister Tachycardia Irregular heart rate	Cardiac dysrhythmias Peaked T waves on ECG	Acidosis Hyperkalemia
Intermediate	Patient warm to touch Cyanosis	Increasing core body temperature Decreasing hemoglobin oxygen saturations	
	Dark blood at surgical site Irregular heart rate	Cardiac dysrhythmias Peaked T waves on ECG	Hyperkalemia
Late	Generalized skeletal muscle rigidity Prolonged bleeding Dark urine Oliguria		Increased creatine kinase concentrations
			Myoglobinuria
	Irregular heart rate	Cardiac dysrhythmias Peaked T waves on ECG	Hyperkalemia

Adapted from: Hopkins PM. Malignant hyperthermia: advances in clinical management and diagnosis. Br J Anaesth 2000;85:118–28.

≡ Table 32–15 • Treatment of Malignant Hyperthermia

Etiologic Treatment

Dantrolene (2–3 mg/kg IV) as an initial bolus, followed with repeat doses every 5–10 minutes until symptoms are controlled (rarely need total dose > 10 mg/kg)

Prevent recrudescence (dantrolene 1 mg/kg IV every 6 hours for 72 hours)

Symptomatic Treatment

Immediately discontinue inhaled anesthetics and conclude surgery as soon as possible

Hyperventilate lungs with 100% oxygen

Initiate active cooling (iced saline 15 ml/kg IV every 10 minutes, gastric and bladder lavage with iced saline, surface cooling)

Correct metabolic acidosis (sodium bicarbonate 1–2 mEq/kg based on arterial pH)

Maintain urine output (hydration, mannitol 0.25 g/kg IV, furosemide 1 mg/kg IV)

Treat cardiac dysrhythmias (procainamide 15 mg/kg IV)

Monitor in an intensive care unit (urine output, arterial blood gases, pH, electrolytes)

2. The use of a combined caffeine-halothane test is associated with a high incidence of false-positive results.

D. **Management of anesthesia.** No anesthetic regimen has been shown to be reliably safe for malignant hyperthermia-susceptible patients.

1. **Dantrolene prophylaxis** for malignant hyperthermia-susceptible patients is provided with oral administration of dantrolene, 5 mg/kg, in three or four divided doses every 6 hours, with the last dose 4 hours preoperatively (provides therapeutic plasma concentrations of dantrolene at induction of anesthesia for at least 6 hours). Alternatively, dantrolene 2.4 mg/kg IV may be administered over 10 to 30 minutes as prophylaxis just prior to induction of anesthesia; for continued protection one-half of the dose is repeated in 6 hours.

2. Large doses of dantrolene administered as prophylaxis may cause skeletal muscle weakness of sufficient magnitude to interfere with adequate ventilation or protection of the lungs from aspiration of gastric fluid. In view of

Table 32–16 • Nontriggering Drugs for Malignant Hyperthermia

Barbiturates
Propofol
Etomidate
Benzodiazepines
Opioids
Droperidol
Nitrous oxide (?)
Nondepolarizing muscle relaxants
Anticholinesterases
Anticholinergics
Sympathomimetics
Local anesthetics (esters and amides)

the potential adverse effects associated with dantrolene therapy, it has been concluded that prophylactic use of dantrolene therapy is not necessary in patients suspected to be susceptible to malignant hyperthermia provided that all known triggering drugs are avoided.

3. **Drug selections.** See Table 32–16.
4. **Anesthesia machine.** No studies confirm that malignant hyperthermia can be triggered by residual concentrations of volatile anesthetics delivered from previously used anesthesia machines (continuous flow of oxygen at 10 L/min for 5 to 20 minutes before using the machine to deliver anesthesia to malignant hyperthermia-susceptible patients).
5. **Regional anesthesia** is an acceptable selection for anesthesia in malignant hyperthermia-susceptible patients (skeletal muscle biopsies).
6. **Postoperative discharge home** is not associated with an increased risk in patients susceptible to malignant hyperthermia.

XI. FAMILIAL DYSAUTONOMIA

Familial dysautonomia is characterized by dysfunction of the autonomic nervous system (lability of systemic blood pressure, decreased pain perception, vomiting crises with pulmonary aspiration and dehydration, hyperthermia) and development of kyphoscoliosis.

XII. SOLID TUMORS

A. Neuroblastoma is the most common extracranial solid tumor in infants and children resulting from malignant proliferation of sympathetic ganglion cell precursors (most often in the adrenal medulla).

B. Nephroblastoma (Wilms' tumor) typically presents as asymptomatic flank masses in otherwise healthy children. Systemic hypertension may be a manifestation of nephroblastoma, particularly if the tumor involves both kidneys. Surgical treatment may predispose to sudden, and excessive blood loss.

XIII. ONCOLOGIC EMERGENCIES

See Table 32–17.

XIV. BURN (THERMAL) INJURIES

Survival after burn injuries depends on the patient's age and percentage of body area burned, with younger patients most likely to survive. Classification of burn injuries and outcomes is based on the depth of the burn (Table 32–18). Definitions of major burn injuries are based on the percentage of body surface area burned and the area of the body burned (Table 32–19).

A. Pathophysiology. See Table 32–20. Mediators released from the burn wound contribute to local inflammation and burn wound edema. With major burns, local injury triggers

---

≡ Table 32–17 • Oncologic Emergencies in Children

Superior mediastinal syndrome (airway obstruction may occur; highly sensitive to radiotherapy; ventilation of lungs may become impossible after the loss of consciousness despite a properly placed tracheal tube)

Spinal cord compression

Tumor lysis syndrome (sudden systemic overload of uric acid following initiation of chemotherapy)

▬ Table 32–18 • Classification of Burn Injuries

Classification	Depth of Burn Injury	Outcome and Treatment
First Degree (superficial)	Epidermis	Heals spontaneously
Second Degree (partial thickness)		
Superficial dermal burn	Epidermis and upper dermis	Heals spontaneously
Deep dermal burn	Epidermis and deep dermis	Requires excision and grafting for rapid return of function
Third Degree (full thickness)	Destruction of epidermis and dermis	Wound excision and grafting required Some limitation of function and scar formation
Fourth Degree	Skeletal muscles Fascia Bone	Complete excision Limited function

Adapted from: MacLennan N, Heimbach DM, Cullen BF. Anesthesia for major thermal injury. Anesthesiology 1998;89:749–70.

▬ Table 32–19 • Definition of Major Burns

Third degree (full-thickness) burn injuries involving > 10% of the total body surface area

Second degree (partial thickness) burn injuries involving > 25% of the total body surface area in adults (at extremes of age, 20% of total body surface area)

Burn injuries involving the face, hands, feet, or perineum

Inhalation burn injuries

Chemical burn injuries

Electrical burn injuries

Burn injuries in patients with serious co-existing medical diseases

Adapted from: MacLennan N, Heimbach DM, Cullen BF. Anesthesia for major thermal injury. Anesthesiology 1998;89:749–70.

≡ **Table 32–20 •** Pathophysiologic Responses Evoked by Burn Injuries

Cardiovascular
Early
   Hypovolemia (burn shock)
   Impaired myocardial contractility
Late
   Systemic hypertension
   Tachycardia
   Increased cardiac output
Pulmonary
Early direct effects
   Upper airway obstruction (burns)
   Effects of smoke inhalation (chemical pneumonitis, carbon
     monoxide)
   Asphyxia
Early indirect effects
   Effects of inflammatory mediators
   Pulmonary edema (complication of resuscitation)
Late direct effects
   Chest wall restriction (thoracic burn injuries)
Late indirect effects (complications of ventilation and airway
   management)
   Oxygen toxicity
   Barotrauma
   Infections
   Laryngeal damage
   Tracheal stenosis
Metabolism and Thermoregulation
Increased metabolic rate
Increased carbon dioxide production
Increased oxygen utilization
Impaired thermoregulation
Renal and Electrolytes
Early
   Decreased renal blood flow
   Myoglobinuria
   Hyperkalemia (tissue necrosis)
Late
   Increased renal blood flow
   Variable drug clearance
   Hypokalemia (diuresis)
Endocrine Responses
Increased serum norepinephrine concentrations
Hyperglycemia (susceptible to development of nonketotic
   hyperosmolar coma)

Table continued on opposite page

≡ Table 32–20 • Pathophysiologic Responses Evoked by Burn Injuries *Continued*

Gastrointestinal
Stress ulcers
Impaired gastrointestinal barrier to bacteria
Endotoxemia
Coagulation and Rheology
Early
  Activation of thrombotic and fibrinolytic systems
  Hemoconcentration
  Hemolysis
Late
  Anemia
Immunology
Impaired immune function (sepsis, pneumonia)
Endotoxemia
Multiple organ system failure

Adapted from: MacLennan N, Heimbach DM, Cullen BF. Anesthesia for major thermal injury. Anesthesiology 1998;89:749–70.

the release of circulating mediators, resulting in systemic responses (characterized by hypermetabolism, immunosuppression, and the systemic inflammatory response syndrome) (Fig. 32–2).

B. **Management of anesthesia.** See Table 32–21.
  1. **Altered drug responses.** See Table 32–21. Immediately after burn injury, organ and tissue blood flow is decreased as a result of hypovolemia, depressed myocardial function, and release of vasoactive substances. Drugs administered by a route other than intravenously have predictably delayed absorption. Pharmacologic alterations may persist after recovery from burn injuries (thiopental requirements may remain increased more than 1 year after such injuries).
  2. **Ketamine,** 1 to 2 mg/kg IV, with or without nitrous oxide provides excellent somatic analgesia for skin grafting procedures. Sevoflurane is the most likely inhaled drug to be used for anesthesia in children with burn injuries.

XV. ELECTRICAL BURNS

See Table 32–22.

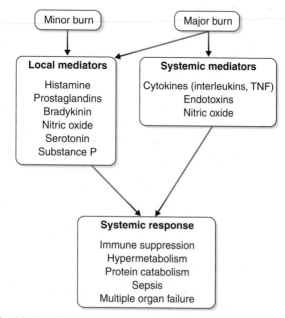

Fig. 32–2 • Mediators released with thermal injuries and responses to their release. (From MacLennan N, Heimbach DM, Cullen BF. Anesthesia for major thermal injury. Anesthesiology 1998;89:749–70. © 1998, Lippincott Williams & Wilkins, with permission.)

≡ Table 32–21 • Anesthetic Considerations for Excision and Grafting of Major Burn Injuries

Preoperative Medication
Provide adequate analgesia
Limit period of fluid fasting
Vascular Access
Establish appropriate intravenous access
Consider invasive monitoring
Airway Management
Consider alternatives to direct laryngoscopy
Consider awake fiberoptic intubation (neck or facial contractures)
Ventilation
Minute ventilation requirements increased (increased metabolic rate, parenteral hyperalimentation)
Mechanical ventilation (smoke inhalation, acute respiratory failure)
Fluids and Blood
Anticipate possibility of rapid, large blood loss
Evaluate coagulation status
Temperature Regulation
Increase ambient temperatures of the operating rooms
Warm intravenous fluids
Anesthetic Drugs
Include opioids
Consider effects of increased circulating catecholamine concentrations
Muscle Relaxants
Avoid succinylcholine
Anticipate resistance to neuromuscular blocking effects of nondepolarizing muscle relaxants
Postoperative Period
Anticipate increased analgesic (opioid) requirements

Adapted from: MacLennan N, Heimbach DM, Cullen BF. Anesthesia for major thermal injury. Anesthesiology 1998;89:749–70.

≡ Table 32–22 • Characteristics of Electrical Burns

Deep tissue injury may be extensive despite limited superficial damage
Cardiac dysrhythmias (cardiopulmonary arrest may have occurred initially, especially with lightening injury)
Renal failure (myoglobin from injured skeletal muscles)
Neurologic complications (direct injury to nerves or subsequent scarring)
Cataract formation a late sequela
Scarring of oral commissures

XVI. SEPARATION OF CONJOINED TWINS

Separation of conjoined twins requires two anesthesia teams, separate anesthesia machines, extensive and invasive monitoring, and consideration of the effects of cross-circulation on responses to drugs. Aggressive efforts are required to maintain normothermia. The need for postoperative support of ventilation is predictable.

33

Diseases Associated with Aging

Aging is accompanied by unavoidable alterations in organ function (physiologic decline) that predispose elderly patients to homeostatic failure, chronic diseases, and loss of independence in the performance of daily activities (functional decline) (Stoelting RK, Dierdorf SF. Diseases associated with aging. In: Anesthesia and Co-Existing Disease, 4th ed. New York, Churchill Livingstone, 2002;739–756). Decreased organ function can often be demonstrated only by stress testing. It is important to recognize that there is not necessarily a correlation between biologic and chronologic age.

I. PHYSIOLOGIC CHANGES ASSOCIATED WITH AGING

Aging is accompanied by unavoidable alterations in organ system function (lack of functional reserve and inability to respond to stress) and responses to drugs. Exercise tolerance best reflects biologic age and is one of the most important predictors of perioperative outcome in elderly surgical patients.

A. **Organ system function.** See Table 33–1.

B. **Management of anesthesia**

1. **Preoperative evaluation** of elderly patients includes consideration of the likely presence of co-existing diseases independent of the reasons for surgery (Table 33–2). Alcoholism may be an unexpected finding in elderly patients. Elderly patients are likely to be taking several drugs that can result in adverse effects or drug interactions (Table 33–3).

   a. **Functional reserve.** Preoperative evaluation of the elderly patient's functional reserve and airway should consider the presence of changes characteristic of aging (Table 33–1).

   b. **Airway.** The potential for vertebrobasilar arterial insufficiency can be evaluated by determining the effect of extension and rotation of the patient's head on men-

---

■ **Table 33–1 •** Organ System Function and Aging

Nervous System
Loss of neurons (cerebral cortex)
Slowed conduction velocity in peripheral nerves (decreased dose requirements for inhaled and injected drugs)
Sleep disturbances (nighttime wakefulness)
Cardiovascular System
Increased myocardial and vascular stiffness
Blunted β-adrenergic receptor responses
Autonomic nervous system dysfunction
Physical fitness associated with maintenance of cardiac output
Congestive heart failure
Atrial fibrillation
Autonomic Nervous System
Increases in sympathetic nervous system activity (results in down-regulation of β-adrenergic receptor responsiveness)
Decreases in parasympathetic nervous system activity (sinus node function)
Decreases in baroreceptor function (heart rate responses to changes in systemic blood pressure)
Respiratory System
Progressive decreases in arterial oxygenation
Sleep apnea syndrome
Renal Function
Progressive declines in renal blood flow and glomerular filtration rate (vulnerable to fluid overload)
Plasma creatinine concentrations often unchanged (decreased skeletal muscle mass)
Decreased urine concentrating ability
Hepatic, Gastrointestinal, and Endocrine Function
Decreased hepatic blood flow (drug clearance)
Decreased rates of gastric emptying may occur
Diabetes mellitus
Hypothyroidism

---

tal status. Cervical osteoarthritis or rheumatoid arthritis may interfere with visualization of the glottic opening during direct laryngoscopy.

   c. **Blood volume.** Elderly patients are often volume-depleted during the preoperative period.
   d. **Skin.** Senile atrophy with collagen loss and decreased elasticity makes the skin more sensitive to injury (tape, adhesive monitoring pads).

Table 33-2 • Co-Existing Diseases Often Accompanying Aging

Essential hypertension
Ischemic heart disease
Cardiac conduction disturbances
Congestive heart failure
Chronic pulmonary disease
Diabetes mellitus
Subclinical hypothyroidism
Rheumatoid arthritis
Osteoarthritis

Table 33-3 • Drugs Commonly Prescribed for Elderly Patients

Drug	Adverse Effects or Drug Interactions
Diuretics	Hypokalemia
	Hyperkalemia
Digitalis	Cardiac dysrhythmias
	Cardiac conduction disturbances
β-Adrenergic antagonists	Bradycardia
	Congestive heart failure
	Bronchospasm
	Attenuation of autonomic nervous system activity
Centrally acting antihypertensives	Attenuation of autonomic nervous system activity
	Decreased MAC
Tricyclic antidepressants	Anticholinergic effects
	Cardiac dysrhythmias
	Cardiac conduction disturbances
	Increased MAC
Lithium	Cardiac dysrhythmias
	Prolongation of muscle relaxants
Cardiac antidysrhythmics	Prolongation of muscle relaxants
Antibiotics	Prolongation of muscle relaxants
Oral hypoglycemics	Hypoglycemia
Alcohol	Increased MAC
	Delirium tremens

MAC, minimum alveolar concentration.

2. **Preoperative medication** in elderly patients may be best achieved with a preoperative visit, describing events that are going to occur during the perioperative period. If additional anxiety relief is desired, benzodiazepines are often selected. Atropine may contribute to postoperative confusion in elderly patients.

3. **General anesthesia.** Selection of drugs and techniques for induction of anesthesia in elderly patients must consider changes in organ system function that are likely to accompany aging and altered responses to drugs because of age-related changes in pharmacokinetics or pharmacodynamics.

4. **Regional anesthesia** is an acceptable alternative to general anesthesia in selected elderly patients (transurethral resection of the prostate, gynecologic procedures, inguinal herniorrhaphy, hip fractures) who are alert and cooperative.

5. **Postoperative period.** Early ambulation is recommended in an effort to decrease the likelihood of pneumonia or the development of deep vein thrombosis. Postoperative confusion and impaired memory may contribute to morbidity in elderly patients.

II. GERIATRIC SYNDROMES

See Table 33–4.

A. **Delirium** is a transient, potentially reversible disorder of cognition and attention that occurs in 10% to 15% of elderly general surgical patients (30% to 50% of elderly patients admitted with hip fractures) (Table 33–5).

1. **Causes.** In elderly hospitalized patients, delirium is most commonly associated with acute infection (pneumonia, bladder infection), arterial hypoxemia, hypotension, and administration of psychoactive drugs (benzodiazepines, opioids, drugs with anticholinergic effects).

2. **Diagnosis.** Delirium should be considered in elderly patients who experience changes in cognitive function (Table 33–5).

3. **Treatment** of obvious potential causes of delirium (pneumonia, arterial hypoxemia, electrolyte derangements, polypharmacy) is the first step in the evaluation and management of elderly patients who develop delirium. Promotion of normal sleep cycles and avoidance of restraints are useful.

☰ Table 33–4 • Examples of Geriatric Syndromes

Cognitive dysfunction
  Delirium
  Postoperative delirium
  Dementia
Gait disturbances
Urinary and/or bowel incontinence
Immobility
Pressure ulcers
Malnutrition
Dehydration
Sensory impairment
  Hearing
  Vision (cataracts, glaucoma, macular degeneration)
Iatrogenic illness
  Polypharmacy
  Nosocomial infections
Progeria

☰ Table 33–5 • Differential Diagnosis of Delirium and Dementia

Feature	Delirium	Dementia
Onset	Abrupt	Insidious
Duration	Hours to days	Persistent
Attention span	Decreased	Normal
Awareness	Impaired	Normal
Alertness	Fluctuates	Normal
Consciousness	Depressed	Normal
Memory	Impaired (especially short-term)	Impaired (especially remote)
Language	Normal to incorrect naming	Aphasia Anomia Paraphasia
Perception	Illusions Hallucinations Misperceptions	Delusions
Psychomotor activity	Increased to decreased	Normal
Sleep-wake cycle	Disrupted (reversed)	Normal to fragmented

Adapted from: Palmer RM. Management of common clinical disorders in geriatric patients. Sci Am Med 1998;1–16.

4. **Postoperative delirium** (postoperative cognitive dysfunction, postoperative confusion) is common in elderly patients especially following orthopedic procedures, cardiac surgery requiring cardiopulmonary bypass, and cataract surgery.

   a. **Signs and symptoms.** See Table 33–5. Postoperative delirium is usually seen on the first or second postoperative day, and symptoms are often exacerbated at night. Increased morbidity, delayed functional recovery, and prolonged hospital stays accompany postoperative delirium.

   b. **Causes.** See Table 33–6.

B. **Dementia** is the clinical syndrome characterized by acquired persistent impairment of cognitive (intellectual) and emotional abilities severe enough to interfere with daily functioning and the quality of life (Table 33–5).

   1. **Signs and symptoms.** Intellectual impairment in patients with dementia may manifest in the spheres of language, memory, abstract thinking, and judgment. Dementia occurs primarily late in life (prevalence about 1% at the age of 60 years, then doubles every 5 years to reach 30% to 50% by 85 years of age). It may be difficult to differentiate dementia from mental depression.

   2. **Alzheimer's disease** is the most common of the progressive cortical dementias, accounting for about 70% of the dementia in individuals over 55 years of age. The characteristic cognitive feature of Alzheimer's disease is progressive memory impairment (predominantly loss of short-term memory).

      a. **Diagnosis** of Alzheimer's disease is probable when the dementing illness is characterized by insidious onset, progressive worsening of memory, and normal levels

---

≡ **Table 33–6** • Causes of
   Postoperative Delirium

Polypharmacy
Preoperative administration of anticholinergic drugs
Intraoperative hypotension
Perioperative arterial hypoxemia
Postoperative use of opioids and/or benzodiazepines
Postoperative surgical complications

of consciousness. Computed tomography typically shows ventricular dilation and marked cortical atrophy.

    b. **Treatment.** There is no proven preventive therapy for Alzheimer's disease, and drugs (anticholinesterase drugs) are not consistently effective. Drugs with anticholinergic effects are avoided. The typical course is one of progressive decline, with an average survival of 8 to 10 years.

    c. **Management of anesthesia** includes avoidance of sedative and anticholinergic drugs. Maintenance of anesthesia can be acceptably achieved with inhaled or injected drugs. Pharmacologic antagonism of nondepolarizing neuromuscular blocking drugs might logically include glycopyrrolate, rather than atropine.

  3. **Vascular dementia.** Permanent cognitive impairment resulting from cerebrovascular disease is the second most common form of dementia.

  4. **Pick's disease** is cortical dementia characterized by an impaired ability to plan and initiate goals and the development of disinhibited behavior.

  5. **Subcortical dementias** may occur in patients with Parkinson's disease.

C. **Gait disturbances.** Disorders of balance and gait increase with advancing age and predispose elderly individuals to falls and injuries (hip fractures, subdural hematomas, cervical spine fractures, soft tissue damage).

  1. **Hip fractures** are major causes of disability, functional impairment, and death in elderly individuals (hip protectors may provide protection).

  2. **Anesthesia for hip fracture surgery.** The literature is conflicting with respect to choice of general or regional anesthesia for repair of hip fractures in elderly patients and subsequent morbidity and mortality.

D. **Urinary and bowel incontinence.** Urinary incontinence results from neurologic defects (stroke) or anatomic defects (prostatic hyperplasia) that interfere with normal bladder function. Chronic constipation and fecal impaction are often associated with inadequate dietary fiber intake and inactivity.

E. **Immobility.** Prolonged bed rest produces many physiologic changes, including decreased circulating plasma volume and cardiac output, orthostatic hypotension, arterial hypoxemia,

☰ Table 33–7 • Manifestations of Malnutrition in Elderly Patients

Weight loss
Low weight for height
Decreases in midarm circumference
Nutrition-related disorders (osteoporosis, vitamin B_{12} deficiency, folate deficiency)
Unexplained normocytic anemia
Serum albumin concentrations < 3.5 g/dl

skeletal muscle atrophy, and generalized skeletal muscle weakness.

F. **Pressure ulcers** occur when persistent external pressure on the skin damages underlying tissues, especially over bony prominences.

G. **Malnutrition** is common in elderly patients, especially in association with congestive heart failure, chronic obstructive pulmonary disease, and cancer (Table 33–7).

H. **Dehydration** is the most common fluid and electrolyte disorder in the long-term care setting and is often associated with infection. Physiologic reasons for development of dehydration include decreased ability of the kidneys to concentrate urine, altered thirst sensations, and relative resistance to vasopressin.

1. **Classification.** See Table 33–8.

☰ Table 33–8 • Classification of Dehydration

Isotonic Dehydration
Balanced losses of water and sodium
Vomiting and diarrhea
Hypertonic Dehydration
Water losses exceed sodium losses (serum sodium > 145 mEq/L and serum osmolarity > 300 mOsm/L)
Fever
Hypotonic Dehydration
Sodium losses exceed water losses (serum sodium < 135 mEq/L and serum osmolarity < 285 mOsm/L)
Diuretics that stimulate sodium excretion

2. **Diagnosis** of dehydration is suggested by rapid weight loss of more than 3% of the individual's body weight (Table 33–9).

3. **Treatment** is with supplemental oral fluids (dyspnea and confusion may reflect developing fluid overload). Vomiting- and diarrhea-related fluid losses are replaced with isotonic saline.

I. **Sensory impairment**

1. **Hearing impairment** is categorized as sensorineural (hearing aids) and/or conductive (cerumen impaction, otosclerosis).

2. **Vision impairment** includes presbyopia, poor night vision (decreased pupillary dilation), cataracts, glaucoma, macular degeneration, and diabetic retinopathy.

a. **Cataracts** are treated by outpatient surgical removal (most common operation in elderly patients).

i. **Preoperative evaluation.** Tests should be ordered only if the history or a medical finding on physical examination indicates a need for the test.

ii. **Management of anesthesia.** Cataract extraction may be performed under local anesthesia utilizing a retrobulbar block with or without intravenous sedation (propofol, midazolam, remifentanil) or under general anesthesia. General anesthesia must ensure immobility (adequate depth of anesthesia with or without skeletal muscle paralysis) of the patient, as sudden movements or attempts to cough when the lens is exposed could result of extrusion of vitreous and ocular damage. It is desirable to minimize the incidence of vomiting during the postoperative period (propofol for induction of anesthesia and avoid postoperative use of opioids).

iii. **Incidence of perioperative myocardial ischemia.** Intraoperative myocardial ischemia is most likely

---

≡ **Table 33–9** • Signs and Symptoms of Dehydration

Orthostatic hypotension (systolic blood pressure decrease > 20 mmHg after 1 minute)
Orthostatic heart rate increases (10–20 beats/min)
Blood urea nitrogen/serum creatinine ratio of 25 or higher

to be associated with tachycardia (> 20 beats/min above the preoperative baseline).

b. **Glaucoma** is an optic neuropathy with peripheral vision loss that occurs before loss of central vision.

    i. **Treatment** of glaucoma is lowering the intraocular pressure by decreasing the amount of aqueous humor produced by ciliary bodies (timolol as topical eyedrops) or by increasing its outflow through the trabecular meshwork (iridectomy, laser).

    ii. **Management of anesthesia** for patients with glaucoma includes maintenance of miosis by continuing topical miotic therapy throughout the perioperative period. Intraocular pressures are lowered by hypocarbia and decreased central venous pressure, as produced by drug-induced osmotic diuresis, opioids, and volatile anesthetic drugs. Bradycardia and exaggerated hypotension have been attributed to β-blockade produced by topical administration of timolol.

c. **Macular degeneration** is deterioration of the central portions of the retina (associated with cigarette smoking).

d. **Retinal detachment** is a separation in the retina between the photoreceptors and retinal pigment epithelium (increased incidence in the presence of high degrees of myopia).

    i. **Treatment** is laser therapy to coagulate holes in the retina and production of a tamponade effect (sulfur hexafluoride gas) until laser-induced adhesions develop.

    ii. Nitrous oxide is avoided for general anesthesia administered to patients undergoing retinal detachment surgery, as this gas could diffuse into any remaining air bubbles in the globe.

J. **Iatrogenic illnesses**

1. **Polypharmacy.** The concomitant use of several drugs increases the risk of drug interactions, unwanted side effects, and adverse reactions. Medications should be used with special caution in elderly individuals because of changes in drug pharmacokinetics and pharmacodynamics (Table 33–10).

2. **Nosocomial infections** (urinary tract, pulmonary, wound infections) are most likely to occur in those with physical

<hr>

≡ Table 33–10 • Age-Related Changes in Pharmacokinetics and Pharmacodynamics

Pharmacokinetics

Drug distribution is altered by changes in body composition (decreases in total body water and lean body mass and relative increases in body fat)

Malnutrition-induced decreases in serum albumin concentrations

Drug metabolism and clearance may be altered (decreases in hepatic blood flow and renal blood flow, slowed hepatic microsomal mixed function oxidase system metabolism)

Pharmacodynamics

Decreased β-adrenergic receptor responsiveness

Increased opioid receptor responsiveness

<hr>

    debility, prolonged hospitalization, and exposure to broad-spectrum antibiotics.

K. Progeria is characterized by premature aging (ischemic heart disease, congestive heart failure, cerebrovascular disease, osteoarthritis, diabetes mellitus).

    1. Management of anesthesia for patients with progeria is based on changes in organ system function that predictably accompanies aging.

    2. The presence of mandibular hypoplasia and micrognathia may lead to difficulty with airway management and tracheal intubation.

III. SKELETAL CHANGES LIKELY TO ACCOMPANY AGING

A. Osteoarthritis (degenerative joint disease), a common form of arthritis in elderly individuals, is characterized by degeneration of articular cartilage (pain and dysfunction of affected joints).

    1. Classification. Primary osteoarthritis is present when specific inflammatory or metabolic conditions known to be associated with arthritis are absent. Secondary osteoarthritis is associated with conditions that cause damage to articular cartilage through a variety of mechanisms (trauma, inflammatory, metabolic).

    2. Risk factors. Age is the factor most strongly associated with osteoarthritis.

    3. Diagnosis. Characteristic radiographic features corroborated by compatible clinical symptoms confirm the diagnosis of osteoarthritis. Rheumatoid arthritis can usually be distinguished from osteoarthritis on the basis of a different pattern of joint disease, more prominent morning stiffness, and soft tissue welling and warmth on physical examination.

4. **Signs and symptoms.** Typical signs and symptoms of osteoarthritis include pain (worse with activity), stiffness, swelling, deformity, and loss of function.

   a. **Specific joint involvement and spinal canal stenosis.** The most commonly affected joints in the hands are the distal and proximal interphalangeal joints. Osteoarthritis frequently involves the knee and/or hips and is a common cause of significant disability. Spondylosis is the term used to describe osteoarthritis of the cervical and lumbar spine. Stenosis of the spinal canal can occur in patients with extensive degenerative changes, resulting in compression of the cervical spine or of the cauda equina in the lumbar region [chronic radicular pain that is worse with activity (neurogenic claudication)].

   b. **Radiographic changes** characteristic of osteoarthritis include joint space narrowing and the presence of osteophytes (bone spurs).

5. **Treatment** of osteoarthritis is based on relieving pain (acetaminophen, nonsteroidal antiinflammatory drugs, intra-articular corticosteroids, joint replacement), exercise, and weight loss.

B. **Cervical spine disease** may interfere with airway management and with direct laryngoscopy for tracheal intubation. Spinal cord compression can be secondary to hyperextension or hyperflexion of the patient's neck in the presence of spinal stenosis. For every decade of life after the age of 30 years, there is approximately 10 degrees of loss in the range of flexion and extension of the cervical spine.

1. **Treatment.** The goals of cervical spine surgery include stabilizing the spine and decompressing the spinal cord or neural roots (Table 33–11).

2. **Management of anesthesia.** Awake fiberoptic tracheal intubation is often indicated in patients with cervical spinal canal stenosis, keeping in mind the importance of avoiding extremes of neck range motion. Monitoring somatosensory evoked potentials is useful for early recognition of spinal cord compression and resulting brain stem ischemia during the surgical procedure.

■ Table 33–11 • Surgical Treatment of Cervical Spine Disease

Anterior Discectomy with Fusion
Complications include damage to the recurrent laryngeal nerve and damage to the thoracic duct
Consider awake fiberoptic tracheal intubation if there is preoperative evidence of cervical spinal cord compression (detect neurologic impairment before induction of anesthesia)
Hyperextension of the patient's head may result in acute spinal cord compression
Prevent reactions to tracheal tube (could expel bone graft)
Posterior Fusion
Treatment for cervical spine instability in the presence of rheumatoid arthritis
Awake fiberoptic tracheal intubation
Laminotomy-Foraminotomy
Enlarge bony openings through which the nerve roots exit the spinal cord

---

    C. Osteoporosis is a systemic skeletal disease characterized by low bone mineral density (lumbar spine) and microarchitectural deterioration with a consequent increase in bone fragility and susceptibility to fracture (acute pain from vertebral fractures).

        1. Risk factors for the development of osteoporosis includes family history, low body weight, inactivity, and cigarette smoking.

        2. Treatment of osteoporosis is with drugs that decrease bone resorption (estrogens, bisphosphanates, calcitonin). Mixed estrogen agonists and antagonists decrease bone resorption and do not stimulate endometrial growth.

Index

Note: Page numbers followed by the letter *f* refer to figures and those followed by *t* refer to tables.